REVIEWER ACCLAIM FOR

Women Afraid to Eat

"Highly recommended to all readers"

"HEALTH AT ANY SIZE!" is this book's emphatic message to American women. Berg argues that the media and society cause women to obsess over the numbers on the scale and subsequently abuse their bodies and minds.

Throughout, she backs up her observations with research and statistics. Recommended for libraries serving consumers, educators, health professionals.

— LIBRARY JOURNAL

THIS BOOK SPEAKS THE PAINFUL TRUTH all women need to hear so that we can come home to our bodies.

— JEANINE COGAN, *PhD, Research Psychologist Washington, D.C.*

WHAT I LIKE MOST ABOUT BERG'S APPROACH is that she flings a coconut cream pie at the contention that thin equals fit. She knows we must make sure our girls start thinking in terms of how they feel more than how they look. The jackpot answer is the better they feel, the better they look.

— MINNEAPOLIS STAR TRIBUNE

SHOWS IN STARTLING DETAIL what the current warped norm for body shape (unachievable by most) is doing to women, how it harms them physically, emotionally, and socially. ... *Women Afraid to Eat* is also a handbook for change at the personal and cultural level. It offers women positive feelings, reaffirming that they can be healthy and attractive at any size.

— MIDWEST BOOK REVIEW

THE GURU OF THE NONDIETING MOVEMENT has struck again. Frances Berg scores a direct hit, plunging an arrow into the heart of the dieting industry... (She) plunks the missing piece into the puzzle with a resounding "clink" — a federal policy that works too closely with the weight-loss industry.

Berg reiterates her theme that weight loss is disproportionately promoted as the means to improve health to the detriment of women.

Well-written, thought-provoking ... a reference as well as an inspiration... belongs on every dietitian's bookshelf.

— TODAY'S DIETITIAN

A DANGEROUS EPIDEMIC is plaguing women desperate to lose weight: They've become too afraid to eat! In her startling new book *Women Afraid To Eat,* Berg warns that the all-too-common end result is damage to the body from dysfunctional eating and to the mind from distorted self-image.

—eDIETS.COM

OFFERS MANY CONSTRUCTIVE SUGGESTIONS for change at both the personal and cultural level. Berg points out how advertising teaches body shame, and how the media offers confusion over foods and health.

Berg believes that dieting can diminish women and keep them playing the anticipation game, instead of enjoying life to its fullest.

— NAPLES DAILY NEWS

WOMEN AFRAID TO EAT offers practical guidelines to help women reclaim control over their bodies by teaching them how to eat for nutrition, exercise for health, and lose their anxieties over weight.

— WAYNE C. MILLER, PhD, George Washington University
Medical Center, Washington, D.C.

EATING DISORDER SCREENING TESTS, lists of help centers, references (including websites) and helpful charts, graphs and sidebars are also provided.

—FITNESS MANAGEMENT

HER PRESCRIPTION IS AN EASY pill to swallow, if we can accept it: Stop dieting; eat in normal ways; listen to internal body signals that tell us to eat when hungry and stop when full; and increase activity level. She advocates "saying 'no' to the diet industry ... to medical and media pressures to be thin and weak."

As a culture, Berg says we need to accept larger people, demand that media stop ridiculing large people and strive for size, shape and age diversity, and be strong enough to make a difference.

—BISMARCK TRIBUNE

A COMPREHENSIVE OVERVIEW of our major weight and eating problems, and a delightfully simple, integrated framework for working to resolve them. ... All of this is packaged in a personal, easy-to-read style.

— GAIL MARCHESSAULT, RD, PhD (Cand.), Winnipeg, Canada

AMERICAN WOMEN ARE CAUGHT UP in a body-image crisis, afraid they'll gain weight, afraid they will not lose down to their goal, afraid to fully nourish themselves. They feel oversized in one part or another and wish they were thinner. *Women Afraid to Eat* probes why this is happening at a time when women have more freedom than ever before. ... How did it happen that a woman's value now is being judged by her degree of slimness, not her talent, insight or generosity?

Berg charges that the risks of obesity are being exaggerated, and the severe risks of eating disorders, malnutrition, and hazardous weight loss are ignored.

All public libraries will want at least two copies, one for the reference desk and a second for the circulating collection.

— PUBLIC LIBRARY QUARTERLY

FRANCIE'S WORK IS CONSISTENTLY on the cutting edge. She asks questions that must be answered if we are to truly assist people in improving health.

— KARIN KRATINA, MA, RD, PhD (cand.)
Eating Disorder Therapist, Cocoanut Creek, Fla.

AN AUTHORITY ON WEIGHT MANAGEMENT, Frances Berg provides the most comprehensive and socially responsible guide to dealing with weight-obsession available to date. Its scope, intensity and integrity is simply unparalleled.

Berg systematically and eloquently argues that women need to know the risks associated with extreme dieting: "It's time to confess we don't know the answers ... Time to get serious about solving weight problems instead of letting weak or unethical leaders, a relentless diet industry, doctors who dispense 'rainbow pills,' advertisers and the media lead us into even deeper trouble."

Highly recommended to all readers — from undergraduates and the general public to faculty and professionals.

— CHOICE, American Library Assoc.

A MUST READ for women ... an amazing read for men!

— NANCY KING, MS, RD, Nutrition Therapist, La Canada, Calif.

WOMEN AFRAID TO EAT is a refreshing antidote to our culture's preoccupation with weight. ... Affirming, liberating, and a must-read for any woman who has ever obsessed over the size of her thighs.

— SALLY E. SMITH, Editor, BBW Magazine

A MUCH-NEEDED BOOK. ... a practical approach to a difficult, multifactorial problem affecting many women in today's society.

The author addresses the problems while providing direction in how to break free with a new approach that helps people and does not harm them. ... She also offers direction to health professionals, educators, and policymakers who see the need to shift towards a health-centered approach to weight loss.

The book includes self-help tools, questionnaires, health-centered resources, websites, references, and an index.

— DOODY'S JOURNAL, Health Sciences Libraries

PACKED WITH INSIGHT AND INFORMATION relevant to the plight of women today living in a weight-obsessed world. Berg exposes the unhealthy collusion between government, pharmaceutical companies, and scientific research in the multi-billion dollar a year diet industry.

The last chapters of her book call for action. She advocates building self-esteem, boycotting products with destructive images, school-based education programs, and using non-dieting weight counseling techniques.

— VENTURES, American Dietetic Association

MS. BERG DOES IT AGAIN, this time for women! ... Her analysis of the images of women reveals great truths that our society has for so long chosen to ignore. ... This book is a must read for women of the new millenium.

— LINDA L. JOHNSON, MS, Director
North Dakota School Health Programs

AN EXCEPTIONAL BOOK that can help high school students improve their health and well-being.

— WHAT'S NEW

SHOULD BE REQUIRED READING for all students in medical, nursing or dietetics programs. Perhaps then they would not be so flippant in recommending weight loss.

— JOANNE IKEDA, MA, RD, State Nutrition
Specialist, University of California Berkeley

FRANCIE KNOWS THE RESEARCH and presents it in a way that the reader cannot but be profoundly changed for having listened to her arguments. *Children and Teens Afraid to Eat* has become a standard text for the nutrition practitioner, and her newest addition to this series is likely to join its predecessor in the libraries of those on the cutting edge.

— MONIKA M. WOOLSEY, MS, RD, *After the Diet Newsletter*

EVERY PAGE IS PACKED with information, support and encouragement for women of all sizes. Bravo!

— PAT LYONS, RN, MA, Co-Author, *Great Shape*

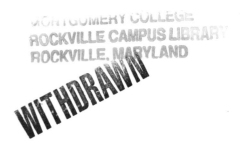
Women Afraid to Eat

Breaking Free in Today's Weight-Obsessed World

■

Frances M. Berg

Edited by
Kendra Rosencrans

Published by
Healthy Weight Network

Acknowledgments

It has been my great privilege and pleasure to network with many outstanding leaders in the fields of nutrition, eating disorders, obesity, and size acceptance throughout the United States and Canada over the years. I thank them for their many valuable contributions to my work and that of others through their research, concern, insight and vision. I thank Kendra Rosencrans for her superb editing, and Ronda Irwin for her dedication and skill in production of this book. Special appreciation also to my family, to my husband Bert, to Kathy and Dennis, Rick and Tracy, Cindy and Todd, Mike and Wendy, and their children for their support and the many ways they inspire me.

Women Afraid to Eat:
Breaking Free in Today's
Weight-Obsessed World
Second printing
Copyright 2001, 2000
by Frances M. Berg
All rights reserved. Reproduction in whole or in part prohibited without publisher's written permission.
ISBN: 0-918532-63-9 hardcover
ISBN: 0-918532-62-0 softcover

Afraid to Eat Series: *Women Afraid to Eat; Children and Teens Afraid to Eat*
ISBN: 0-918532-70-1 hardcover
ISBN: 0-918532-69-8 softcover
Printed in USA

Edited by Kendra Rosencrans
Layout and production by Ronda Irwin
Published by
Healthy Weight Network
402 South 14th Street
Hettinger, ND 58639
Tel: 701-567-2646; Fax: 701-567-2602
hwj@healthyweight.net
www.healthyweight.net

Foreword

Getting dressed for work in the morning, I catch a glimpse of my body in the mirror. Familiar waves of self-loathing and anxiety begin to wash over me, but this time it is different. I step forward, look at myself squarely in the mirror, and smash the waves before they can drown out the joy and creativity in my day. Today is different because I have just finished reading *Women Afraid to Eat: Breaking free in today's weight-obsessed world*.

Francie Berg's new book delivers what the title suggests — tools women can use for "breaking free." The tools are delivered in two forms — information and specific techniques. The powerful opening chapters give a stirring overview of the many forces acting on women to make them feel defective if they are not thin. It is explained how it came to be that, in our American society, a woman's value is judged by her degree of slimness. Intellect, competence, generosity — none of these matter unless a woman meets the warped norm for body shape — a norm that is biologically unachievable by most people.

The reader comes to understand the subtle ways in which the weight loss industry sells body dissatisfaction in order to sell products, and the way pharmaceutical companies marketing weight loss drugs can manipulate scientific opinion and public policy. The role of sexual harrassment and sexual abuse of young women in the initiation of disordered eating is clearly described.

The tremendous human costs of our cultural imperative for thinness are put into sharp focus. For example, there are predictable personality changes accompanying caloric deprivation that researchers have documented among cultural groups subjected to famine and among volunteers in laboratory studies of human starvation. These characteristics — irritability, apathy, depression, self-centeredness are typical of women who severely curtail their food intake.

The statement "Well-nourished women cannot be stereotyped but malnourished women are all alike" is typical of the thought-provoking perspective of this book.

Women Afraid to Eat offers one of the clearest descriptions in print of how it feels to have an eating disorder, as well as how eating disorders are promoted by our bizarre cultural values. The phenomenon of overuse of exercise as a form of eating disorder is also fully described. The inevitability of eating disorders given the prevailing medical paradigm for weight and health is shown with frightening lucidity. In fact, Ms. Berg's explanation of the intrinsic inter-relatedness of obesity, eating disorders, dysfunctional eating, and size prejudice leaves no doubt that these four phenomena must each be addressed, but cannot be addressed separately.

The second part of the book is a manual for profound change in how we deal with weight and health — change at both the personal and societal level. Very specific techniques are offered to women to help them stop looking at their bodies through lenses that have been distorted by cultural depravity.

Suggestions have been gathered from a number of clinicians for refocusing energy away from incessant, doomed efforts to be less than we are, toward getting on with lives that are rich and rewarding.

A new paradigm is presented, where women help themselves become healthier at any size, with a broad definition of health that includes positive feelings toward our bodies. Tried and true techniques from the field of psychology for healing self-damaging thoughts are thoroughly explained. Interesting, accurate, detailed explanations of what constitutes healthy eating and life-enhancing physical activity are offered.

The concept of "healthy lifestyles" is removed from the realm of moralistic thinking and placed into a larger perspective: "... Consider the many large, wonderful, capable volunteer community leaders who give generously, cheerfully and enthusiastically of their time and energy, day after day ... Shall we allow them to be compared unfavorably with others who focus on their own health, work out daily, diet, stay slim, and do nothing for anyone else?"

For women who have decided to "get on with their lives," practical suggestions are given for dealing constructively with size discrimination from a number of fronts. Approaches are proposed for defusing prejudice in a job interview, dealing with rude sales staff, and selecting a physician who will focus on health at any size. For women (and men) who would like to do something at a policy level, realistic ways to constructively work toward change in the political realm are offered.

There is nothing dry or dull about *Women Afraid to Eat*, because every page of the book is infused with the author's passion. Francie Berg has spent sixteen years searching for the truth about weight and health. Her unique position as editor of the *Healthy Weight Journal* has given her access to information that would not be available to most individuals. She has listened to obesity experts all over the world. She has listened to the most respected researchers and policy makers. She has listened to clinicians treating eating disorders. With equal attention and intelligence, she has listened to the people on the other side of the conventional "wisdom" on weight — to women who have lost and regained 1,000 pounds over their lifetimes, to families whose lives have been shattered by "accepted" weight loss treatment, and to courageous clinicians who have pioneered new ways of dealing with weight issues.

The result of sixteen years of searching for truth is this book, an expression of Francie Berg's conclusions as to where the truth lies. Her conclusions will resonate with women everywhere.

KAREN PETERSMARCK, PhD, MPH, RD
Public Health Consultant
Division of Chronic Disease and Injury Control
Michigan Department of Community Health

CONTENTS

PART II: BREAKING FREE, LIVING FREE

Enjoy Health at Any Size

LIVE ACTIVELY

- Be active your way, every day
- Move for the sheer joy and power of it, for time spent with family, friends, nature
- Celebrate activity as a natural part of life — fitness feels good
- Pace yourself; choose fun activities
- Be creative — increase activity throughout the day
- Enjoy the benefits — meet new people, increase your energy, lower stress, sleep better, and improve health, bone strength, and resistance to illness. Take time to care for yourself
- Add years to your life, and life to your years
- Share the benefits with family and friends
- Have more fun!

EAT WELL

- Take pleasure in eating a variety of foods
- Think of food as a friend — celebrate, enjoy, taste, savor
- Meet your body's energy and nutrient needs
- Enjoy a nondiet lifestyle; keeping stable weight is worthwhile
- Listen to your body: eat when hungry, stop when full and satisfied
- Eat at regular times, typically three meals and one or two snacks
- Eat in a balanced way — enjoy all five food groups
- Trust your body to make up for mistakes
- All foods can fit; there are no good foods/bad foods
- To improve, make small changes over time
- Enjoy home cooking, eating with friends and family

RESPECT YOURSELF AND OTHERS

Beauty, health and strength come in all sizes ♡ Celebrate and enjoy your unique characteristics ♡ Like yourself and others in spite of imperfections ♡ Make peace with your genetic blueprint (avoid unrealistic goals, perfectionism, all or nothing, body bashing, guilt, body shame) ♡ Wear clothes that fit comfortably and look good now ♡ Wear what you want, including shorts, swim suits or sleeveless tops no matter what your size or shape ♡ Think critically of media messages that portray unrealistic standards or suggest that happiness is based on appearance ♡ Accept, respect and celebrate diversity

Have confidence in your ability to make choices for better health ♡ Change your lifestyle gradually ♡ Nurture yourself ♡ Enjoy increased self-esteem ♡ Be flexible, go with the flow ♡ Keep in tune with your body ♡ Focus on quality of life, health and well-being ♡ Use positive language ♡ Embrace joy, pleasure, freedom, and self-discovery ♡ Nourish, listen, empower, explore, encourage, motivate, inspire, counsel, guide, validate, accept, respect, appreciate, self-care, heal, celebrate ♡

"I can if I choose"

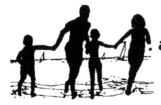 *a health centered approach*

for the 21ˢᵗ century

Developed by Frances M. Berg with adaptations from *Vitality*, Health Canada, and Linda Omichinski's HUGS programs, and credits to dietitians Ellyn Satter, Dayle Hayes, Nancy King, Karin Kratina and Gail Marchessault. Copyright 2001, 2000, by Frances M. Berg, *Afraid to Eat* series. All rights reserved. May not be reproduced without written permission from the publisher. Healthy Weight Network, 402 South 14th Street, Hettinger, ND 58639 (701-567-2646; fax: 701-567-2602). Website: www.healthyweight.net

HEALTH AT ANY SIZE
A new paradigm

Beauty, health and strength come in all sizes. Health at Any Size affirms this truth with a health-centered approach that focuses on health and well-being, not weight.

It's about wellness and wholeness, eating in normal, healthy ways and living actively. It's about acceptance, self-respect and appreciation of diversity. It's health at any size.

Everyone qualifies!

— FRANCES M. BERG

PART I

CHAPTER 1

Fear of food,
fear of fat

■

*The number one wish of brilliant, ambitious young women is
not to save the rain forests or succeed in a career, but to lose
weight.*

Why do modern women in the most affluent countries in the world
live like starving people in a primitive land? Why do they choose to be
weak, apathetic and unable to fully contribute to their families, their
careers, and their communities? Why, when instead they could be strong,
capable, and caring women?

It's simple. They are terrified of being fat.

Women today are afraid to eat. From girlhood to adulthood, they're
afraid to gain weight and terrified of failing to lose it. They're afraid
their bodies will be unacceptable in a society obsessed by thinness. It's
a fear that consumes, shatters lives, even kills.

These same fears inhibit women throughout the modern world. In
England, gaunt models are recruited from eating disorder clinics. In
Argentina, thin, compliant women feed into that country's macho values.
In Japan, small women seek to be thinner and hollow-cheeked. In
America, the brightest and best young college women are faltering in
the steps of their dieting mothers.

Where is all this taking us?

In the thinness obsession that grips our culture, many women are
making their bodies their life's work. They keep themselves undernour-

ished to stay thin and as a result, they become less able to contribute to the wider community. As girls and women eat in increasingly disturbed ways, problems like overweight, eating disorders, and dysfunctional eating multiply, affecting more children at younger and younger ages.

Americans have never been healthier or had longer life expectancy than today. Our food supply is the envy of the world. Yet our culture has developed an unhealthy fear of overweight, and food terrorism in the media about "unhealthy foods" or high-fat foods adds to these fears.

The damaging effects are seen everywhere. They start at a very young age and continue throughout life.

Almost every day I hear new horror stories: A daughter-in-law who lives on cigarettes and coffee; a 15-year-old who skips breakfast and lunch and never eats meat; a mother who eats and feeds her family only diet foods; a grandmother who fasts a day before daring to visit her doctor for a cold; a girl whose mother keeps a scale by the refrigerator door and weighs herself every time she eats anything.

Four-year olds are asking, "Mommy, am I too fat?" Seven-year-olds have full-blown eating disorders, and as many as 81 percent of 10-year-old girls are eating in dysfunctional, disturbed ways.[1]

The number one wish of brilliant, ambitious young women is not to save the rain forests or succeed in a career, but to lose weight.

I'm especially concerned about what is going on in our colleges today. Young women learn that appearance is all-important, more critical than the careers they had planned. Female bodies must be perfect and extremely thin. Young men are taught to demand thinness of women, to revere muscles and to scorn fat. Men are the new targets of the thinness message, learning body dissatisfaction from a thousand advertisements and muscle magazines that demonstrate the perfect male physique. These messages affecting men have a powerful impact on women and relationships between women and men.

University professors tell me how often they see malnourished and undernourished female students who sit with blank faces in their classes, unable to concentrate on school work because they feel dizzy, weak, nauseated, depressed, and are consumed with thoughts of food, hunger, weight and body image.

Many of these women are in health and physical science fields. Their teachers tell rueful stories about young professionals who have not resolved their own eating and weight issues, yet go forth to teach others what can scarcely avoid being mixed messages of health and wellness.

All this work at being thin comes at a stiff price.

The dieting, fat-phobic woman pays for her dysfunction and nutrient deficiency with a loss of energy — she feels fatigued, weak, lethargic, apathetic, dizzy and faint. Her bone health suffers and her risk for osteoporosis skyrockets. She may suffer chest pain, abdominal pain, constipation and hair loss. She may feel cold all the time and she loses her interest in sex. Her periods stop, her muscles cramp, her sleep is disturbed and she may develop heart abnormalities.

Even more dramatic are changes to her mind and her emotions. A woman in a state of semistarvation becomes moody, depressed, and anxious. She is often irritable, critical, intolerant of others, preoccupied with her body, and unable to concentrate. She may suffer decreased alertness, have difficulty with comprehension, experience memory loss. Her interests get narrower, she feels like doing little other than think about food and weight. She becomes self-centered and may lose the capacity for kindness, compassion, and generosity.

These changes can happen quickly.

And sudden death is a real possibility.

I was once a guest on a segment of *Inside Edition* that focused on dieting deaths. The tragic story that day featured photos of a bride in her coffin wearing her satin and lace wedding gown. The young woman, 23-year-old Patti Allen of Mobile, Ala., had died of a heart attack while watching a movie with her fiance just weeks before her wedding.

Patti's stunned father told viewers in a hurt, puzzled voice that her death was "Just impossible ... Patti was in perfect health." His daughter was happy and excited about losing weight for her wedding, he said, and had lost 21 pounds in five weeks at a local diet center.

Another bride-to-be who wanted to lose 20 pounds for her wedding was 29-year-old Mary Linnen, who died in Boston after taking the prescription diet drugs, fen-phen.[2]

Closer to home, I know of three people just in North Dakota, population 640,000, who died from medically supervised weight loss attempts. These deaths seldom hit the newspapers and are not recorded as dieting deaths. Two of the patients were on very low calorie liquid diets, the third on prescription diet pills.

These costs are too high. We are severely, dangerously out of balance.

Ideal woman cut by one-third

When a girl or woman looks at her body and then to the mirror of society, she sees an ever-thinner image of the ideal female. In the United States, the ideal woman has been reduced by one-third over the past 30 years, as shown by studies of Miss America contestants and Playboy centerfold girls.

The 1950s screen goddess, Marilyn Monroe, had, at a size 12 to 14, the curvaceous body of the average American woman. But today's gaunt models come in size 1 or 2, or even zero — setting forth an ideal body size that most women and girls cannot meet in a healthy way. Yet they are desperately trying.

Attempts to meet these unrealistically thin expectations have devastated the health of women and girls so severely that the results can no longer be hidden. Many women of all ages and sizes are undernourished or malnourished. Teenage girls have the poorest nutrition of any group in the United States. At least two-thirds are deficient in iron, calcium and other important nutrients. Starting off with this poor history, young women have many of the same deficiencies, according to the Third Report on Nutrition Monitoring in the United States. The nutrient deficiencies of the hungry one-fourth of women at the bottom are severe.

One in 10 young women struggles with the most serious kind of abnormal eating — potentially fatal clinical eating disorders. Some are consumed by their eating disorders for most of a lifetime. Others die. Singer Karen Carpenter is one famous example.

Another tragic example of this terrible disease is Kansas City gymnast Christy Heinrich, who died in 1994 of anorexia nervosa. She was 22 years old and weighed 60 pounds.

Heinrich had been weight-conscious as long as she'd been competing. But in 1988, a judge at an international competition told the then 16-year-old Heinrich that she needed to watch her weight if she wanted to continue winning. Her offending weight: 93 pounds.

More than half of women and girls in the United States are trying to lose weight at any one time, often using hazardous methods to do it.

For the first time ever, white high school girls are now smoking more than boys, of any ethnic or racial group. These percentages are even higher in Canada, with a similar breakdown of girls higher than boys. These habits will persist, as we find that — with their terrible fear of weight gain — women are less likely to quit smoking than men.

At the same time that more women are dieting, more are obese.

To be overweight is to fail in the diet wars. This message is so pervasive in our culture that larger women face severe discrimination in health care, career, college, and personal relationships. Too often shamed, stereotyped and rendered invisible, their wisdom may be untapped and ignored. Discrimination and disrespect have sidelined many competent, compassionate large women. What a loss, when we badly need their unique talents — all the more in today's world where so many thin women are too wounded to fully participate.

This is an international crisis.

All of this searching for the culturally acceptable, starving body has given rise to four major weight and eating problems: dysfunctional eating, eating disorders, overweight, and size prejudice. I've seen alarming increases in all four problems in the 15 years I've been writing and publishing *Healthy Weight Journal,* reviewing worldwide research on eating and weight, networking with leaders, and observing the social scene.

At first I was appalled at the disarray in the health field. Then I grew hopeful, believing that once weight- and eating-related problems were better understood and put into perspective, they might be solved.

It hasn't happened. Instead, the problems have only gotten worse, exacerbated by a federal policy that works all too closely with the weight loss industry. I have watched eating and weight problems intensify through a manipulative system of funding, power, and the desire of obesity experts to maintain their authority. I'm still hopeful, but it's not a happy picture.

Unchecked, these four problems are intensifying among women and girls at younger and younger ages. Closely interrelated, they need to be dealt with in sensitive, health-focused ways, so that some aspects are not made worse by attempts to solve others.

Unfortunately, this is what is happening today: Eating problems are growing more disruptive as people try harder to lose weight.

The four problems that make up this crisis are:

- **Dysfunctional eating.** This is characterized by irregular and chaotic eating patterns — dieting, fasting, bingeing, skipping meals, overeating, undereating. Millions of Americans are engaged in these eating patterns. The National Center for Health Statistics finds that 40 percent of women and 24 percent of men are trying to lose weight at any given moment, and that 62 percent of teenage girls and about one-quarter of boys dieted in the previous year. Many of the methods they use are dangerous, and cause injury and death every year.[3]

- **Eating disorders.** An estimated 10 percent of high school and college students, most of them female, suffer from debilitating clinical eating disorders. They may undergo profound physical and mental changes, some irreversible. Death rates for anorexia nervosa and bulimia nervosa are estimated at 10 to 20 percent, according to the Canadian National Eating Disorder Information Centre in Toronto. Eating disorders are extremely difficult to treat — research suggests that less than half of those afflicted recover. Clearly, prevention is critical. Yet eating disorders and their prevention have been largely ignored in U.S. public health policy. "The public is silent when young women die" of eating disorders, charges Naomi Wolf, author of *The Beauty Myth*.[4]

- **Overweight.** Overweight is rising throughout the world, and is associated with higher rates of diabetes, hypertension, heart disease and other conditions. New federal guidelines recently changed the definition of overweight so that now 55 percent of American adults are considered overweight (an estimated 97 million), up from 43 percent in 1960. Unfortunately, every type of obesity treatment has failed to help people lose weight in a lasting way. Because the false promises of easy weight loss are widely believed, prevention efforts have not moved ahead, and are not viewed as important in the health community.[5]

- **Size prejudice.** A cruel fact of our culture, size prejudice hurts not only large people, but everyone, because no woman is ever thin enough to feel safe. Many large people live with vicious bigotry at work, school, community, home, and in health care. Size prejudice promotes body shame, and effectively keeps women in line, keeps them dieting. Even young children feel the stigma of obesity and fear being a target.

There's a great deal of confusion within health care on how to deal with these problems. Some of our public health policies seem to cause even more confusion and conflict. Currently, U. S. health policy exaggerates the risks of obesity, and ignores or minimizes the risks of undernutrition, disruptive eating, eating disorders, and hazardous weight loss. It often repeats the false and misleading media messages that thin people live longer and larger people are unhealthy, that we should enjoy only low-fat and no-fat food, that most Americans should keep dieting and trying to lose weight.

Is it only coincidence that increases in all four problems parallel an increase in dieting, weight cycling, and disruption of normal eating?

Risks overblown

The risks of being moderately overweight have been exaggerated by health professionals and the media, causing people to turn to diets that are more risky than the few extra pounds they carry. One example is a study of elderly people that found undernourished men and women anxiously cutting out meat, eggs and dairy products, and subsisting on diets that were nutritionally poor and severely deficient, and as high in fat as ever.[6]

In fact, the risks of moderate overweight are almost negligible, especially for women, if they exist at all. With severe obesity, the risks are higher (as they are for severe underweight), and yet as women grow older, most weight-related risks seem to disappear.

So why do we have such a cultural fear of fat?

It's probably a combination of things. Elizabeth Whelan, president of the American Council on Science and Health, blames the tobacco industry for spreading health terrorism about non-risks as a smoke screen over smoking issues. In obesity research, scientists with vested interests in the weight loss industry often shape and publicize their reports in ways that promote profitability.

In 1995, a Harvard scientist made the shocking announcement that almost any weight over 119 pounds for a 5-foot-5 woman can be dangerous. A closer look at the study showed this was not really the case, but that data were grouped in a special way to suggest these results. In truth, the lowest mortality was not at 119 pounds, but with a weight gain of nine to 22 pounds after age 18. Further, the study was self-reported and non-representative. Later, it was revealed that the lead author had vested interests in a drug company that was seeking Food and Drug Administration approval of its diet pills.[7]

Analysis of large nationally representative studies shows the lowest mortality is at about a body mass index of 25 for white men and women and 27 for African American men and women. Some studies show Native American men can carry BMIs of 35 to 40 without increasing their risk of death, and for the women there's no relationship.

This area of lowest risk is a rather broad range, especially for women. And as women grow older, if they are in good health, there is almost no relationship between weight and health risk. On the other hand, the evidence suggests a higher risk of death for those at a lower weight, with a BMI under 20. (A 5-foot-5 woman who weighs 119 pounds has a BMI of 19.9; at 160 pounds she has a BMI of 27.)[8]

Further, the evidence suggests that weight loss for women of every size is linked to higher death rates, particularly as women grow older. This may be because the harm caused by loss of lean body mass, including muscle, organ and bone, exceeds the benefits of fat loss.

Enjoy your good health

Americans have never been healthier, or longer lived than at this moment in time. Yes, most of us probably could improve our lifestyle one way or another. But even if we don't, we will likely live long and healthy lives.

Many weight-related risks are actually trivial. Even when risks are legitimate or measurable, they may be small, especially compared to smoking or a sedentary lifestyle. Some which have been widely publicized actually only shorten a person's life by two to three days. Sometimes these minimal risks are deliberately stated in fear-producing ways.

For example, "double the risk" sounds ominous, but may in fact be of little importance. It depends on the comparison. If one person in a room of 100 average-weight people has heart disease risk factors, and two people in a second room of 100 overweight people have these risks, then statistically the risk is twice as high for everyone in the second room, even though 98 people, compared with 99, have no risks at all.

Other so-called risks are more related to size prejudice than to health.

It's time to bring a reasonable perspective to weight issues.

It's time for women to break free from all this and to find for themselves a sounder path to wellness and wholeness that will bring personal benefits and allow them to help others.

Let's get real here.

Current confusion

The traditional paradigm, or control model, holds that all bodies should be at an "ideal" weight and large people must lose weight to be healthy, even though they cannot do this in a healthy and lasting way. It's clear these old ways of dealing with weight and eating problems haven't worked.

The crisis continues to grow. The crisis diagram on the next page summarizes the current crisis, and demonstrates how health providers, educators, family and friends, depending on their area of concern, give out conflicting messages and allow the negative aspects of culture to exert a powerful influence. The risks of losing perspective by focusing on one or two problems to the detriment of others cannot be overemphasized.

This is the case today.

Most professionals deal with only a few elements of the problems, often giving advice that conflicts with that of others, equally well-intentioned. For instance, obesity specialists sometimes focus so narrowly on making weight loss happen that they seem unaware of the consequences of their actions. Eating disorder specialists are keenly aware of the dangers of promoting weight loss, but sometimes discount the problems of excessive weight gain. Size acceptance groups are advocating for civil rights, and pressing health professionals to get off their backs. Few specialists have seemed willing to stand back and view the whole picture, bringing all problems into perspective. Few have examined the broad tragic network of weight issues that holds so many lives hostage.

Current weight and eating crisis

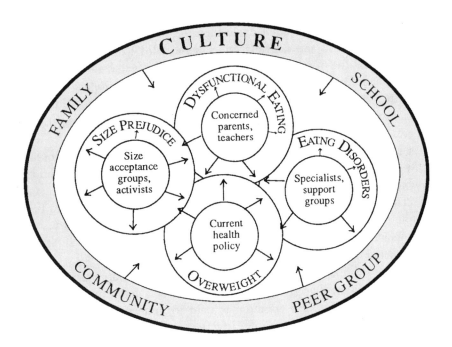

People today are caught in a weight and eating crisis in which national health policy, health care providers, teachers, family, peers and the media give out conflicting messages, working at cross-purposes and allowing the negative aspects of culture to exert a powerful influence that makes problems even worse.

AFRAID TO EAT 1997/WOMEN AFRAID TO EAT 2000

We need to do it now.

It is a concern that overweight is increasing, but we need to be more careful to do no harm while trying to solve that problem. Many obesity specialists are emphasizing the risks of obesity and want to jump right in with a major campaign that would first hit schools, by identifying and trying to treat large children. If they do this, what happens to eating disorders, dysfunctional eating and size prejudice?

I think they'll get worse. In fact, that's just what's happening now. As our culture emphasizes thinness these problems are increasing. And of course, obesity specialists are having no success in helping people lose weight, but only weight cycle them up and down. Currently they offer no long-term safe and effective methods of losing weight.

However, the official health policy view today is that all large people can and should lose weight. Health and medical professionals who promote this view assume that any excess weight over a narrow "ideal" is unhealthy, dangerous, and expensive. They believe that weight loss is always desirable and healthy for persons over this ideal, no matter how it is accomplished; and that all large persons can successfully lose at least 10 to 15 percent of their weight and maintain it. These assumptions are not supported by research.

They further assume that emphasizing the risks of obesity will help people lose weight, despite a great deal of evidence to the contrary. And they fear that warning about eating disorders or the risks of weight loss will discourage people from trying.

In the official view, there is more concern over large people who don't lose weight than over dangerous treatments being prescribed for high risk patients. Little attention is paid to underweight and normal weight women and teens who are severely restricting their nutrition, or to the young women and girls who smoke because of their fear of fat. Eating disorders, dysfunctional eating and size prejudice are regarded as unimportant, or at least irrelevant to anti-obesity messages. The fact that the policy itself might be contributing to these problems is ignored.

This thinking needs to be challenged.

Those who set national health policy, in particular, need to take a broader view of weight and eating problems, since national health policy sets the agenda for what happens throughout the country, and profoundly influences how the media responds.

Undue influence from the industry

Many who set national health policy appear to be influenced unduly by the powerful weight loss industry that pulls in $30 to $50 billion a year in the U.S. alone.

For example, when the nine members of the federally-funded National Task Force on the Prevention and Treatment of Obesity, which sets obesity policy in the United States, were required to disclose their financial affiliations, the list read like a who's who of the diet industry. They are company consultants, serve on advisory boards, conduct industry research, and receive honorariums and grants from weight loss companies and drug manufacturers of diet pills.[9]

This disclosure of vested interests illustrates the charges Thomas J. Moore makes in his book, *Lifespan,* that it is "almost impossible to find any boundary between the government, the industry and the medical elite. ... (It's) a closed circle of medical insiders operating without the normal checks and ethical barriers."

This is certainly true of obesity research. It's even more true in this time of tightening budgets when industry funding is avidly sought by scientists and their universities, and when partnerships are forged with huge multi-national pharmaceutical companies, now that diet drugs loom so tantalizingly on the horizon.

Many health officials and researchers do not share the official view of emphasizing weight loss, and refuse to support its policies. However, it is the one that currently determines U.S. health policy in regard to weight and eating issues.

The truth is, we do not have any safe way to effectively treat obesity, including prescription diet pills. Over the past 16 years of reviewing worldwide research, attending international conferences, reporting to health professionals and educators, I've watched a steady stream of miracle cures come and go.

It's all too clear that everything works short-term — and nothing works long-term. Every weight loss treatment and product I know causes people to weight cycle or yo-yo their weight down and up. Often it ends up higher than before.

It has been my mission to investigate and report the truth about these miracles that weren't. Most have been promoted with a full measure of misinformation and false promises. Many have killed.

One cult after another, as one scientist complained.

Another likened it to groping in the dark. "The public must understand that all current methods from thigh creams to stomach staples are like gropes in the dark," said Jules Hirsch, MD, an obesity researcher at Rockefeller University in New York. "An endless set of new products, new diets, and drug interventions that play legal tag with regulatory agencies while reaping profit from a public desperate for answers."[10]

Our health and medical specialists should be as candid, and stop pretending that these failed methods work. It's time to confess we don't know the answers. Time to get serious about solving weight problems instead of letting pretense, half-truths and manipulation of data get in the way of meaningful answers.

Why can't obesity be dealt with in the same way as other health problems, honestly, in a straightforward manner, without this hidden agenda? No one has pretended cancer is cured, then worked secretly backwards to see what went wrong with the cure. We haven't burdened heart patients with the onus of curing themselves. But in the weight field it's standard, it happens all the time.

Shifting to health at any size

Clearly this nation needs to deal with weight issues in healthier ways than it has in the past. We can do better than this.

Women hold the key to turning these problems around. As women we can live up to our rich potential as strong, capable, loving, generous individuals, and inspire others to do the same.

It's time to develop a vision and a new direction.

The good news is that in the midst of this crisis, a new and sounder approach is struggling to emerge. Leaders in this new approach say it is time to promote the health and well-being of every individual at every size and to put an end to our fear of fat.

This new approach advocates a paradigm shift from the old, failed weight-centered model, to a new health-centered model that helps people and does not harm them. This is about wellness and wholeness for everyone. It's about eating well, living actively, and feeling good about yourself and others. It embraces the intellectual, physical, emotional, social and spiritual well-being of the whole person, and every person.

Everyone qualifies.

Health at any size keeps eating and weight issues in perspective. It recognizes that the four problems of overweight, eating disorders, dysfunctional eating and size prejudice are all part of the big picture. Understanding this helps people realize they can't rush in to "fix" one problem without affecting, and perhaps doing harm in, other areas. We can't diet without disturbing normal eating patterns — and normal eating is not easily restored after the diet ends. It reminds health professionals of the Hippocratic oath to "do no harm," and emphasizes that much harm has been done trying to help large people lose weight. It rejects the false notion that thin people are healthy and large people unhealthy.

The new approach asks: How can we be healthier at the weight we are now? How can we gradually shift to healthier habits that will last a lifetime? How can we prevent eating and weight problems? How can we move to health at any size?

Four guiding principles help us make the shift:

1. Eat well. This means eating normally, at regular times, responding to internal signals of hunger, appetite and satiety. It means making healthy food choices based on the three principles of sound nutrition: balance, variety, and moderation. Balanced eating ensures us of getting a balance of the many nutrients needed for health, energy, and the protective immune system, through five groups: grains, vegetables, fruits, milk and milk products, and meats and alternates. Eating in variety promotes choosing many different kinds of foods from each group. Eating moderately reminds us to avoid extremes, neither overeating nor undereating, neither overindulging in high-fat, high-sugar foods nor rejecting them entirely — many may be favorites that can certainly fit in with healthy eating.

2. Live actively. Enjoy physical activity, take pleasure in being active in your own way, every day, as a normal part of your life. Engaging in regular activity is important for many reasons, only one of which is its beneficial effect on weight. It's a mistake to hold out weight loss as the primary reason for women to be active. Live actively because it's a great and wonderful way to live.

3. Feel good about yourself. Respect, accept and trust yourself. Each of us is unique, with special talents and traits, and this is a marvelous thing. Self-acceptance may be a first step in getting on with life. This can be very freeing. It liberates the larger woman from "waiting to be thin," and helps her move on with health-centered changes that improve her life and well-being. Keep up your positive self-talk and avoid negatives.

4. Feel good about others. Respect and appreciate the size diversity and special qualities of others, and be non-judgmental about their appearance. Everyone needs to feel accepted, and deserves a sense of well-being, peace and tranquility. It's important to instill policies of zero tolerance for size bias in the workplace, schools and colleges. Family members need to support each other by giving unconditional love: "I love you no matter what."

Following these guidelines shifts the focus from thinness to being healthy and happy at the weight we are. It puts these issues into perspective, and prevents eating and weight problems from looming too large. It helps people get on with their lives.

A word of caution: If you're a traditional thinker or a dedicated dieter — still waiting to be thin, or keeping thin by living in the starvation mode — making this mental shift may take time, so don't expect to do it overnight. It may even involve a grieving process, the giving up of misplaced hopes. But once you fully embrace it, you'll never go back.

Sometimes it's enough to plant seeds, and after a time they begin to grow and flourish. I've seen this happen many times in the last 10 years as health and nutrition leaders gradually shift to this new way of thinking. And once they've tasted its freedom and soundness, I've never known any to shift back to the old way of thinking.

A healthy people goal

People come in different sizes and shapes. And that's okay.

Just as in height, some people are very short, others very tall, with most of us in between. So in weight, some people will be naturally thin, others naturally large, and most of us in between.

The goal is to be healthy at the weight you are.

The healthy people diagram on the next page demonstrates this new approach.

The goal in the center is to promote health and well-being, wellness and wholeness for women, men and children at every size.

To achieve this goal, we need to take a comprehensive approach in which family, teachers, health providers, the media, and the culture itself, on the outside of the circle, consistently reflect healthy messages: Eat well, live actively, and feel good about yourself and others. In this way, the four problems in the smaller circles — dysfunctional eating, eating disorders, overweight, and size prejudice — can be diminished, or even eliminated. Special programs developed to prevent these problems will keep within this context.

With this new approach, people can develop and grow in normal ways, without fear, working with their natural regulatory abilities to maintain a stable weight through life. They can freely develop their unique potential as lovable, capable, valuable individuals, take pride in themselves and their bodies, without stigma or apology.

The first step is to stop harmful programs and practices, especially those that promote dieting, food restriction, and weight loss. Empowering our half-starved daughters to feed themselves is an urgent health issue. For many, their nutrition deficiencies are having severe effects on their bones, growth and mental functioning.

The next step is to encourage healthy, normal eating and physical activity for everyone, at appropriate and pleasurable levels. Finally, we need to develop, test, and implement safe and effective preventive programs.

Canada has already initiated this sound and integrated approach in addressing weight issues. I've been much inspired by Canadian leaders and Health Canada's public awareness Vitality campaign. I love Vitality's

Healthy people

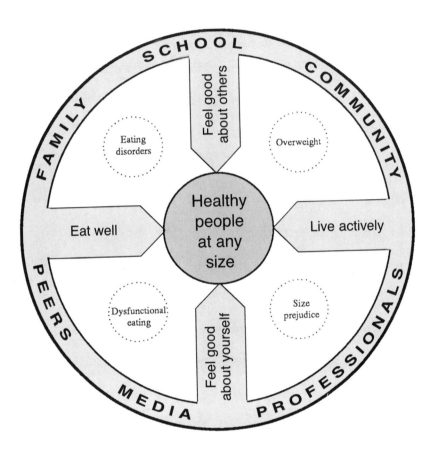

To achieve the goal of healthy people at any size, a comprehensive health approach is needed, whereby all receive consistent messages that encourage eating well, living actively, and feeling good about yourself and others. If family, teachers, health professionals, peers and the media consistently give these messages, then the four major weight and eating problems (dysfunctional eating, eating disorders, overweight and size prejudice) will be diminished.

simple and eloquent message and have incorporated its philosophy into this book: Eat well, be active and feel good about yourself.[11]

At the same time, larger women must not sit back and allow prejudice to discourage them. They are needed in leadership roles, not just as the wonderful community volunteers they have always been, but in political, social and entertainment arenas. They are desperately needed as successful role models for young girls in a world that seeks to constrict their ambitions to narrow appearance standards.

CHAPTER 2

Our culture fails
to nurture women

■

*"The tyranny of the ideal image makes almost all of
us feel inferior. We are taught to hate our bodies,
and thus learn to hate ourselves. This self-hatred
takes an enormous toll ... (in) feelings of inferiority,
anxiety, insecurity and depression."*
— *Jean Kilbourne*

How did we get to this point?

Why do we need to readjust our thinking back to sound, nutritional eating, active living and positive self-esteem?

The answer lies in our culture. At no time in history have women been so pressured to be thin. Thinness is sold on every street corner, and the wonderful diversity of women, their inner beauty and well-being, is rejected. Women — even those of below average weight — look at themselves and see a body that is too big or is oversized in one part or another.

Our culture is deeply ambivalent about women and their bodies.

"Women are idealized and denigrated, protected and abused, encouraged and discriminated against. By the time most girls become women, they have confused and conflicting feelings about their place in the world. This confusion manifests itself in a dissatisfaction with their bodies and their appearance. Before long, their confused and conflicting feelings boil down to one issue: Fat," write Jane Hirschmann and Carol

Munter in *When Women Stop Hating Their Bodies.*[1]

Perhaps in decades to come, our culture will place less importance on the "ideal female body" — the term should be an obscenity — and women can feel good about themselves in their natural sizes and shapes.

But not now.

The distorted media mirror

Page through almost any magazine, look at almost every television show. Notice anything about the women there?

It seems as if there is literally one model — one who is thin, youthful, beautiful and who, in reality, represents perhaps five percent of women in America.

Where are the other 95 percent? We need to be seeing women in a wider range of shapes, sizes, ages, and attractiveness on television, in advertising, magazines, and the movies. We need lots more role models for the 95 percent of girls and young women who will never achieve that "ideal look" — which of course is often reshaped through plastic surgery, or retouched, airbrushed, and computer-enhanced on the page.

But how can we expect girls and women to know what a normal, healthy body looks like when all they see are the victims of starvation being praised and glorified for their skeletal structures?

Women on television seem to get thinner each year. Their fashionable faces are now gaunt and hollow-cheeked, reflected everywhere in real life. It hurts to see a lineup of thin girls from the side — high school cheerleaders, for instance — their stomachs caved in, bony clavicles and hip bones protruding. Where are the bodies they have worked so hard to perfect? There's no body. Only bones, arms, legs, hair and that frightening skeletal face, screaming out cheers — or maybe, screaming for help from a society that has abandoned them.

Media — in all its forms — is a powerful messenger.

Here's how *Newsweek* described the look of the 1990s — which has only intensified as a new decade begins: "It is a slimmer, more dissipated vision ... reedy, women with hollow curves and sinewy lines ... small, frail-looking ... wan and disengaged ... austere as the times ... human coat hangers ... Clothes fall off them."

These images have toppled the "curvaceous supermodels" of the past decade, the writers proclaim. The magazine leaves unexplained its odd conclusion that this is a "return to reality ... down to earth" and proves that "men and their appetites" don't rule the world.[2]

Along those lines, the two institutions of the "ideal woman" — the Miss America Pageant and Playboy — are being represented by women who are thinner and thinner every year and proportionately smaller in the hips, as a 30-year survey vividly illustrates. Now the typical contestant or model weighs in at 13 to 19 percent below expected weight, and has almost no curve at the hip. The clinical criteria for anorexia nervosa is 15 percent below expected weight.[3]

\"Pathologically underweight women are being held up as cultural ideals," laments Dr. David Greenfeld, medical director of the Yale-New Haven Hospital Adolescent and Young Adult Treatment Unit.[4]

This distorted picture of reality portrayed through the media adversely affects girls and women in three ways, says Karin Jasper, PhD, of the Women's Center Toronto.[5]

The distortions include:

1. Frequently propagating myths and falsehoods
2. Normalizing or even glamorizing what is abnormal or unhealthy
3. Creating the false impression that all women are alike by failing to represent whole segments of the real world

These false messages contribute to the confusion of women, thinness obsession, and prevalence of eating disorders, says Jasper.

Women and girls believe them, respond to them.

Devastating spotlight

Even veterans of the movie and media scene have been devastated by these distortions.

Mary Evans Young, the English author of *Diet Breaking*, describes what body image issues have meant for four famous women, two Brits and two Americans. She says their treatment by the media and the public regarding their size, shape and weight, serve to remind all women that their bodies are open to comment, and that any deviation carries the risk of public disapproval.[6]

Princess Diana. Before she became Her Royal Highness, Princess of Wales, Lady Diana's image was that as seen in one famous photograph — wearing a long, flowing, semi-transparent skirt and holding a child. She is "probably a size 12." As her relationship with Prince Charles became official, the media scrutiny of her clothing and body size intensified. The press hounded Princess Diana as she lost weight. She lightened her hair and she grew image-conscious.

Once, Princess Diana lost too much weight for the media and "there was mock concern" when it was suspected that she might be suffering from anorexia or bulimia. She was criticized for playing with her food and for her faddish eating. "Diana had gone too far. ... She couldn't win. It was a pointed reminder to all of us that our margin of acceptability is very narrow and nonnegotiable, and that failure invites a heavy penalty."

Sarah Ferguson. Before her marriage to Prince Andrew, there is an early impression of Sarah in another photo. "She had just finished a day's work at a publishing firm and was happily skipping along, smiling at the photographers and film crews ... wearing a gathered, calf-length skirt and a navy blue top, probably a size 12 to 14. She looked so ordinary and so happy ... a living contradiction of the thin edict — she had escaped the tyranny."

But as Evans Young tells it, the press soon started hounding Sarah and pulling her apart, criticizing her size and shape, her hairstyles, her dress sense. Sarah seemed to reel, and there followed a well-publicized series of exercise and reducing scenes. While the world watched, the new princess turned into a thin and very different person. But her new, waif-like figure did not ensure a happy marriage.

"She has since regained much of that weight and is again a target for comments about her size and shape, while Andrew largely escapes hurtful comments about his size."

Later, Sarah came to the United States, a well-trained dieter, and became a spokeswoman for Weight Watchers.

Elizabeth Taylor. Over 30 or 40 years, in countless pictures and articles the press chronicled Liz Taylor's relationship with food, dieting, fat farms and up and down cycles of weight. "A photograph of a 'fallen star' — which means 'fat' — fetches a premium price in the press. So long as she is thin, we will all want and love her ... and aspire to be like her. This message is not lost on ordinary women. Already feeling a bit insecure, we know we need to be loved."

Oprah Winfrey. If ever we needed an example of the way women are tyrannized into being thin, Oprah Winfrey is that example, says Evans Young. She has lost weight, regained, lost again, regained, and shared with the public her experiences, successes and failures around food, weight and size. Oprah is a warm, caring, compassionate woman who has accomplished much, yet she has said her greatest achievement was losing weight.

Evans Young asserts that the treatment dealt famous women like these "serves to chastise and tyrannize the rest of us." It is a reminder that women are targets for being sized up in a way that brings other women into line.

For women, she says, "Our bodies are perceived as public property — up for scrutiny and debate, rather than a personal matter. Because ll have to be very thin, it stands to reason that the fatter ones will be pressured most. I believe if we accept that even one uld be oppressed for her body size and shape we are all by body size and shape — because that is the gauge by which we are all being measured."

In a more recent example, Alicia Silverstone, slim s
fame, was ridiculed by the press at the Academy Awards because she
had gained five or 10 pounds since making her last movie.

Headlines read "Batman and Fatgirl," and "Look out Batman, here
comes Buttgirl." She was called "More Babe than Babe."

The power of advertising

But who has the power to resist the bombardment?

Advertising expertly conveys the message that "you're not okay —
and here's what you need to buy to fix what's wrong." Advertising sells
body dissatisfaction a thousand times a day to women and men who are
being set up by the constant stream of gaunt images in the media. The
perfect model guarantees our desire to fix our "ugly fat" or other "ugly"
features through buying product X.

We buy the product; it doesn't work. We're left with dissatisfaction about a feature we hadn't even noticed before, and the belief that
there is one more thing wrong with us. Then we go out and buy more.

It's a wildly successful strategy.

Advertising is a $130 billion industry and the most powerful educa-
tional force in America. It has designed the cultural ideals of the last
two or three decades.

Media pressure to be thin is stronger now than at any time in the
last 19 years. A recent study found that television diet promotions,
nonexistent in 1973, now comprise about five percent of TV advertisements.[7]

Jean Kilbourne, EdD, author of *Still Killing Us Softly: Advertising and the Obsession with Thinness,* argues that advertising over-
powers almost every other cultural message through sheer force. The
average American sees 1,500 ads per day and spends a year and a half
of a lifetime watching TV commercials.[8]

"The tyranny of the ideal image makes almost all of us feel inferior," Kilbourne says. "We are taught to hate our bodies, and thus learn
to hate ourselves. This self-hatred takes an enormous toll ... (in) feelings
of inferiority, anxiety, insecurity, and depression."

The thinness craze is lucrative for the fashion and tobacco industry; for the makers of body products, weight loss products and services,
diet drinks, and for every industry from trucks to whiskey that advertises
with striking models posed with the product.

Advertisers are "killing us softly," warns Kilbourne. Yet she says
they will never voluntarily change, because it is "profitable for women
to feel terrible about themselves."[9]

Women's magazines sell readers

Women's magazines have become so dependent on promoting their advertisers that many are little more than catalogs selling products."

"Women's magazines are controlled by advertisers in ways that other magazines aren't," *Ms* co-founder Gloria Steinem told a gathering of writers. She said 85 percent of women's magazine copy is really "unmarked advertorial."

Extremely thin models are used almost exclusively to illustrate the pages of women's magazines. One senior-level editor told a writer I know that it's absolutely taboo to run photos of women who are not slender. Even articles with the message that it's perfectly healthy to be heavier than the ideal are invariably illustrated with very thin women.

The desire to please the magazines' lifeline is one reason trivial or incorrect nutrition advice appears so often in these publications. They want feel-good nutrition stories without much substance, especially next to their ads.

This is why food-as-medicine stories are so popular, explains Marilyn Larkin, a New York free-lance writer. For years she wrote what she now calls lopsided viewpoint articles. These feature food-of-the-month, or food-as-magic-bullet angles — carrot power, the grapefruit diet — single foods touted to fight cancer, strengthen the immune system, stave off heart attacks, burn fat, reduce stress, or improve your sex life. A single food is lauded all out of perspective.[10]

Diet articles need to be a quick read and entertaining, so women's magazines continually recycle easy-to-swallow stories like "Seven secrets every thin person knows." or "Myths that keep you fat." Sidebars, boxes, cute little quizzes, and "starter menus" are favored.

Larkin was asked to write articles for weight loss centers, for which she'd be paid twice, by the magazine and the company. She considered this unethical and refused, but it's clear that other writers don't.

Beauty divides, isolates women

Consumerism is at stake. Industry benefits when women's bodies fail the test. When women fail, keep striving, and continue to be dissatisfied, ideally, they'll keep buying and competing.

In a searing account, author Naomi Wolf charges that the power structure, acting largely through the media, especially women's magazines and their advertisers, unites to force women into a competition of continual striving for thinness and beauty. It's a cruel struggle they can't win.

In this struggle, every woman is made to feel a failure in her attempts to perfect her body and face. No matter what her successes in other areas of life, she falls short. She feels her body is constantly on display and being judged unfavorably.

The goal of a perfect appearance is divisive for women, says Wolf. Since it is impossible, a woman always falls short, feels inadequate and counts herself a failure. Yet she stands alone, pitted woman against woman. Thinner and more beautiful, another woman is disliked; less thin and beautiful, she is discounted. It's a competition in which there are no winners, except the political and corporate power structure which sells the products of supposed perfection.

This competition and divisiveness is clearly seen among white teen-age girls in an Arizona study that compared their body images with those of African American girls.

The study of 300 adolescents found the white girls were dissatisfied with their bodies and wanted to lose weight as a way to be popular and "perfect." Almost as one they described a rigid and fixed image of their ideal. She weighed 120 pounds, had very long legs and long blonde hair. Perversely, these girls did not support their peers who were closest to this ideal, but felt envious and competitive with them. Comparing themselves to their ideal, the girls were very dissatisfied with their own weight and appearance. Over 90 percent were dissatisfied even when their weight was normal. Younger girls were most severely affected.

By comparison, the African American girls held images of beauty that were flexible, fluid and unrelated to size. Beauty was based on each girl's sense of self, style, confidence, and "looking good." Looking good meant a girl was projecting her self-image, establishing a presence, presenting a sense of style, and "making what you have work for you."

Unlike the white girls, they felt supported in their efforts to look good by other girls and by family, friends and community.[11]

With more wholesome attitudes like these, it is no coincidence that African American girls are dieting at only two-thirds the rate of white and Hispanic girls, or that their suicide behavior is only two-thirds as high. Nor is it surprising that for women, as well, African American culture defines beauty in broader terms than white values. Studies show women of many sizes feel acceptable, and African American women don't have to be thin to be thought beautiful.

While all this sounds positive for the African American community, many of these women, too, are feeling the intense pressures of our weight-obsessed culture. Despite research that indicates less serious concerns on average, we cannot make light of the anguish over weight that many of these women and girls feel. Their feelings about weight run the gamut from self-acceptance to dissatisfaction to desperation. New research suggests they are starting to develop similar or equal rates of eating disorders as white women.

Hollow-cheeked images

Pressures to be thin are especially acute on college campuses today. Food restriction is taking its toll as young women struggle to attain an emaciated ideal.

"Instead of being strong and creative and full of resilience, so many young women I speak to on college campuses, again the best and the brightest, are barely making it through at a level of survival," warns Naomi Wolf. "Because they're exhausted. And they're exhausted because they're starving or vomiting compulsively. This generation's voice is diminished, their reasoning powers are blunted. And this is America's future leadership."

But the passion for thinness is by no means confined to younger women — a phase they pass through, and then outgrow as they mature. In today's world women of all ages are threatened by body dissatisfaction, and older women are not exempt.

Studies show that even after age 70, a great many women are still dieting. Among women over age 60 who are not overweight, more than 22 percent are trying to lose weight, according to national statistics from the Centers of Disease Control. This includes nearly 25 percent of Mexican American women, 22.4 percent of white women, and 14.4 percent of African American women — all of them within normal weight range.[12]

In the fitness industry, the body-shaping goal being promoted for women is getting thin, lean and hard, but not necessarily gaining muscles or strength.

The current ideal of female beauty is "anorexics with barbells," notes Roberta Seid, PhD, of the University of Southern California.

Kilbourne agrees, "The fitness craze co-opts the whole idea of power for women, reducing it to narcissism ... A woman who lifts weights and is also starving herself will have significantly decreased energy and power. Thus, in the guise of offering health, fitness, and expanded opportunities to women, the culture restricts all of these things."

These contradictions can be seen throughout women's sports. High rates of eating disorders and nutrient deficiencies are documented on women's athletic teams.

Medicine, too, endorses thinness. The health community, medical establishment, and federal government are all doing their share to promote skeletal images for women. In the medical view, health equals thinness — period.

Seid writes that in the past, excesses of fashion were severely criticized by social authorities, including doctors, teachers, clergy, parents and feminists. Moralists stressed that there were values more important than outward appearance. But no more.

"In the late 20th century all these authorities, especially physicians, seemed to agree that one could never be too thin, " she says.

Credibility on the job

For many women, their appearance is a yardstick by which their ability on the job is measured. Having the right figure is important for women in getting and keeping a good job in most of the business world. "

Laura Fraser points out that many women join diet groups not just for the traditional reasons of romance or a happy marriage, but to land a successful career, supposedly available only if they are thin. In these groups, women try to gain power by becoming more attractive and seeming more disciplined, controlled, and health-conscious.

"But it is the kind of power parceled out by a society that is profoundly distrustful of women: the power and privilege that come from attaining a body that fits the socially approved mold. It's the power derived from living up to society's expectations of women as objects, and of behaving in a manner — restraining one's desires and appetites — that fits the confining rules of proper female conduct. In other words, it's not much real power at all."[13]

Demands of the workplace reinforce the need for women to conform to slender ideals, charges Naomi Wolf. These can be rigidly enforced as in the case of flight attendants, who have won discrimination lawsuits. But often they are more subtle.

"Even if you think you are free to be at your own weight or your own size, very often there's what I have called the Professional Beauty Quotient in the workplace," says Wolf. "In retail, in sales, not to mention the media, and television work, many women find this operating. Many women find they are expected to fit a rigidly thin ideal to stay employed."

This is illegal, Wolf warns: The occupational qualification to be thin and conventionally attractive is a different expectation for women than men, and this is an illegal employment issue.

The employment issue is important, particularly if we have developed a society in which a young woman can be anything she wants to be — as long as she is thin and pretty.[14]

Even on the opera stage, robust women with voices to match may be in less demand, as television dominates the cultural scene. It's getting harder for great singers to get roles unless they are attractive and slender. Both opera and record companies are feeling the pressure to value appearance over the sound of the voice. "Heaven forbid that Don Jose would sacrifice his honor and life for a full-figured Carmen," comments one reporter.[15]

In politics, a woman needs to look right before she can run for office. She'll wait until "she's down to a perfect size 10, and the kids are out of school," says New York Times editorial writer Gail Collins, commenting on why so few women are in high political office today, long after the promise of the 1970s.[16]

For women, it's hard to win. They can comply with thin body prescriptions, but may need to lower career goals in the effort needed to tend the body, especially when it involves semistarvation. Or they can focus on career and other personal fulfillment issues and let the pounds fall where they may, but risk losing the support of others if they gain too much weight.

The thin among us are the saints of the system, says Margaret Visser, writing in the *Journal of Gastronomy,* "They fulfill our ideals while demonstrating impressive dedication and willpower in the process; their physical shape constitutes proof of guiltlessness."[17]

Thinness has taken the place of virginity in representing the goodness of women since the 1960s sexual revolution, says eating disorder therapist Catherine Steiner-Adair. As a result "obesity is regarded with the scorn previously reserved for sexuality."[18]

Historical cultural targets

Unfortunately, cultures have long defined their "feminine ideal," dictating the way a woman should look, dress and act.

Preferred shapes have varied from "round as a ball" in African fattening rooms that rendered young girls plump and beautiful before marriage, to the tummy-centered maternal European woman of the 1500s, to today's "steeples of bones."[19]

In the 10th century China, foot-binding gave women the "lotus" or "lily" foot, crippling them for life in the name of beauty and femininity. Little girls had their toes bent under and tightly wrapped until the bones eventually broke, causing deformed clubfeet.

A Chinese woman recalled: "I was inflicted with the pain of foot binding when I was seven years old. I was an active child who liked to jump about, but from then on my free and optimistic nature vanished ... I wept and hid in a neighbor's home, but mother found me, scolded me, and dragged me home. She shut the bedroom door, boiled water, and from a box withdrew binding, shoes, knife, needle and thread. I begged for a one-day postponement, but mother refused ... Mother would remove the bindings and wipe the blood and pus which dripped from my feet. She told me that only with removal of the flesh could my feet become slender."

Why did mothers continue a custom that inflicted such suffering, asks Sharlene Hesse-Biber, associate professor of women's studies at Boston College. Because the bound foot, symbol of feminine beauty and male authority, represented a woman's best prospects in life, the chance for a prosperous marriage.[20]

In the 19th century, European and American women laced their corsets far past the point of pain. Worn all night, they were cinched in tighter next morning. Stays of whalebone, and later steel, constricted women's waists to as small as fourteen or fifteen inches, which a proud husband could encircle with his hands, subtly exerting his power and control. Again, there were handsome rewards for women who could marry well.

The 1920s brought the right to vote and more freedom for American women, and with it came straight, thin, boyish figures. Even though women were urged into factories during World War II, society reversed itself for the postwar 1940s and 1950s. Women were urged to give up their jobs for returning servicemen after their "Rosie the Riveter" stint for the war effort, and return to the kitchen. Body styles blossomed with feminine curves, full breasts and hips, set off by tiny cinched waists. It was the Gibson Girl hourglass look.

In the 1960s, with rapidly expanding political and sexual freedom for women, the feminine was again drained from the female body. Fashion lauded Twiggy and the lean, boyish, broad shouldered and slim hipped figure. And like the Victorian corset lacings pulled tighter each morning, the ideal shape for women has become thinner, more gaunt, and more painful every decade since.

Present-day "beauties" are women with faces gaunt and angular, their necks resembling steeples of bones, as described by Seid. Their arms and legs are unfleshed, full of sharp angles, gangly and disproportionately long.[21]

"Each era has exacted its own price for beauty, though our era is unique in producing a standard based exclusively on the bare bones of being, which can be disastrous for human health, happiness and productivity," she writes. "Indeed the lean body looks as repressed and controlled as the spirit that must have gotten it that way ... it offers no softness, no warmth, no tenderness, no mysteries," she writes.

Seid wonders if future historians might think we Americans had fallen in love with death, or if a terror of nuclear destruction had made "fashion play with cadavers and turn them into images of beauty."

Women as objects

There's a fine line between the pressures directed at women to be thin and young and beautiful, and the message that women are merely decorative objects.

Susan Kano, author of *Making Peace with Food,* writes that women are dehumanized by beauty contests, bodybuilding contests, and pornography, as well as by advertisers and the fashion industry. "Beauty contestants are paraded across stages like so many units of flesh, bone, and fashion, and judged on purely aesthetic grounds. With the exception of token 'talent' and 'question' portions of the contests, they are glorified lessons in the practice of objectification," she says.

Pornography is another form of the objectification of women. "Much pornography portrays women as defenseless objects to be used and abused for the pleasure of another person or group of people (almost always men). What lies within those beautiful bodies is irrelevant ... Sexual slavery and abuse is celebrated," says Kano.[22]

Men's magazines are fighting it out these days to show ever more breasts, skin, and sensual female bodies, *Newsweek* reported in 1999. "One thing is sure, more guy mags are coming."[23]

Kano points out that the most insidious offenders are less obvious and more widespread. The way women's bodies and body parts are treated in advertising, draped over cars or appliances like pretty decorations. Most movies, she believes, objectify women to some extent.

Women's clothing, which is often tight and has an ornamental purpose with little regard to ability to move, is part of this objectification. Woman's comfort and ability to function is secondary to her appearance.

And then, there is the woman as an accessory. Esther Rothblum, PhD, professor of psychology at the University of Vermont, cites research that suggests a man's social status depends more on having attractive female partners than on his own physical attractiveness. He is judged by his "quality toys" and his playmates.[24]

When Coca Cola launched a marketing campaign for Diet Sprite, they chose a bony model listlessly nursing her diet drink and boasted in the advertisement that her nickname was "Skeleton." Public protest forced the company to pull the ad.

"There's something very sick going on here," complained the mother of an anorexic daughter in a Boston consumer group that boycotted Diet Sprite as a result of the ad.

Yes. There is a cultural sickness when emaciated, vulnerable, passive, childlike women are idealized as the role models for our daughters.

Sexually provocative ads also send potentially harmful messages.

Take the Calvin Klein ads that feature pathetically young, thin, vulnerable waifs in sexual poses in upscale magazines and billboards. These cultural messages seem to promote child sexual abuse.

The adult version of this sexual message often shows models doing nothing at all but displaying themselves while males reinforce ownership of them by towering over or grasping them, points out Rothblum.

Sexual harassment, abuse

The dark side of our culture, and every culture, is the sexual abuse and violence against women and children. How does our culture allow — and even promote — sexual harassment and sexual abuse of women and girls?

When girls and women are treated as objects, in advertising, television, men's magazines, and pornography, and at the same time rendered weak, dependent, and self-critical – they are especially vulnerable.

Harassment, sexual violence, and stigmatization are three interrelated traumas that can lead to eating and body struggles. They influence the way women feel about their bodies, and how they eat and nourish themselves, especially when they occur during childhood.

Three Canadian researchers think sexual harassment may be one of the important ways in which young girls learn to feel shame, embarrassment, rejection and hatred toward their developing bodies. June Larkin, Carla Rice and Vanessa Russell, Women's Studies specialists at the University of Toronto, organized focus groups in schools in which girls recorded in their journals and shared incidents of sexual harassment.[25]

They suggest that sexual harassment or teasing is a tool of oppression that can alienate girls from their developing bodies and give them a distorted sense of self.

"We have heard countless accounts of this contempt being expressed by their male peers: the girl who is afraid to walk home from school because she is forced to walk past a gang of adolescent boys who routinely call her a 'fat bitch' while they pelt her with stones; the girls who do not want to walk down a certain hallway in their high school because they are afraid of being publicly rated on a scale of one to 10 and coming out on the low end; the girls who are subjected to barking, grunting and mooing calls and labels of 'dogs,' 'cows,' or 'pigs' when they pass by groups of male students; those who are teased about not measuring up to the buxom, bikini-clad girls that drape the pages of various newspapers; and the girls who are grabbed, pinched, groped and fondled as they try to make their way through the school corridors."

Having to ward off these kinds of comments created a growing uneasiness about their developing bodies for many of the girls.

The Toronto researchers charge that harassing words thrown at girls do not slide harmlessly away as the taunting sounds dissipate. "They are slowly absorbed into the child's identity and developing sense of self, becoming an essential part of whom she sees herself to be. Harassment involves the use of words as weapons to inflict pain and assert power."

Sexual harassment is so commonplace it is often perceived as normal, an integral part of female development, and gets largely ignored. Yet it is one of the more pervasive ways that teenage girls are reminded of the hazards of living in a woman's body. Larkin, Rice and Russell see harassment as a pervasive form of violence that contributes to young women's uneasiness about their bodies and results in a disruption of healthy female development. It's a process that brands girls as defective, inferior, and inadequate.

Stigmatizing girls (and boys) who don't measure up is a way of marking them as different, defining that difference as inferior, and using it to justify oppression. Stigmatizing large girls not only hurts them, it's also a way to keep thinner girls in line, continuing to focus on diet and weight.

Leering finds its target

The Toronto writers say ogling by males quickly teaches girls the risks inherent in their maturing bodies. They find leering can be a process used by males to select those females who will be the target of their future sexual and abusive comments and behavior.

They quote Marian Bosford Fraser, "At some point in their physical development, all female children lose the protection of baby fat and barrettes and become prey in a game in which there are rules only if the laws are broken ... The worst messages come from men. I have watched the way that grown men feel free to look at young girls ... lets his eyes slide all over the body of a pretty teenage girl walking by ... grunts when he encounters two teenagers young enough to be his daughters ... mutters, 'check out the hot blonde' to his buddy; the hot blonde is not yet 16."

Some young women attempt to take control of their bodies by shrinking them until the self seems to disappear.

Sexual abuse

If it is true that one-third of women were sexually abused during childhood, as these experts report — and most subjected to some kind of sexual harassment or shaming of their sexual bodies — this is a tremendous burden.

Sexual violence is the most graphic and oppressive tool for subordinating women. Often women and girls report they use bingeing and purging as a way of expelling the frightening feelings that come from being sexually traumatized. They may develop eating and weight struggles, cut or burn themselves, or disassociate from their bodies as a way of disconnecting from the source of their vulnerability, eating disorder specialists Larkin, Rice and Russell suggest.

Rape, incest or sexual abuse in childhood is reported by 30 to 40 percent of women, but is much higher in eating disordered patients. Symptoms can include nausea, vomiting, eating disorders, fatigue, headaches, and sexual dysfunction.[26]

It's about shame

The consequence of this abuse is shame, often felt as the result of humiliation and failure to measure up to high standards of appearance. Shame is the response to being violated, harassed and stigmatized, the overwhelming sense of being inadequate and wrong. Shame as a result of harassment and oppression can make women want to disappear, become invisible, disconnect from their bodies while engaging in "relentless body criticism and improvement in an effort to bolster their shattered self-esteem," say the Toronto specialists.

Rice says this can make them vulnerable to chronic dieting and eating disorders, "For someone faced with unrelenting discrimination in the form of blatant public hostility and disgust, demeaning and dehumanizing jokes, and unwanted advice ... losing weight becomes an attractive means of attempting to retrieve lost self-esteem as well as gaining and achieving success."

Sexual abuse makes women want to escape their bodies, to deprive and punish and control their bodies, or to become more perfect to wipe out the shame.

We need to help strengthen women and girls, encourage their emotional toughness and self-protection, support and guide them, but this is not enough. Most important is to change our culture.

Socializing young girls

Where does it all start? By age 2, girls are watching television and starting their daily exposure to messages that show successful women are are thin. They are hearing their mothers, teachers, older sisters, and women in general objectify, distrust, and battle their bodies in order to make them acceptably thin. They are hearing their fathers, brothers, and important males in their lives talk about and judge women's bodies.

As preschoolers, they learn that certain types of foods will make them fat. Six-year-olds know eating fat is bad, and that people who are fat should diet and exercise. More seriously, a substantial number of girls in primary grades are so concerned about their bodies, they have already tried to lose weight. Weight preoccupation and body dissatisfaction are occurring earlier and earlier. By fourth grade, 40 percent or more of girls "diet" at least occasionally. Those who do not are gathering information and forming values and opinions.

Modern culture is youth-centered, yet in many ways it does not provide an environment that is nurturing or supportive for the healthy growth and development of girls. In fact, it nurtures serious problems.

"A girl-poisoning culture ... a girl-destroying place," psychologist Mary Pipher brands our society in her book, *Reviving Ophelia*.[27]

Pipher says that in early adolescence girls are expected to sacrifice the parts of themselves that our culture considers masculine on the altar of social acceptability. They have to shrink their souls down to petite size.

With nearly all the messages about thinness aimed at girls and women, some researchers see strong ties between the American public health crisis over weight and eating disorders and an intentional cultural oppression of women. The attack messages work best when the target is young. And young adolescent girls are most vulnerable.

"I am deeply concerned about what is happening to young girls in our society today," says Paula Levine, PhD, former president of Eating Disorders Awareness and Prevention. "Young girls up until the age of 11 are confident, unafraid of conflict, and willing to say exactly what is on their minds. As they enter puberty, however, they adjust to society's messages about what young women are 'supposed' to be — nice, kind, caring, self-sacrificing, agreeable and compliant."

In classrooms across the country, girls are encouraged to speak quietly, defer to boys, avoid math and science, and to value popularity and appearance over integrity and intelligence.

I have clipped a set of Doonsbury cartoon strips in which a small girl keeps waving her hand in the classroom, signaling that she knows the answers, but is repeatedly overlooked in favor of boys. In the last frame, still ignored by the teacher, she comes to a forlorn conclusion, "Maybe I should go on a diet."

"If it is true that by the time young girls in this country reach puberty, they are voiceless, their self-esteem is at a low ebb, and they feel anxious, inferior and out of control, is there any more fertile ground for the development of an eating disorder? I think not," says Levine.

She says teenage girls need to recapture the time in their lives when they were confident, courageous, and critical thinkers. It seems that many women need to do this, too. "Only when they begin to value themselves as worthy human beings and not as objects of beauty will we begin to win the war on eating disorders."[28]

But the odds against that are incredibly high.

Setting the stage

Why are so many young girls in therapy in the late 1990s? asks Pipher. "They are coming of age in a more dangerous, sexualized and media-saturated culture. They face incredible pressure to be beautiful and sophisticated, which in junior high means using chemicals and being sexual. As they navigate a more dangerous world, girls are less protected."

Yet, this is happening at a time when women have more freedom and independence than ever before. They can command companies, lead hospitals, hold public office and make millions.

Women have never had more opportunities than now, yet they grow up feeling as though their bodies are being constantly watched. They learn to feel disconnected from their bodies, as if observing themselves from the outside, and this is especially likely when they have been sexually abused or harassed, say these experts.

Girls do not simply live in their bodies but become aware of how their bodies appear in the eyes of men and boys. By seeing themselves as images in male eyes, they begin to observe rather than to experience their own bodies, say Deborah Tolman, EdD, and Elizabeth Debold, MEd, of Harvard University. "Their bodies become 'Other' to themselves."[29]

Some are asking: What is "normal" and what is "disordered," for women growing up in a culture that forces them to live as if their bodies are being "watched, desired and judged?" A culture that encourages women to use "the power of weakness"; that allows high rates of violence and sexual assault on women, at the same time it demands that the female body be highly attractive and sensual?

Is it about women's freedom?

What kind of culture would require its women to remain hungry and half-nourished?

The answer, some would say, is a culture that has given women more freedom than it is comfortable with.

Is this, then, about women's freedom? That's one explanation.

In this view, women entering the marketplace in such large numbers threaten the power of corporate and political institutions, as well as threatening male power. Keeping women physically small, immature, semi-starved, and diverted from life's real issues diminishes their power as competent individuals, and reduces their chances of building strong careers.

This travesty is not being perpetuated on women by individual men, for the most part — men, after all, have female friends, lovers, wives, sisters, daughters they care about — but by the political power structure and multinational corporations bent on shaping women into the ultimate consumers, perennially dissatisfied with their appearance.

From a feminist perspective, the selling of thinness and the ignoring of the diversity of real women is seen as a manipulative tool to prevent women from gaining power in the work force. The adverse effects of self starvation in the ceaseless quest for a thin body keeps women passive, preoccupied, dependent, and off track from career ambitions. It keeps them in their place as objects to be viewed or pleasured, or used as recreational toys or playmates.

Dieting and thinness came to be female preoccupations when women got the right to vote around 1920. Never before had there been idealized "the look of sickness, the look of poverty, and the look of nervous exhaustion." The new, leaner form replaced the more curvaceous one with startling rapidity, Wolf says, in a great weight shift that must be understood as one of the major historical developments of the century, a direct solution to the threat posed by the women's movement and their newly-won economic and reproductive freedom.

"Prolonged and periodic caloric restriction is a means to take the teeth out of this revolution ... so that women just reaching for power would become weak, preoccupied, and mentally ill in useful ways and in astonishing proportions," says Wolf.

The cultural fixation on female thinness is not about beauty but female obedience, Wolf charges. It's "about how much social freedom women are going to get away with."

The "good girl" today is a thin girl, one who keeps her appetite for food (and for power, sex and equality) under control, agrees Kilbourne. Girls are still being admonished to keep their place, to not compete too seriously.

Both men and women are conditioned and socialized to feel that women must be controlled, kept in their place. Women, of course, internalize these messages, says Kilbourne. "Ironically, what is considered sexy today is a look that almost totally suppresses female secondary sexual characteristics, such as large breasts and hips. Thinness is related to decreased fertility and sexuality in women."

Kilbourne argues that women are allowed success in the workplace if they focus on being thin, maintain a fragile, waifish image, and do not take up too much space. "The pursuit of thinness is a way to compete without threatening men."

Another explanation for the idealization of the lean boyish female figure is that as women have moved into previously male-dominated activities, the traditional feminine shape has developed negative connotations, while the masculine shape symbolizes self-discipline and competency. Thus the rejection of the maternal body can be seen as women's revolt against the sometimes impossible demands of trying to fill both career and reproductive roles.[30]

Kilbourne warns, "This is not a trivial issue; it cuts to the very heart of women's energy, power and self-esteem. This is a major public health problem, one that endangers the lives of young girls and women."

Women's movement silent

One would think the woman's movement would be outraged by these issues, picketing and parading on the Capitol mall, making headlines. But most feminist leaders do not seem interested. They have little to say on these topics. The lesbian professional literature is similarly silent on eating disorders and the problems of fat.

Some have asked, what has happened to the women's movement? Why are they not speaking out against the thinness obsession that holds so many women and girls hostage?

"The women's movement has clearly failed young girls in this country," Levine says.[31]

Most protest in the literature seems to come from eating disorder professionals, therapists and nutritionists who see first hand the devastating effects of our culture's obsession with thinness.

But maybe the problem goes deeper. The women's movement has become silent on numerous issues. Where is the vigor of new young leaders?

My theory is not a happy one. I'm thinking far too many of these silent younger and older leaders, like the college girls, are at work reshaping their bodies, deeply immersed in body dissatisfaction, dieting, turning inward, weak and withdrawn, choosing to disempower themselves. Each woman struggling alone with her weight issues, her appearance, her place as a woman.

Certainly, the women's movement seems to endorse the thin body. Size acceptance is not an issue these groups have embraced. Few of their leaders have objected to the sidelining of large women, who have so much to offer.

"Why haven't feminists focused on hatred of fat in our society?"

asks Rothblum. Obesity is highly stigmatized even in feminist groups, she says.

That the power of culture is affecting these women as strongly as others demonstrates that no one is immune to it. Women everywhere, of all ages and all persuasions will need to actively work through their own body issues.

CHAPTER 3

Dysfunctional eating disrupts normal life

■

"Diets teach people to ignore the natural biological signals of hunger and satiety. ... Then when they go off the diet they don't know when to stop eating. The best way to stop people from overeating is to stop them from restraining their eating."
— *Janet Polivy*

When you diet, that's dysfunctional eating. You're not listening to those hunger and fullness signals from the tummy, but to your mind which is counting calories and fat grams or checking off the diet sheet that says a half cup of pasta is what you get, no matter if you want more — or less.

"Dieters are people who get up in the morning and the first thing they say is, 'Mirror, mirror on the dresser, do I look a little lesser?'" so says a bit of *Readers Digest* humor.

That's the goal — to look lesser. To be lesser. Be less than you are, less than you could be. And, sadly, many young women are less than they could be in their desperate efforts to be thin. They eat, not to nourish, but to be as thin as possible, so they eat less food than their bodies need.

Dysfunctional eating is chaotic eating — dieting, fasting, bingeing, skipping meals — or it may be consistently undereating less or overeating more than the body wants or needs.

This kind of eating hasn't been investigated in much detail. Yet, concerned leaders have been writing about various aspects of it for more than a decade. It's been called restrained eating, disordered eating, disconnected or emotional eating, as well as chronic dieting syndrome. Professionals often use the term disordered eating; however, since this is easily confused with eating disorders in general conversation, it is not being used here.

Dieting starts in children as young as age 7. Even infants are forced to eat dysfunctionally. By age 11 this kind of eating is so common some researchers are calling it the norm for girls today. Children are growing up with skewed attitudes toward food, eating, and weight, because of fear of fat. They are turning away from normal eating and mealtimes with family to a restricted, restrained and chaotic form of eating.

Where are they learning this? Often at home. A lot of chaotic eating is going on in homes these days. Their mothers are the first generation of serious dieters with an intense thinness drive. Dads are dieting as well. Foods may be restricted. Frequent dinner table talk focuses on calories, fat grams, the "good" and "bad" foods. Comments may deplore the size of hips, stomachs, and thighs. A growing number of studies reveal how this disturbing trend affects kids. My earlier book in this series *Afraid to Eat: Helping children and teens in today's weight crisis* documents these problems. For example, up to 81 percent of 10-year-old girls in a California study had disturbed eating, restricting their food, trying not to eat fat, and feeling guilty when they ate.[1] More than half of 14-year-old girls in a study of 1,000 suburban Chicago girls had already been on at least one weight loss diet.[2]

If dysfunctional eating behavior is so prevalent, why don't we know more about it? It's time to take a closer look.

What is dysfunctional eating?

Dysfunctional eating is separated from its normal function of nourishing the body, providing energy, health and good feelings, and from its normal controls of hunger and satiety. Instead it seeks to reshape the body or relieve stress, and is regulated by external and inappropriate internal controls.

Dysfunctional eaters try not to eat. Or they eat and binge to relieve anxiety, anger, loneliness, boredom, to numb pain, for comfort or adventure, or to gain pleasure. Their eating is regulated by a 1,000-calorie diet, what their scale tells them, counting fat grams, "will power," or emotional or sensory cues.

But instead of relieving pain, it often makes the situation worse. It is common afterward to feel guilty, ashamed, uncomfortably full, regretful, or, if still unsatisfied, to feel ravenously hungry and fear triggering a binge. There may be a sense of loss of control and the inability to stop eating.

One woman said she felt intense remorse after eating. "When I'm eating, I feel good. But when I finish, I really hate food. After I've eaten, lots of times I feel sick."[3]

Dysfunctional eating charts

Dysfunctional eating exists on a fluid continuum between normal eating and clinical eating disorders. It may be of mild, moderate or severe intensity. The charts on pages 56 and 57 are designed to provide a better understanding of these differences in eating behavior, their effect on functioning, and the value of normalizing eating behavior. They are not intended as a diagnostic tool and should not be used to label children or adults.

You might move back and forth across the continuum, moving into mild dysfunctional eating by going on a diet on Monday morning, then breaking it on Friday and returning to normal eating. But after a few bouts with dieting, it may be harder to return, and eating patterns may shift over, between mild and severe intensity. In this model, some women develop and sustain certain types of dysfunctional behavior, relatively unchanged, for long periods of their lives. Still others may develop increasingly severe dysfunctional behaviors, perhaps leading to severe clinical eating disorders from which they cannot recover alone.

The question of whether dieting can cause eating disorders is controversial. But there is increasing evidence that dieting may be a common pathway for the vulnerable individual in the context of our thinness-

---

Dysfunctional eating: a definition

Dysfunctional eating is eating in irregular and chaotic ways — dieting, fasting, bingeing, skipping meals — or it may mean consistently undereating much less or overeating much more than your body wants or needs. Dysfunctional eating is separated from its normal controls of hunger and satiety, and its normal function of nourishing the body, providing energy, health and good feelings. Instead, it is regulated by external and inappropriate internal controls, and seeks to reshape the body or relieve stress.

WOMEN AFRAID TO EAT 2000

obsessed culture. Eating disorders almost always start with a diet, and many consider dieting a necessary, but not sufficient, cause of eating disorders.

Normal eating

By contrast, normal eating is having regular eating habits, typically three meals a day and snacks to satisfy hunger. It is regulated by internal signals of hunger, appetite and satiety — we usually eat when hungry and stop when satisfied. Normal eating enhances our feelings of well-being. We eat for health and energy, sometimes for pleasure and social reasons, and afterward, we feel content and satisfied.

Dysfunctional patterns

The harmful effects of dysfunctional eating and benefits of normal eating have received little attention. Yet studies suggest dysfunctional

Are you a dysfunctional eater?

1. Do you regularly restrict your food intake?

2. Do you skip meals regularly?

3. Do you go on diets?

4. Do you count calories, fat grams, weigh or measure your food?

5. Are you "afraid" of certain foods?

6. Do you turn to food to relieve stress or anxiety?

7. Do you deny being hungry or claim to feel full after eating very little?

8. Do you avoid eating with others?

9. Do you feel worse (anxious, guilty, overfull) after eating?

10. Do you think about food, eating and weight more than you'd like to?

A *yes* answer to more than three of these questions indicates a pattern of dysfunctional eating.

and disturbed eating is extremely prevalent and increasing, especially among girls and women. It may include at times the 50 to 80 percent of girls and women in the United States who say they're trying to lose weight. Increasingly, they are joined by about one-fourth of teenage boys and men who are changing their eating habits in response to new advertising pressures that advocate lean, muscular bodies.

Dysfunctional eating includes three general patterns:

1. Chaotic eating. Irregular and chaotic eating — fasting, bingeing, skipping meals, snacking, grazing — in today's world is often aimed at reshaping the body. In addition, increases are coming through a disturbing trend in which many children and adults no longer eat regular family meals, but adopt chaotic ways of eating.

2. Consistent undereating. Many women and girls concerned with maintaining a thin body successfully override their hunger signals, and regularly eat less food than meets their daily needs. They exist in a starvation mode, and even though they do not meet the clinical criteria for eating disorders, they likely have some rather severe disruptions of their lives.

3. Consistent overeating. Consistently eating more food on a daily basis than one's body wants or needs means a person is overriding normal satiety signals. Some individuals overeat from emotional or stress-related reasons, such as for comfort, or to relieve anxiety, anger, or boredom. Others overeat from habit, perhaps in response to family habits of overeating. Body size cannot identify this type of dysfunctional eating. People's needs differ, and it cannot be assumed that just because a woman is large, that she is eating abnormally, or past the point of satiety.

Cultural pressures encourage dysfunction

Modern culture encourages dysfunctional, disturbed and disruptive eating patterns, shaped by billions in advertising dollars. We have lots of inexpensive, good-tasting foods, easily available. In advertising and the media, instead of encouraging normal eating, we are being urged to overeat.

Advertisements for Pringles Right Crisps show people eating 10 or 20 chips at a time. Ritz Air Crisp ads implore people to "inhale them." Baked Lays Potato Chips challenge, "Betcha can't eat just one — bag."

People are eating out more, and they favor fast food chains and restaurants where they seem to get more for their money. Restaurants are offering larger servings, larger meals, more abundant buffets with many food choices. A study in Restaurants USA found customers expected larger quantities of food in 1993 than in 1991, and that people

Dysfunctional eating: a description

Contrasted and compared with normal eating and eating disorders

	Normal eating	Dysfunctional eating *mild moderate severe*	Eating disorders
Eating pattern	Eating at regular times, having regular habits. Typically may be three meals a day and one or two snacks to satisfy hunger.	Irregular, chaotic eating — individual often overeats or undereats, skips meals, fasts, binges, diets. Or usual pattern is of undereating much less, or overeating much more than the body wants or needs.	Patterns typical of anorexia nervosa, bulimia nervosa, binge eating disorder, other eating disorders.
How eating is regulated	Eating is regulated mostly by internal signals of hunger, appetite and satiety. Individual usually eats when hungry, stops when full, is hungry at mealtime.	Eating often separated from normal controls of hunger, appetite and satiety. Often regulated by inappropriate internal and external controls such as "will power," a planned diet, calories or fat grams, emotional or sensory cues, sight or smell of food.	Eating regulated predominantly by inappropriate external and internal controls, not hunger and satiety.
Function/ purpose of eating	Eat for nourishment, health, energy. Also for pleasure and social reasons. Eating enhances feelings of well-being, makes one "feel good."	Eating often for reasons other than nourishment: to shape body, improve body image, seek comfort or pleasure, numb pain, relieve stress, anxiety, anger, loneliness or boredom. May feel uncomfortable after eating, and have feelings of remorse, guilt, shame or insatiable desire for more.	Eating almost entirely for purposes other than nourishment or energy, as for body shaping, to numb pain, relieve stress. Eating may cause distress.
Prevalence	Infants, small children, persons who don't diet or interfere with normal eating. At this time, likely higher rates for males, lower for females.	Chaotic eating and undereating affect many girls and women in U.S., perhaps at times as many as 50-80% age 11 and over who say they are trying to lose weight; also increasing numbers of boys and men. Consistent overeating may occur for both genders.	Estimated prevalence is 10% of high school and college students, 90-95% of female, 5-10% male.

Dysfunctional eating: effects and relationships

	Normal eating	Dysfunctional eating *mild moderate severe*	Eating disorders
Physical	Promotes health, energy, strength, healthy growth and development of children and youth.	May typically feel tired, apathetic, lacking in energy, chilled, with undernutrition. Decreased bone development or bone demineralization and higher risk of fractures. Delayed puberty, decrease in sexual interest and libido. Increased risk of eating disorders.	Physical effects may be severe. Mortality reportedly as high as 10-20% for anorexia nervosa and bulimia nervosa.
	WEIGHT: Normal weight for the individual, expressing genetic and environmental factors. Any weight within wide range, usually stable.	WEIGHT: Any weight within wide range depending on genetic potential. Eating pattern may cause weight to decrease, cycle up and down, remain stable, or increase.	WEIGHT: Any weight within wide range, depending on genetic potential and the disorder and its expression.
Mental	Promotes clear thinking, ability to concentrate.	Risk of decreased mental alertness and ability to concentrate, narrowing of interests, loss of ambition, and a turning inward.	Diminished capacity to think, memory loss, extreme narrowing of interests.
	FOOD THOUGHTS: low key, usually at mealtime. For women, 15-20% of time awake may be spent thinking of food, hunger, weight, 10% if no food preparation, in one estimate.	FOOD THOUGHTS: Increased preoccupation with food. Thoughts often focused on eating, weight, planning when and what to eat, counting calories or fat grams. Thoughts of food, hunger, weight may occupy 30-65% of time awake, according to one estimate.	FOOD THOUGHTS: Thoughts focused most of time on food, hunger, weight. For untreated anorexia reportedly as much as 90-110%, bulimia 70-90%, of time awake (extra includes dreaming).
Emotional	Promotes mood stability.	Potentially greater mood instability — highs and lows. May be easily upset, irritable, anxious, have lowered self-esteem. Increasingly preoccupied and concerned with body image.	Greater risk of mood instability and functional depression.
Social	Social integration; promotes healthy relationships with family, peers, and community.	Less social integration, may be withdrawn, self-absorbed, more risk of feeling isolated, stigmatized, disconnected from society, lonely. May lose interest or see less value in generosity, sharing, affection, community service, volunteer activities.	Social withdrawal, isolated from family and friends, avoidance of and by peers, alienation, often eating alone; may be worsening family relations.

think of large servings as getting better value for their money when they eat out.[4]

Recently a *Healthy Weight Journal* subscriber in London sent me a newspaper clipping titled "Portions out of all proportion" that decried America's "elephantine cuisine." The writer compares calories in a serving of food in the two countries: hot dogs (350 calories in the U.S., 150 in Britain), cookies (493 vs 65), ice cream cone (625 vs 160), muffin (705 vs 158), nachos (1,650 vs 569), and a meal of steak and fries (2,060 vs 730). Until recently, our large muffins were called "jumbo muffins," now they are simply "muffins." The Cheesecake Factory heaps food "practically a foot high on its plates and proudly serves up a 12-ounce burger. As for the cheesecake, each slice has about 700 calories. It claims it tried to serve lower-calorie slices but nobody wanted them," he reported.

We probably deserve the writer's concluding remark, "Europeans are a lot more quality conscious ... Americans just want value for their money, and base value on size."

At the same time we are urged to overeat, the same media hold dieting and thinness as the saintly ideal.

Both extremes, under- and overeating, promote eating for purposes other than to nourish the body for optimal health and performance. They ignore and override the fact that our bodies are wonderfully designed to maintain balance through natural regulating systems.

Moreover, there is an intense fear of supposed risks related to food today. People are confused and worried about the foods they eat. No wonder, with the contradictory scare messages in the media. We read the food terrorist message of the day with morning coffee.

"I've never known so many people to be so worried about what they eat, or so many who think of the dinner table as a trap that's killing them," laments Julia Childs, the noted chef and author.[5]

Out of touch with hunger

Hunger means the body has spoken. It is a request to eat. But dysfunctional eaters and those with eating disorders try to silence this voice, keep the body numb, quiet and contained. Instead of feeding hunger as an act of self-care and healing, they may perceive hunger as a potential betrayal of their determination not to eat.

Nutrition therapists Karin Kratina, MA, RD, and Nancy King, MS, RD, say that the woman on a food plan operates from a dieting mentality, out of touch with her body. Her diet is based on overriding or ignoring the body's cues and messages as a way to control weight, and results in a restrained eating style. She learns to distrust her body, and when she goes off the diet she continues to distrust and ignore her internal cues. She becomes more dependent on external cues to eat such as time of day, proximity to food, feeling states, and a belief system regarding good foods and bad foods. They point out that this style of eating is prone to disruption, to eating less than needed on the one hand, and eating out of control, on the other.[6]

Family battlegrounds

Family attitudes can set the stage for disturbed eating early in life.

The uneasy relationships that mothers have with food and their bodies are mirrored in daughters at very young ages, says Ellyn Satter, RD, an eating disorder specialist. She advises parents to model normal eating.[7]

Parents disturb children's normal eating patterns when they insist on rigid rules and give children frequent instructions, such as to clean their plates, eat their beans before they can have dessert, eat more, eat less, or by investing food with emotional value, giving food as comfort or instead of affection. Remember your long-term goal is to get your kid to listen to and trust her inner signals. It's not to get her to eat those beans now.

Satter says parents should purchase, prepare and serve the food, but then allow the child to choose what and how much he or she will eat. Unfortunately this natural division of responsibility is often violated by parents with rigid or restricting eating styles, who try to take over their children's eating. This sets the stage for disruptive eating styles.

"Even the fat child is entitled to regulate the amount of food he eats," Satter insists.

Making meals a battleground contributes to eating problems for children. In a Canadian nondiet program, teens shared these family battles:

- "My mom knows I hate mushrooms and I told her I would throw up and she made me eat it and I threw up."
- "My grandmother serves me, so I can't pick."
- "Cooked peas and carrots make me gag and my parents wouldn't let me eat anything else until I was finished."
- "If we eat too much, we get this story about being greedy."
- "My mom won't give me any more, even if I'm hungry."
- "If you breathe through your mouth, you don't taste it."
- "We used to stuff our mouths with the foods we didn't like and then ask to go to the bathroom."[8]

Disruption of normal eating may also occur when parents fear a child is gaining too much weight and they begin to restrict food.[9]

A new medical term coined to describe the stunted, underfed babies being seen at the North Shore University Hospital in Long Island, New York, is the "fear-of-obesity syndrome," related to the fat phobia of parents who are so afraid a child will grow too large that they keep them half-starved.[10]

Never put a child on a diet, Satter advises. "Restricting food intake, even in indirect ways, profoundly distorts developmental needs of children and adolescents."

Eating behavior diminishes personality

Many of the effects given in the dysfunctional eating charts on these pages are associated with undernutrition and weight loss. However, it also may be that dysfunctional eating patterns, of themselves, can alter mental and physical functioning. Indeed, it is amazing how powerful these associations reveal themselves when we look at the big picture.

Women with dysfunctional eating often feel tired, apathetic, listless, lacking in energy, and chilled. Girls risk stunted growth and poor bone development. Bone demineralization may begin early, leading to stress fractures and osteoporosis.

Normal sexuality may be arrested. As weight drops, so do female hormone levels, sexual feelings, and interest in the opposite sex. I have a clipping of "The 100 world's sexiest women," a foolish article about celebrities, models, and jet setters, each one pictured as extremely thin and hollow-cheeked. These women may be sex objects and pose in sexual ways, but it's not likely they feel sensual. Assuming that most are half-starved, as they appear to be, they will have very low female hormone levels, and may not even menstruate. Their shrunken breasts are probably augmented by implants, or "push-up" bras. Calling them sexy is as absurd as making this claim of starving Holocaust victims. It's not without logic that some say the Viagra pill for women is called "food."

Dysfunctional eating affects weight, yet in its various forms it is associated with a wide range of weights as genetic potential interacts with environmental lifestyle factors. Associated with dieting, weight will often cycle up and down in "yo-yo" fashion. Consistent undereating can be expected to result in a stable weight lower than normal for that person, or below setpoint. Overeating will probably result in higher weight than normal, likely increasing year by year.

Even in moderate dieting, personality changes can be dramatic. Often a woman becomes depressed, moody, anxious, irritable, apathetic, intolerant and rigid, with highly controlled behavior. She may be unable to concentrate, have decreased mental alertness, memory loss, narrowing of interests, decline in ambition, and difficulty with comprehension. She may feel a sense of hopelessness and lack of control, along with lowered self esteem. Socially, she may withdraw, becoming lonely and self-absorbed. Preoccupation with eating drives her day, and she may spend as much as 65 percent of waking hours thinking about food, hunger, weight and her bodies. This food preoccupation is one of the most striking changes for a dieting person.

The other side of the dieting coin is bingeing. Once the diet is broken, bingeing may be a natural survival trait that helped early people recover quickly from famine.

Before they go on a diet many people binge in anticipation of the deprivation to come. In a "last supper" study at Stanford University 86 women and men were tested on eating patterns two weeks before a diet. When the diet began, those who said they overate when angry had gained an average of 5.2 pounds. Those who ate from depression gained 3.6 pounds, and those who ate from anxiety had lost 1.5 pounds.[11]

Dieting shrinks a woman's world

"Dieting is not just about eating, it is an entire way of life," warns Janet Polivy, PhD, a University of Toronto professor who has researched the harmful effects of dieting for over 20 years. "Life has a different meaning for people when they become dieters. Their self-image and self-esteem is all tied up in this."

Polivy's research shows chronic dieters respond differently than non-dieters in a range of situations. They are compliant and have a need for perfection, are preoccupied with weight and body dissatisfaction, have lost touch with internal signals. They salivate more when faced with attractive food, and have higher levels of digestive hormones and elevated levels of free fatty acids in their blood. They can go longer without food and eat less under "ideal" circumstances than nondieters, but once started, they binge or eat more, then experience guilt.[12]

Ellyn Satter says dieting causes a woman to cross the line into regulating food through external restriction. She may not cross back. Even so, the internal processes will not be denied. Satter warns, "You have to invest more and more time and effort in overcoming the physical and emotional symptoms of energy deficit: hunger, increased appetite, fatigue, lethargy, irritability and depression."[13]

One chronic dieter says dieting made her less of a human being. "What I resent about dieting is that it makes one so terribly self-centered, so much aware of oneself and one's body, so preoccupied with things that apply to oneself only, that there is scarcely any energy left to be really spontaneous, relaxed and outgoing. It starts with thinking about what to eat and what not to eat, and gradually goes over to other fields, and it is this aspect that makes me resent dieting; it makes me less of a human being."[14]

Others say if you deprive yourself of food, you probably deprive yourself of other equally important sources of nourishment — avoiding taking stands for yourself, speaking the truth, forming interpersonal bonds. If you feel you can't be trusted with food, you tend to mistrust your overall judgments, abilities, and feelings as well.[15]

"Dieting shrinks a woman's world," agrees Merryl Bear, coordinator of the National Eating Disorder Information Centre in Toronto.[16]

Dieting is abnormal

Dieting doesn't work because it's abnormal, says Mary Evans Young, founder of No Diet Day. "Dieting is based on deprivation, sacrifice and guilt, which are difficult to sustain."[17]

The diet industry has the perfect product, Evans Young observes. "It promises so much, and when it doesn't deliver the consumer blames herself and then goes on to the next diet." Dieting can make women feel they are doing the right thing. They feel good just having made the decision to go on a diet. Pursuing thinness is widely perceived to be the same as pursuing good health.

"That feeling of self-sacrifice can hook us into wonderful feelings of purity and goodness. The diet becomes a kind of fanatical religion, requiring you to abide by a set of stringent rules or pay the penance of guilt. It's a guilt that starts by slowly nibbling and then steadily gnaws away at your body, spirit and confidence. Give yourself a break. You deserve much, much more," she says.

The milkshake study

The classic milk shake studies at the University of Toronto by Polivy, Peter Herman and colleagues show how dieting disrupts a person's sense of normal eating.[18]

In one test, a group of dieters and nondieters were asked to compare ice cream flavors. But first they were divided into three groups. Those in the first group were asked to drink two milk shakes before eating the ice cream, the second group was told to drink one milk shake each. The third group got no milk shake. Then the groups were given three flavors of ice cream and told to rate them and eat as much as they liked.

What happened next was bizarre, but revealing. While the nondieters responded in logical ways — they ate less ice cream when they had one milk shake and much less with two milk shakes — the dieters acted just the opposite. Dieters in the no-milk shake group ate only small amounts of ice cream — they had maintained their control. Those in the one-milk shake group ate a lot more. And the floodgates came down for the two-milk shake group — these people ate the most ice cream of all. It was as if they lost all control once they had breached their own set limits.

The Toronto researchers call this disinhibition, and find a dieter can be disinhibited by anxiety, distress, depression, alcohol, actual or antici-pated consumption of a "diet-breaking" food such as a milk shake, or exposure to smells or thoughts of tempting foods. As long as no disinhibitors hit, they can maintain their diets.[19]

In another study nondieters were put on an intermittent fast-or-feast diet for a month. On four days a week they consumed only 600 calories; the other three days they ate freely. By the end they were eating more total calories, had a worsening of mood, irritability, fatigue and impaired concentration, and had lost no weight. Although they tested as normal eaters, this severe restricting of food had caused feelings of deprivation and great stress.

Other experiments showed that when dieters indulged in a high-calorie food they perceived as bad, they went overboard on other "bad" foods, such as cookies, ice cream, and candy, believing they had "blown it" anyway. But when they were eating "good" foods like a salad they did not overeat, even though it contained the same number of calories as the "bad" food.

Do dieters eat less?

Most people believe dieters eat less. Some do. But others, although they may appear to eat less, and often report and believe they eat less, eat as much or more than normal eaters. One study found that in a natural setting, dieters ate slightly more than nondieters. Two laboratory studies found that dieters significantly underreported what they ate, while nondieters were very accurate in what they reported.[20]

Polivy and colleagues report that dieters eat less when they are in a state of increased awareness, either in private, or in public when they feel that others may be monitoring what they eat. For instance, having another person in the room identified as a confederate, or as a "dieter" who eats lightly, will cause the dieter to carefully monitor what she eats. But dieters usually follow their rules only temporarily, until interrupted by a diet-breaking trigger.

There are two kinds of non-hunger overeating, says Francie White, MS, RD, a specialist in eating and body image. The first comes when a person overvalues "forbidden" foods, and the desire for them builds until control snaps. Then an internal rebel seems to take over and she goes on an eating binge or resorts to sneak eating.

The second type is addictive eating, in which food acts like a mood-altering drug. The person with this kind of eating comes to depend on food for a state of numbness or calmness that is emotionally comforting and stress relieving.[21]

The binge

The amount of food people eat and call a binge varies greatly. For the person who restricts food severely or has anorexic nervosa, a binge may be only 200 calories. Another with binge eating disorder or close to it may eat 20,000 or more calories. There is always the sense of being out of control and unable to stop.

One study showed one third of 125 patients coming for gastric bypass surgery had severe binge eating problems. About 60 percent reported bingeing two or more days a week. About the same number "grazed" two or more days each week; they ate small portions of food continuously or larger amounts of food over an extended period.[22]

In a Duke University study, the obese women most often binged when alone and their binges were related to negative emotions such as sadness, anger, loneliness or conflict. On the other hand, obese men tended to overeat in social situations when they felt happy, excited or were encouraged to eat.[23]

The downward dieting spiral

When you diet it's easy to get caught in the downward spiral of repeated dieting and more intense body dissatisfaction, warns Janet Polivy. Dieters begin their diets feeling dissatisfied with their bodies, but for a time they are buoyed by a false sense of hope. Then hopes are dashed once again by the inevitable transgressions and weight gain. Their self-image drops lower. Yet as one diet fails, another beckons them on, again with false hope. It's a downward spiral of negative self-esteem marked by repeated failure, depressed mood, loss of hope, worsened self-image, and commonly, an even stronger resolve to begin another, better diet.[24]

Typically, dieters hold to the belief that dieting will make them happier. They feel exhilarated as the drama of a diet begins. Excitement builds as they see their stomachs flatten and clothes fit more loosely. But this soon gives way to problems. There's the inconvenience of not being able to eat where, when and what they want. Socializing is restricted. Worse is the distress to emotional well-being. Dieting is significantly related to depression, social anxiety, stress, neuroticism, insecu-

Top 10 reasons not to diet

1. Diets don't work. You lose weight and gain it right back (weight cycle), often regaining more than you lost.

2. Dieting is dangerous. It causes many deaths and injuries every year.

3. Diets are expensive and without value.

4. Dieting causes fatigue, lightheadedness, saps your energy and strength.

5. Dieting disrupts normal eating, causes bingeing, overeating and chaotic feeding patterns.

6. Dieting increases food preoccupation, so half your day or more is spent thinking about food and weight.

7. Dieting diminishes women, subverting their dreams and ambitions, keeping them playing the anticipation game. There's a lot more to life than this.

8. Dieting decreases self-esteem, feelings of well-being. Instead, accepting and respecting yourself as you are brings confidence, health and a sense of wellness and wholeness.

9. Dieting stunts the growth and development of young people, mentally and physically.

10. Dieting increases size prejudice, makes people more judgmental and critical of themselves and others.

WOMEN AFRAID TO EAT 2000

rity, maladjustment, and emotional instability, notes Polivy. Dieters get more upset than nondieters in the same situation. The frustration that comes from deprivation and restricting natural eating behavior leads to irritability and hostility as the diet proceeds.

The lonely voice of Marian Fineman of Philadelphia, testifying in an early Senate hearing on the weight loss industry, hints at these deep emotional scars. Fineman told of her repeated weight loss attempts and weight fluctuations between 138 and 183 pounds, over a period of 34 years, "No one knows the anguish, the feeling of worthlessness, the guilt and the shame that I feel every time I regain the weight I have lost."[25]

After the diet

Depression is higher for women who diet. While this may be related to malnutrition, one telephone survey found the more diets women had been on, the more severe were their symptoms of depression. Women in this survey of 2,000 adults had been on an average of 1.2 diets during the past year.[26]

Many physicians agree that the aftermath of very low calorie liquid diets, fewer than 800 calories per day, cause some of the most difficult disruptions they have seen for their patients. Recovery from this extreme diet seems to be especially difficult. In the fallout from the very low calorie diet popularity of the late 1980s and early 1990s — when Oprah Winfrey announced on her show that she had lost 67 pounds on an Optifast liquid diet, and later confessed to gaining it all back — many women coming off these diets were entangled in a destructive relationship with food, terrified of eating, alternately starving and bingeing. They felt hopeless, depressed, defeated and desperate about their weight.

Some of these women and their providers called me and wrote long impassioned letters about their resulting health problems. A dietitian told me was convinced some of their patients had compromised their immune systems because of health problems that began with that diet.

Ex-liquid dieters had a distinct profile, said Alan Wayler, PhD, director of a women's residential program for weight and health management in Vermont, where some came for help. They were obsessive about food, afraid to eat real food, ate compulsively, and engaged in a binge-starvation-binge cycle. They seemed paralyzed by the experience, and were feeling extremely angry. These women had much greater anger, desperation, and fear of food than any he had ever seen before.

The women had to re-learn how to eat real food, and seemed unable to regulate their eating. And they had an aversion to exercise.[27]

A study in the Netherlands treated 260 obese women in two groups over a year, one with a regular low calorie diet and the other group with six weeks of a very low calorie diet. While both groups had disturbed eating patterns five years later — skipping meals, preferring sweets, eating alone, thinking a lot about food, bingeing, and regularly losing control over eating in an emotional situation — the rates were much higher for those treated with the liquid diet.[28]

Weight cycling research threatens industry

One consequence of chaotic eating patterns is weight cycling, or yo-yo dieting, which may have serious, even fatal, consequences. This is an important health issue.

There is no question that weight cycling is extremely prevalent in the modern world. Sixty to 80 million people in the United States are trying to lose weight. Most lose some weight and almost all of them regain it fairly quickly.[29] In one study, 80 percent of college women had dieted, about half were currently dieting, and one-third had dieted six or more times.[30]

One study that tracked the weight of 153 middle-aged adults over six years found the women lost an average of 27 pounds and gained 31 pounds in that time. This was a loss of 19 percent and a gain of 21 percent of body weight.[31] Another study of patients planning stomach reduction surgery found that most of them had lost and regained 20 pounds or more at least five times.[32]

What are the risks of weight cycling? Most research focuses on three questions:

1. Does weight cycling increase health and mortality risk?
2. Does it lower psychological well-being?
3. Does it slow down metabolism and make weight loss more difficult the next time?

The research is controversial with some evidence in support of both views for these questions. Definitions, and how to measure weight cycling have been unclear. However, answers appear to be "yes"to the first question, to the second "maybe," and to the third, possibly "no."

Weight cycling research is extremely controversial for the diet industry, because this is what it does — it weight cycles people up and down. (It could be called the *weight cycling industry*.) This industry does not want "yes" answers to surface for any of the three questions, and has largely succeeded. The National Task Force on the Prevention and Treatment of Obesity, an arm of NIDDK (National Institute of Diabetes and Digestive and Kidney Diseases), often considered an ally of the industry, went along with this and placed an article finding no negative effects from weight cycling in the *Journal of the American Medical Association*. The article focused only on the metabolism question, which the evidence said slows down with decreased calorie intake and rises again with increased calories, which seems harmless enough, although some have faulted the research for being of short duration. The article largely ignored the two more serious questions and went on to urge obese individuals to not "allow concerns about hazards of weight cycling to deter them" from weight loss efforts.[33]

Weight cycling increases health risk

However, potential health risks from weight cycling cannot be ignored. An impressive body of evidence consistently shows an increase in death from all causes and death from coronary heart disease with weight cycling.

In a 32-year analysis of weight fluctuations in 3,130 men and women in the Framingham Heart Study, those with high weight variability, many weight changes or large changes, were 25 to 100 percent more likely to be victims of heart disease and premature death than those with stable weight. They had increased total mortality, and also increased mortality and morbidity due to coronary heart disease. These risks were seen in all weight categories, whether the individuals were initially thin or obese. They held true regardless of physical activity, smoking, and health risk factors. And risks were higher at ages 30 to 40, the group most likely to diet.[34]

Similar research in Sweden found an increase in death rates with body weight variability for 2,317 middle-age adults, measured five times in 25 years.[35]

The Harvard Alumni studies reported by Steven N. Blair, an epidemiologist at the Cooper Institute for Aerobics Research in Dallas, show that men risk heart disease, hypertension and diabetes by "always dieting." Of 12,025 men, average age 67, regardless of their initial weight, those who said they were always dieting had a heart disease rate of 23.2 percent, compared to 10.6 for the men who never dieted. Hypertension rates and diabetes were higher for the always dieting versus the never dieting men. The more often these men dieted, whether always, often, sometimes, or rarely, the higher their rates of disease. This held true even among the leanest men and was basically unchanged by physical activity, smoking, or alcohol intake. In view of these results, Blair advises people to keep a stable weight and avoid either weight loss or gain.[36]

Weight cycling can predispose animals to diabetes, according to a study that tested 64 female rats over a period of one year. Findings were that rats fed high-fat diets and weight cycled showed significantly more insulin resistance than did non-cycled rats fed high-fat diets.[37]

Kelly Brownell, PhD, obesity specialist at Yale University, concludes that the harmful effects of weight cycling are about the same as for obesity. He finds weight fluctuation increases risk about 1.25 to 2.00 times, similar to the risk attributed to obesity.[38]

Psychological well-being may drop

As for psychological health, several studies do not find any differences between wieght cyclers and non-weight cyclers. Others do.

Researchers at Baylor College of Medicine in Houston found more pathological traits and distress among people who weight cycled than those with stable weights. And they were surprised to find a weight loss of only five pounds could affect mental health. Losing five pounds over a year was significantly related to lower feelings of well-being, more out-of-control eating, and higher stress levels, regardless of body weight. The weight cycling seemed to be causal, they said.

"People whose weight fluctuates up and down had many more emotional problems. It didn't matter whether they were thin or large, if their weight was stable they were much better off," concluded John Foreyt, PhD, the study director.

Brownell and Judith Rodin, PhD, also report weight cycling as consistently linked to increased psychopathology, lower life satisfaction, more disturbed eating in general, and perhaps increased risk for binge eating. They cite research on runners that linked weight cycling to higher levels of disturbed eating.[39]

Distressing trends

Looking ahead, there are few signs our culture will promote normal eating without a major change in direction. The opposite seems more likely.

Fewer families are eating meals together. American families eat together an average of only 4.8 times per week, according to a 1995 survey by the Food Marketing Institute. Less than half of Americans eat dinner together every night. Conflicting schedules are the major obstacle, especially with teenagers. Yet families value these times together, and nearly all say they appreciate talking over the day's events at mealtime. One study found the number of family meals eaten together was predictive of whether a teenager was doing well in academic motivation, peer relationships, substance abuse and depression factors.[40]

Instead, Americans are moving toward eating fast and alone, says nutritionist Margaret Reinhardt of Minneapolis. Some of the ominous

road signs she sees are:
- Fewer family meals and foods eaten together
- More food sold in single serving packs means not sharing meals
- Fast, hot convenience foods moving into gas stations
- Over half of fast food being purchased from drive-through windows
- More all-you-can-eat and super-size servings at restaurants and take-out.[41]

The will to change

We need a national effort to help people normalize disturbed eating at earlier stages, instead of waiting for a clinical eating disorder diagnosis, as today. Recovery from an eating disorder is extremely difficult and death rates are high. If we can prevent dysfunctional eating, I believe we can prevent thousands of women from suffering eating disorders.

But in fact, it is probably even more urgent to prevent the harmful effects of dysfunctional eating itself, since this behavior affects so many people in such detrimental ways. We need the will to change.

More research, too, is needed in these areas. How can we identify and measure the patterns of dysfunctional eating? What are its effects? How can it be prevented? Normal eating, too, needs study. How can healthy eating be measured and encouraged?

Numerous testing scales are available to assess eating behaviors and attitudes.[42] If you'd like to test yourself, the Eating Disorder Screening measures are reprinted in the appendix.

CHAPTER 4

Eating disorders
shatter women's lives

■

"I have many regrets. I lost a number of friends, hurt a lot of people I care about. ... My memories of the last 16 years are spotty and dim. ... My behaviors overtook my life and I essentially lost 16 years of living — years that I can't have back."

— A recovered patient

Struggling with an eating disorder is an unpleasant full-time occupation.

Eating disorders are so terrible in the way they take over girls' and women's lives and the lives of their families that if you suspect someone, or yourself, of being at risk for getting caught in that downward spiral — get help. The sooner, the better. In early stages, eating disorders are treatable. You *can* help a friend. But the longer the disorder continues and the more firmly embedded the behaviors become, the more difficult it is to extricate oneself or a loved one, and the more severe the long-term consequences can be.

No one in their right mind wants to go into this place, or to subject their families or loved ones to this nightmare.

Yet we have reached the point in modern society where young college women look at the skeletal forms of anorexic students hovering at the edges of their classes and murmur in envy, "I wish I could control my eating like that. Wish I could be that thin!"

Sadly, for some people there is an aura of glamour about eating disorders, in the look that has been called "heroin chic," a kind of sick pseudo-sophistication. It's the look of the lean, gaunt, hollow-faced fashion model — vulnerable, weak, vacant, self-absorbed, infantile, emotionally traumatized, sexually available, a toy — that for some people holds an attraction, that perhaps at a distance may seem sophisticated.

In truth, this is far from sophistication. In fact, it is the opposite: the raw, awful, exposed state of advanced starvation, of a human being at its lowest survival level, the haunted state of the starving person who is losing the sense of humanity, of compassion and love. How can it be called attractive or desirable?

How the disorder takes over

An eating disorder takes on a life of its own.

For Claudia K of Morristown, N.J., it began with a diet that gained unstoppable momentum near the end of her senior year in college, fueled by self-doubt, "my boyfriend's worship of skinny thighs," and a painful sexual encounter. Thirty pounds fell off in six months, and by age 25 she weighed only 70 pounds.

"Starvation numbed me; my new body seemed cleansed. I felt childlike, fragile and innocent. The pain of a sexual encounter that had caused me to question my self-worth was obliterated. Food became bad; in resisting it, I became good ... Small, ritualistic meals sustained me, and I knew I would soon have to live solely on air ... But I didn't die. Instead I deteriorated into a brooding, pallid stranger with toothpick thighs, stringy hair and snappable arms. My pulse slowed to 57 beats per minute. My face sprouted fuzzy down, while the hair on my head fell out in clumps. My period stopped; my sex drive died.

"I gave up a wonderful job in advertising sales, the kind of perfect entry-level job new grads dream about. At first, I could survive the commute to work. My fuel was the sheer thrill of being thin — possibly even the thinnest person on the train! In the store! At the bar! But then the two-hour train ride became too much for me. I took a leave of absence and retreated to my parent's house. I lied and sneaked to protect my habit ('No thanks, I had a late breakfast'; 'I ate a big lunch'; 'I'm a vegetarian'). I carried my meals to my bedroom, then flushed them down the toilet ... I hid in my room for days on end."[1]

Eating disorders are often triggered by stressful or disruptive events.

Her life was turned upside down when her parents divorced, and she had to change high schools. For the first time 17-year-old Mona Nottveit of British Columbia, Canada, failed a class. A dancer, she injured her leg and gained weight at about the same time. All compliments and approving comments seemed to stop, and she believed her weight gain was to blame.

"This realization sent me into a six-year battle with anorexia nervosa and bulimia. It was by far the loneliest and darkest period of my life ... The ironic thing about my battle with eating disorders is this: the whole time I was looking for love and acceptance from my peers and family, but I became so enmeshed in my own body that I drove away the very thing that I wanted most ... When I did exercise, my focus was on burning calories. Time used to fly when I danced, with great music and my own creativity to energize me; time now stood still as I fervently monitored the calorie counter on the treadmill."

Nottveit blames the diet industry for preying on the uncertainties of young women. "Advertising has stolen away our self-esteem and attempted to sell it back to us via weight loss products ... I wish I could tell everyone to love themselves the way they are and live life to the fullest."[2]

Shortly after they were engaged Prince Charles reached out to his bride-to-be, writes Diana's biographer, patted her stomach and chided, "A bit chubby here, aren't we?"

It was enough. Diana took the hint.

"The bulimia started the week after we got engaged," Diana later said.

By the time of their marriage, Diana's waistline had shrunk from 29 inches to 23½ inches. But she reported her husband as unsympathetic of the purging methods that accomplished this. "If I ate a lot of dinner, Charles would say, 'Is that going to reappear later? What a waste.'"[3]

Often the initiating event will be sexual abuse or trauma. Some specialists see eating disorders as survival strategies developed in response to harassment, racism, homophobia, abuse of power, poverty, or emotional, physical or sexual abuse. A brief incident of sexual harassment at age 16 triggered an eating disorder for Jeannine A. of Brooklyn. "I had never minded my breasts until a man in the subway pushed up hard behind me, whispering ... and grabbed them when no one was looking. That day, I made myself throw up."

Hospitalized later on, she shared a room with Allison, a 56-pound anorexic patient who was too weak to walk. "She was shrunken and shriveled, and she had extra hair all over her body that grew there to keep her warm. At first, I thought she was a boy, with a mustache and a little beard. Allison taught me all about laxatives. A couple isn't enough, she said; you have to take the whole box."

Jeannine put that knowledge to use later as she vomited, took laxatives by the box, "bicycled for hours on the darkened streets," and bought speed from a boy on the corner to keep away hunger — "all because I'd eaten a potato chip."

It took seven years to undo the damage, she says. And yet, "Even now, I sometimes stop eating. When I can't think straight or I fall too much in love, I still do it. Each hunger pang I withstand proves that I'm in control. Going to bed hungry makes me feel focused, strong and disciplined."[4]

One girl said she broke through her denial when she read Hilde Bruch's *The Golden Cage*. "The phrase that stuck with me was the one that said a person with anorexia nervosa spends all of her time and energy in pursuit of something that accomplishes absolutely nothing of eternal value. This changed my life. I did not want to die and have it say on my tombstone, 'She was thin and she threw up.'"[5]

A need for love, yet hard to love

Sufferers of this illness can be extremely determined to keep their own small rituals and rules. They become rigid, manipulative, exasperatingly stubborn.

Hospitalized for her malnutrition, one young woman wrote, "I quickly learned that there were three things I could do to the doctors who imprisoned me: fool them, shock them, or fight them. Fooling them could mean drinking eight glasses of water before a weigh-in, or running in place when their backs were turned. Shocking them was even better. I laughed silently when the nurse took my blood pressure three times, then looked at me in disbelief and asked, 'Are you alive?' Open warfare wasn't so effective. Returning my meals untouched meant a nurse appeared to watch me eat them. That's when they hooked up the feeding tube. 'Next time,' the nurse said, 'the tube goes down your throat.'"

The ever-elusive quest for thinness becomes a warped, cruel competition. In eating disorder therapy groups, as professionals seek healing for troubled sufferers, the victims eye each other to rate who is thinnest — and compete for that title, even as they struggle to extricate themselves from their lonely prison.

Child-like women bring their therapists pictures of gaunt, hollow-faced British models Kate Moss and Trish Goff and tell them, "This is how I want to look."

In many ways, those who suffer from eating disorders are not sympathetic figures. Lonely and withdrawn, they seem to others anti-social, inflexible and devious. They practice bizarre rituals that make no sense to others, and refuse to give them up. They feel low self-esteem, but exhibit little interest in or compassion for others. Family and friends express their frustration: Why won't they just eat? Why won't they just stop making themselves vomit?

Women with eating disorders do want to stop, in a way. They feel lonely and separated, and wish they could be a part of the happy, laughing groups they see around them. They truly want to feel better. But first — just to be safe — they need to lose a few more pounds.

They are not always easy to love.

I hear anger in the voices of fellow athletes on a basketball team, "We tell her to eat! Even the coach jumped her yesterday for not eating. She's not a team player anymore — she's either a wimp on the court or a frenzied whirlwind."

I hear anger in families. The husband or parent who has tried everything, been rebuffed, watched the loved one progress in treatment, only to have those hopes dashed once again by a reversal. The significant other who throws up his hands and walks out, "I can't help her. She just clams up, won't listen to reason."

The sister of a girl who died from anorexia recalls her feelings of anger and sadness. "At times I felt overcome with anger at my sister and blamed her for the painful discord my family was experiencing. Stronger though was the sadness I felt for my parents as I watched them be blamed, suffer, and hope, only to be repeatedly disappointed."[6]

Families of people with eating disorders are in crisis. They see their child or spouse behaving in destructive ways and feel helpless and frustrated. They may try to gain control over what and how much she chooses to eat. Some police washrooms and search through drawers to throw out diet pills or laxatives. They despair over the loved one's "all or nothing" thinking, her seemingly irrational perfectionism, as the eating disorder threatens to take over their own lives, as well as hers.

Bizarre behaviors

Many of the physical and mental abnormalities of eating disorders are known to chronic dieters and people who severely restrict their food intake. The bizarre eating behaviors common to anorexia nervosa are also typical of those described under other starvation conditions. In Ancel Keys' well-known Minnesota Starvation Study with volunteers who reduced their food intake by half for six months and lost one fourth of their weight, the men exhibited many similar behaviors.[7]

One of the most important advancements in the understanding of eating disorders is the recognition that severe and prolonged dietary restriction can lead to serious physical and psychological complications, says eating disorder specialist David Garner, PhD.[8] Many of the symptoms once thought to be primary features of anorexia nervosa are

Eating disorder diagnosis

■ Anorexia nervosa

Patients with anorexia nervosa refuse to maintain weight at what is minimally normal for age and height (they weigh less than 85 percent of expected weight), and have an intense fear of weight gain or becoming fat. They have disturbance in body image, causing undue influence on self-esteem, and amenorrhea if female, defined as the absence of at least three consecutive menstrual cycles.

Two types are:

- **Restricting type**: severely restricts food without regularly binge eating or purging.
- **Binge eating/purging type:** severely restricts food and binges or purges (vomiting, laxatives, diuretics, enemas).

■ Bulimia nervosa

In bulimia nervosa the individual has recurrent episodes of binge eating. An episode includes eating, in a discrete period of time, an amount of food larger than most people would eat, and a sense of lack of control over what or how much one is eating during the episode. It includes recurrent inappropriate compensatory behavior to prevent weight gain, such as induced vomiting, misuse of laxatives, diuretics, enemas or other medications, fasting or excessive exercise. Both binge eating and the compensatory behavior occur on average at least twice a week for three months. Self-evaluation is unduly influenced by body shape and weight. (The disturbance does not occur exclusively during episodes of anorexia nervosa.)

Two types are:

- **Purging type:** uses regular purging behavior (induced vomiting, misuse of laxatives, diuretics, enemas).
- **Nonpurging type:** uses other inappropriate compensatory behaviors, such as fasting or excessive exercise, but does not regularly engage in purging.

■ Eating disorder not otherwise specified

The largest category is *Eating disorder not otherwise specified.*

Individuals in this category do not meet the definitions for either anorexia nervosa or bulimia nervosa.

Examples are:

- All criteria met for anorexia nervosa except amenorrhea.
- All criteria met for anorexia nervosa except, despite weight loss, current weight is in normal range.
- All criteria met for bulimia nervosa except frequency of binges is less than twice a week or for a duration of less than three months.
- An individual of normal body weight who regularly engages in inappropriate compensatory behavior (such as induced vomiting) after eating small amounts of food.
- Repeatedly chewing and spitting out large amounts of food, without swallowing.
- Binge eating disorder.

Binge eating disorder

A subtype under the category *Eating disorder not otherwise specified,* binge eating disorder is defined as having recurrent episodes of binge eating, which includes eating in a discrete period of time an amount of food larger than most people would eat, and a sense of lack of control over eating it. The individual has marked distress regarding binge eating, and engages in binge eating on average at least two days a week for six months. (The binge eating is not associated with regular use of inappropriate compensatory behaviors and does not occur exclusively during the course of anorexia nervosa or bulimia nervosa.)

At least three of the following must be part of the binge episode:

- Eating much more rapidly than normal.
- Eating until uncomfortably full.
- Eating large amounts of food when not hungry.
- Eating alone because of embarrassment about how much is eaten.
- Feeling disgusted with oneself, depressed, or very guilty about eating.[1]

Diagnostic and Statistical Manual, Fourth Edition, 1994. American Psychiatric Association
WOMEN AFRAID TO EAT 2000

actually symptoms of starvation.

Restoring full nutrition brings dramatic improvement to both the mind and body for sufferers of anorexia nervosa. But the fear of fat goes deep.

"I can't stop throwing up. I try, I really do. Yesterday, I promised myself I wouldn't do it anymore. I tried to keep myself busy. I cleaned house, played with the cat, prayed ... But I don't want to gain weight. I can't do that! I never want to be fat again. I'll never go back there. Nothing is worse than that pain ... My joints even hurt. I feel so old. My hair looks horrible; and it keeps falling out. I find it all over the place. My mouth is so full of sores, it's gross! I can't even walk around the house standing straight any more. I'm in a daze. I can't focus. But I can't stop. I feel so trapped. Please help me ..." said a bulimic patient from Lemon Grove, California.[9]

"I have many regrets. I lost a number of friends, hurt a lot of people I care about," laments one woman who recovered from anorexia nervosa and bulimia nervosa. "My memories of the last 16 years are spotty and dim. In fact, there have been many major events, such as my sister's wedding, that I have no recollection of. Eighty to 90 percent of my time was spent in (eating) behaviors. My behaviors overtook my life and I essentially lost 16 years of living — years that I can't have back."[10]

Food preoccupation

One of the most striking features of eating disorders is how intently the person is preoccupied with food, often to the exclusion of other interests or time spent with friends.

Eating disorder pioneer Hilde Bruch observed that for a woman with an eating disorder, "food thoughts crowd out their ability to think about anything else."[11]

In his studies of the amount of time patients with eating disorders spend thinking about food, Dan Reiff, MPH, RD, a therapist and nutritionist specializing in eating disorders and depression in Mercer Island, Wash., finds that untreated anorexia patients, who may weigh only half their healthy weight, say they spend 90 to 110 percent of their waking hours thinking about food, hunger, weight and body image. (The extra 10 percent that some report comes from recurring eating dreams or night wakening from hunger.) People with bulimia who have a lower weight than healthy report being preoccupied with these thoughts 70 to 90 percent of the time.

With few exceptions, the lower their weight, the higher their food preoccupation. Although less well tested, dieters and other food restricters are likely food preoccupied 20 to 65 percent of the time, he says.[12]

Reiff says that patients with eating disorders quite easily come up with their percentage score. "They can tell you precisely the time — that summer, or just after a certain event — when they lost weight and began to think so much about food," he said.

They admit to spending an inordinate amount of time thinking about what they ate last, and will eat next, or avoid eating. They think about hunger and that hollow ache in their stomach, but distract themselves with diet drinks, gum, and frenetic activity. They think about their bodies, weigh themselves, look in the mirror, ponder and plan how to take off a pinch of fat or another pound. They eye the bodies of other women and judge rather harshly, with envy or contempt those who are thinner or fatter.

One student recovering from anorexia nervosa, explains, "When I was at my lowest weight, I thought about food, weight, and hunger 99 percent of the time. I'd sit in my classes and figure out how many calories I'd had so far and how many I was going to have at lunch. I'd worry about what I was going to eat, when ... and how I could look like I was eating more than I really was when in front of Mom and Dad."

Another said, "While anorexic, my body not only anticipated eating, it reveled in it. Being starved and hungry makes the experience of eating more intense — almost sensual. The feeling is analogous to what is experienced when drinking water when extremely thirsty, sleeping after being totally exhausted, or urinating after one's bladder has become overly full. What is usually somewhat ordinary becomes exciting — something to look forward to in an otherwise painful and lonely world. This made changing behaviors so that I no longer experienced intense hunger extremely difficult."[13]

A crisis being ignored

As American adults continue to obsess about weight and diet, it is hardly surprising that eating disorders among women and girls have risen to crisis levels. Many specialists in the field are convinced that the current high rates of eating disorders in the U.S. are the inevitable result of 60 to 80 million adults dieting, losing weight, rebounding, and learning to be chronic dieters.[14]

Neither health officials nor the public has come to grips with the severity and extent of eating disorders. Perhaps this is in part because of the unsympathetic nature of the illness, and the anger that sufferers engender. Perhaps it is also because the victims are nearly all women.

Therapist Susan Wooley, PhD, has charged that the field of eating disorders would be very different if it were young men instead of young women who were being hospitalized and dying at the height of their educational and career aspirations.

Death rates compiled by experts suggest the severity of eating disorders. They range from estimates of 10 to 20 percent of anorexia and bulimia nervosa patients who die of their illness,[15]

Eating disorder survivors find the road to recovery difficult. While in the grip of the disorder, health, jobs, school and relationships all suffer — and rebuilding one's life can seem a nearly insurmountable challenge. Some have irreversible damage with chronic deterioration of the body accompanied by severe psychological problems, due to malnutrition and purging. Even with treatment, 25 percent of patients have poor recovery or do not recover. About 31 percent have some or intermediate recovery, and fewer than half, about 44 percent, recover well.[16]

Rachel, a college teacher from Oak Park, Illinois, recovering from bulimia, remembers, "I got this disease at age 23 when it dawned on me that my looks would someday fade, that all my boyfriends had left me for thinner women and that hours of exercise would tone my body, not shrink it."

As she shrunk to fit into size-four jeans, she earned lavish praise from her father, friends and the boys she dated. She knew how to hide the signs, "Concealer, foundation and powder hide broken blood vessels around your eyes. You'll lose clumps of hair, but, with luck, you've got enough to spare."

Is she cured? Hardly. "Don't think it's not a battle. It will always be a battle ... Don't think that because a boyfriend complimented my body daily, I was healed. The day he broke up with me, I stared at a picture of his bone-thin ex-girlfriend and threw up five times ... Some days are better than others. Some days, I don't throw up at all. Other days, I eat entire packages of Oreos, Doritos, Froot Loops — and I throw up six, seven, eight times."[17]

The father of a young woman with an eating disorder is in despair. "She has withdrawn into her own world. She's lonely and is missing out on all the fun and exciting things during her teenage years ... I have cried many times over this."[18]

Eating disorder sufferers are not necessarily young. They range from age 5 to over 70.[19]

The fabulously wealthy Woolworth heiress Barbara Hutton, called the "poor little rich girl," had seven husbands, including Cary Grant, and suffered anorexia nervosa for many decades. She died in 1979 at age 66 of a heart attack brought on by malnutrition and her illness. Her last years she spent at the Beverly Wilshire Hotel, heavily sedated and weak from subsisting on Coca-Cola and the liquid diet food, Metrecal.[20]

Prevalence increasingly common

An estimated 8 million people in the United States suffer from eating disorders, including one in 10 high school and college students, 90 to 95 percent of them female. Therapist Michael Levine, PhD, recently compiled figures from published sources for a conservative estimate that shows 5 to 10 percent of post puberty females are affected by eating disorders severe enough to cause significant misery and disruption in their lives.[21]

Of the three types, anorexia nervosa affects about 1 to 4 of every 400 girls, according to Levine, although the Canadian Eating Disorder Information Centre gives somewhat higher figures of up to 3 percent for North American women. Bulimia nervosa affects 1 to 3 percent of middle and high school girls, 1 to 4 percent of college women, and 1 to 2 percent of people in community samples, in Levine's figures. In the category called *other eating disorders*, Levine finds prevalence rates of 2 to 13 percent of middle school and high school girls, and 3 to 6 percent of post puberty women in the community.

Many experts suggest the real figures are actually much higher. They say they are seeing an overall increase in the last ten years, and eating disorders striking at ever younger ages and affecting many more males.

Nancy King, MS, RD, a dietitian who works with disordered eating in southern California, says she now sees 7- and 8-year-old children with nearly full-blown eating disorders. "Many pediatricians are not recognizing it's an eating problem when a child this young loses 12 pounds over the summer — they're not yet in puberty!"

Harold Goldstein of the National Institute of Mental Health suggests that cases of anorexia and bulimia have doubled in the past decade. Sharp increases have been found among females age 15 to 24, and a study in Scotland found the incidence of anorexia increased over six times between 1965 and 1991 in that country.

A Canadian review finds that anorexia more than tripled among women in their 20s and 30s between 1950 and 1992, but increased only 10 percent for teenagers. However, they report that all eating disorder statistics are based on small, incomplete studies, the largest included only 166 cases, and not a single large population-based study has been reported in the scientific literature.[22]

About 9,000 people are hospitalized annually in the U.S. for treatment of eating disorders, according to one source.[23] An estimated 1,000 women die each year of anorexia nervosa, according to the National Eating Disorder Screening Program.

Why are there no adequate statistics on eating disorders? I've oft~

asked this question, and found the answers unsatisfactory.

Granted, prevalence (but not mortality) is a difficult area because of the denial and extreme measures sufferers take to hide their disorder. Yet screening on campuses and in malls during Eating Disorder Awareness Week has been very successful in bringing new cases to treatment.

The reason seems to be due, in part, to apathy of health officials and the public. It is likely there is also resistance from the diet industry. Certainly we would have more accurate statistics by now if eating disorders had been on the nation's Healthy People 2000 agenda. It is being included in Healthy People 2010, but only as a mental health issue, despite heroic efforts from nutritionists and eating disorder specialists to have eating dysfunctions and undernutrition of teenage girls addressed in a broader way.

Eating disorders have gone global and become known for the first time in developing countries. They've now spread to women of all socioeconomic and ethnic backgrounds in Seoul, Hong Kong, and Singapore. Cases are reported in Taipei, Beijing, and Shanghai, and even in countries where hunger remains a problem, such as the Philippines, India, and Pakistan. First documented in Japan in the 1960s, anorexia now afflicts an estimated 1 percent of young Japanese women.

"Appearance and figure have become very important in the minds of young people," says Dr. Ken Ung of the National University Hospital in Singapore. "Asians are usually thinner and smaller-framed than Caucasians, but their aim now is to become even thinner."[24]

Widely regarded as a modern problem, eating disorders have been known for centuries. Earlier belief had it that they strike the middle and upper socioeconomic levels. But it is now clear that they know no barriers, affecting both females and males of all ages, races, religions and economic backgrounds.[25]

Roots of eating disorders

What causes eating disorders? The traditional view held that the roots of eating disorders lie mainly with pathological traits of patients and their dysfunctional, enmeshed families.

Today our cultural emphasis on thinness, widespread body dissatisfaction, and the great numbers of women and girls dieting is believed to have a powerful effect. Further it has been shown that many of the psychological traits once thought to cause anorexia nervosa may instead
't of starvation. Specialists today say they are seeing many
ı what seem to be normal, loving families.

disorders are extremely complex. They arise out of emotional problems and eating disturbances related to food, body image and relationships with oneself and others.

Factors that increase vulnerability may be genetic, biological, psychological, sociocultural and familial, as well as a history of sexual or physical abuse. Other risk factors are body dissatisfaction, control issues, pressures to achieve or please others.

Having type 1 diabetes may be a risk factor, too. It is reported that one third of adolescent girls with diabetes avoid taking insulin to prevent weight gain, and up to 25 percent suffer from clinical or subclinical eating disorders.[26]

Some problems may be rooted in families that are overly controlling or disengaged, or who have problems they can't acknowledge or deal with openly. One study found parents of patients with anorexia sometimes gave a double message of nurturing affection combined with discouraging the daughter from expressing herself.[27]

Yet, eating disorders may not be so very different from dysfunctional eating, some experts say. It may be a matter of degree. It is no longer possible to dismiss patients with severe eating disorders as having pathological roots, as was often done in the past. Women who suffer from eating disorders may be simply expressing what many other girls and women are feeling, say feminist specialists.[28]

Eating disorders may begin long before puberty, however adolescence is a critical time. Accepting their rapidly-changing bodies at puberty is difficult for some girls when placed against the cultural backdrop. Not only are their female role models extremely thin and usually dieting, but males in their homes, schools and communities often praise thin women and openly denigrate large women.[29]

Strong evidence of the media's powerful influence comes from Fiji. Within 38 months from the time satellite television came to the island in 1995 and began beaming in images of thin actresses, the number of teens at risk for eating disorders more than doubled to 29 percent. The number who vomited for weight control went up five times.[30]

For the vulnerable person, it can start with a diet. Dieting is a necessary — but not sufficient cause — for eating disorders, experts say.

Whether or not dieting can lead to eating disorders is still controversial. Yet, increasingly, dieting is being regarded as an important risk factor in both eating disorders and binge eating.[31] A study of 15-year-old girls in London linked dieting to the development of eating disorders. Those initially dieting were significantly more likely than nondieters to have developed an eating disorder one year later.[32]

The American Dietetic Association warns against promoting weight loss to persons with binge eating disorder or other eating disorders. When young people come for help with weight loss, the ADA recommends counseling on body image issues and how to stop the pursuit of thinness. It may be healthier to suggest they accept themselves at or near their present weight, stop binge eating and learn how to prevent future weight gain, says ADA. This official recognition of the value of normalizing weight is a major step forward in the nutrition field.[33]

Links to sexual abuse, violence

Childhood sexual abuse is a common experience of many eating disorder patients. Until very recently, a history of sexual abuse was minimized and ignored by the mostly male therapists who dominated the field. Discussion was a "concealed debate" that women therapists held for years in the hallways during eating disorder conferences, says Susan Wooley, PhD, professor of psychology and co-director of the Eating Disorders Clinic at the University of Cincinnati Medical College.[34] Finally, it is recognized as an important precipitating factor.

The National Women's Study, a national random sample of 4,008 women who were interviewed at least three times over the course of one year, found that women with bulimia nervosa were twice as likely to have been raped (27 percent vs 13 percent) or sexually molested (22 vs 12 percent), and three times as likely to have experienced aggravated assault (27 vs 8 percent) as women without an eating disorder. Twelve percent of women with bulimia nervosa had been raped as children, at age 11 or younger, compared with 5 percent of women without an eating disorder. The age at the time of rape predated the age of the first binge episode in all cases, suggesting the childhood sexual abuse was a causal factor.[35]

This unmasking of sexual abuse at long last was due to the efforts of feminist writers and clinicians, Wooley affirms. In a similar way, Freud's deliberate suppression of sexual abuse among his women patients was not widely revealed until the early 1980s. And it is only in the past 20 to 25 years that the social institutions which help female victims of sexual abuse and domestic violence came into being.

Until recently, most professionals believed childhood sexual abuse was rare and likely harmless. Mark Schwartz and Leigh Cohn, editors of *Sexual Abuse and Eating Disorders*, found that the rate of sexual abuse was estimated at only 1 in 1,000 in a major psychiatric textbook of the 1960s. But by the 1980s many publications were reporting the incidence of sexual abuse at one in three females and one in seven males.[36]

Even so, the true extent of sexual abuse is unknown due to the silencing of victims and their reluctance to disclose abuse even to therapists trained to help them in this area. Wooley cites as an example one report that found 33 percent of patients who later disclosed their abuse, had earlier denied it during five weeks of hospitalization at a center highly experienced in abuse treatment and sensitized to its importance. She says another one of the clear findings of the past decade is the extremely long delay that may precede disclosure even among patients in extensive therapy.

Many of today's eating disorder specialists say they have learned how important it is to be silent and listen to girls and women, rather than to take the role of an authority figure.

Excessive exercise

One of the fastest growing eating disorder behaviors in the past few years is exercise dependance or activity disorder aimed at losing weight or sculpting the body. Physical activity takes priority over everything else for the exercise-dependent individual. She follows rigid, stereotyped patterns, and insists on continuing exercise even when it causes or aggravates a serious physical disorder. She may suffer severe withdrawal symptoms if unable to exercise.

"Stress injuries are common, and frequently the person exercises right through an injury so it can't heal properly," reports Karin Kratina, MA, RD, a clinical outreach coordinator at the Renfrew eating disorder center in Florida.[37] She says at least half her patients with anorexia and bulimia probably deal with some form of exercise dependency.

Traditionally, the drive to exercise of the person with anorexia was viewed as a way to burn calories and lose weight, but it may actually occupy a more central role.

In one study, 75 percent of a group of anorexic patients reported that as they became more physically active, they ate less. They suggested that their exercise, being linked to food restraint, became more and more compulsive and ritualized, until it was driven and out-of-control. Studies similarly show that rats with access to a running wheel will increase their running at the same time they decrease food intake when feeding time is brief. They literally run themselves to death. The researcher suggests that susceptible individuals, with perfectionist personalities, may get caught up this way in an activity-starvation syndrome that increases their risks of developing a full blown clinical eating disorder.[38]

A key to when exercise becomes a problem is often when goals shift from enjoyment and becoming fit and healthy toward body reshaping. It is important for teachers and coaches to emphasize health-promoting goals, and to question weight loss and muscle building goals. Young women may exercise compulsively in efforts to fix what's "wrong" with their bodies. Boys and men, too, are responding to a new emphasis on body sculpting and muscle building, conforming to advertising that is now teaching body dissatisfaction to males.

Kratina describes the typical scenario of a young woman with exercise dependence. "She rises each morning at 5:30, hits the pavement for a brisk three miles, rain or shine, works out 45 minutes at the fitness center on lunch break, and goes to another health club after work for an hour of aerobics, half an hour on the Stairmaster and a half hour on the Lifecycle. She appears to be a motivated, fit and happy person but her legs ache constantly as she continues to work out, despite shin splints. When she stops for a time her depression and anxiety become so overwhelming, she can't wait to get back to her workouts."[39]

Athletes at risk

Eating disorders among women athletes have risen tragically in the last 10 to 15 years. The "female-athlete triad" that links eating disorders, amenorrhea and osteoporosis is a known risk for elite women athletes. Fragile bones and stress fractures are common symptoms.

The highest risks are in appearance sports, where judges reward thinner athletes, such as gymnastics, dancing or figure skating, and performance sports where coaches and athletes believe that lower body fat enhances their performance, such as running, cross country, and swimming. Risks are intensified for elite athletes, who tend to be highly goal-oriented by nature, even fanatical, and they gain enormous social and financial rewards by being successful.[40]

As many as 13 to 22 percent of young women in selected groups of elite runners and dancers have eating disorders. Two studies of female dancers found between 5 and 22 percent had anorexia nervosa, with even higher incidence among elite women athletes competing in national performances.[41]

Amenorrhea is associated with scoliosis and stress fractures in ballet dancers. Delayed menarche, as late as age 19 or 20 for very thin female athletes and ballet dancers, usually with a restrictive diet, is linked to osteoporosis and bone fractures.[42] Trying to control weight while focusing on training and performance may lead to a sense of frustration, guilt, despair and failure, and to unhealthy eating and eating disorders.

Ballet dancer Heidi Guenther, who died unexpectedly of an apparent eating disorder while riding in a car on a trip to Disneyland with her parents in 1997, had been urged three years earlier by the Boston Ballet's assistant artistic director to lose weight — a tacit threat to her position in the company. Later she was cautioned she was getting too thin, but it was too late. "We often tell dancers that they'd look a little better if they lost a little weight," acknowledged Bruce Marks, artistic director emeritus. Guenther had complained for months about a pounding in her chest.

Dancers who come to his practice often are so thin, says Richard Bachrach, MD, president of the Center for Dance Medicine, that "you look at them and you say, 'My God, buy the poor girl a meal.'"[43]

Coaches and trainers are important role models who may subtly or even overtly encourage dysfunctional eating or unhealthy attitudes about body weight or bodybuilding. In one study of college women gymnasts, 67 percent reported being told by their coaches that they were too heavy, and 75 percent of these resorted to dangerous weight control methods including vomiting and laxative or diuretic abuse. In some instances coaches and trainers have eating difficulties themselves.[44]

Bodybuilding and anorexia are similar problems for women, points out David Schlundt, PhD, an eating disorder specialist at Vanderbilt University. "There are special diets, use of diuretics, steroid use, obsessive exercise, very low fat diets, and so on. An obsession with changing size and shape of the body leads to extreme and sometimes dangerous changes in diet, exercise and substance abuse."[45]

One of the reasons eating disorders are increasing among young men is likely a result of this obsession with muscles and body sculpting, and a new dissatisfaction with their natural bodies.

Vegetarianism and eating disorders

Eating disorders are disproportionately common among vegetarian women. Guilt, shame, asceticism, the desire to do penance, sexual abuse, anger, perfectionism and the need to be perceived as "good" may be issues for some involved in the vegetarian choice, and also increase the risks for eating disorders.

Some eating disorder specialists are seeing in their practice so many young women who are vegetarian converts (when this is not a part of their culture) that they consider it a marker for an eating disorder. They suggest that perhaps being a vegetarian is becoming an acceptable way to have an eating disorder. Indeed, it may be an increasingly frequent way that an eating disorder progresses in modern culture, as a major step along the way.

Because food choices are so restrictive and limiting, the girl or woman who is both vegetarian and eating disordered is also more likely to be malnourished, leading to more severity in the illness. The more rigid the vegetarian behavior, the more severe the individual's psycho-

Eating Disorder Warning Signs

Anorexia nervosa

- Significant or extreme weight loss (at least 15 percent with no known medical illness)
- Reduces food intake
- Develops ritualistic eating habits such as:
  a. Cutting up meat into extremely small bites
  b. Chewing every bite a large number of times
- Denies hunger
- Becomes more critical and less tolerant of others
- Exercises excessively (hyperactive)
- When eating, chooses low to no fat and low calorie foods
- Says he/she is too fat, even when this is not true
- Has highly self-controlled behavior
- Does not reveal feelings

Bulimia nervosa

- Makes excuses to go to the restroom after meals
- Has mood swings
- May buy large amounts of food and then suddenly it disappears
- Unusual swelling around the jaw
- Weight may be within normal range
- Frequently eats large amounts of food (a binge), often high in calories, and does not seem to gain weight
- May decide to purchase large quantities of food and eat it on the spur of the moment
- Laxative or diuretic wrappers found frequently in the trash can
- Unexplained disappearance of food in the home or residence

hall setting

Binge eating disorder

- Frequently eats a large amount of food that is larger than most people would eat during a similar amount of time
- Eats rapidly
- Eats to point that is uncomfortably full
- Often eats alone
- Shows irritation and disgust with self after overeating
- Does not use methods to purge

Additional signs of related eating disorders

- Makes excuses to skip meals and does not eat with others
- Develops a tendency to be perfect in almost everything
- Conversation is mostly focused on foods or around body shape
- Often hears other people's problems but does not share her own
- Is highly self-critical
- Worries about what others think
- Thinks about weight and body shape most of the day
- Begins to isolate more from friends and family
- The odor of vomit is in the bathroom regularly
- Repeatedly chews and spits out food — does not swallow large amounts of food
- May purge and yet not binge eat.[2]

NOTE: The more warning signs a person has, the higher the probability that the person has or is developing an eating disorder.

NATIONAL EATING DISORDERS ORGANIZATION 1994/WOMEN AFRAID TO EAT 2000

ⱯⱭthology often turns out to be, says Monika Woolsey, a dietitian who specializes in eating disorders in Glendale, Arizona.

Definitions

Anorexia nervosa. In anorexia nervosa, by definition the individual is more than 15 percent under expected weight, fears gaining weight, is preoccupied with food, has abnormal eating habits, and has amenorrhea, or if male a decrease in sexual drive. Of the two types, one simply restricts food, the other restricts food and either purges regularly, or binges and purges both.[46]

Bulimia Nervosa. By definition, the person with bulimia nervosa goes on an eating binge at least twice a week, eating a very large amount of food within a discrete period and then tries to compensate either by purging or nonpurging behavior. As the disorder progresses it develops into a complex lifestyle that is increasingly isolating, with depressed mood and low self-esteem.

The binge usually progresses through four stages: first, the trigger, often a stress or negative event; second, the active stage of eating avidly and privately, which continues until the binge seems complete; third, the ending, when the person is full, nauseated, or in pain, and stops eating; and fourth, the consequences, which may at first bring relief from stress, soon replaced by shame, guilt, disgust and feelings of loss of control.[47]

Other eating disorders. Some eating disorders don't fit neatly into these diagnostic criteria. They may have many features of anorexia or bulimia, but involve some different eating behaviors. The category for these is *Eating disorder not otherwise specified,* and they are sometimes called atypical eating disorders.

Binge eating disorder is included in this group. This disorder meets the criteria for bulimia nervosa except that individuals do not regularly engage in purging behavior and do not meet the criteria for being unduly concerned with weight and shape. They eat large amounts of food at least twice a week, in a relatively short time, with a sense of loss of control. They may be of average weight, but most often are overweight. This disorder is similar to what has been called compulsive eating.[48]

A Belgium study suggests that large women with binge eating disorder are more likely to have had traumatic childhood experiences, such as physical or sexual abuse. The study compared 29 obese women with binge eating disorder with 35 obese women without it. Of those with the disorder, 41 percent reported a traumatic experience compared with 14 percent of the others.[49]

Complications of eating disorders

Following are mental and physical complications or traits commonly associated with anorexia nervosa and bulimia nervosa, compiled from *Medical Issues and Eating Disorders* by Kaplan and Garfinkel.[50]

Mental complications

Anorexia nervosa

Many of the mental and emotional symptoms common to anorexia nervosa are directly related to the physical effects of starvation. Other traits have to do with attitudes and behavior toward eating and weight.

- **Energy level.** Fatigue, weakness, lassitude, lethargy, apathy, decreasing energy, persistent tiredness, dizziness, faintness, lightheadedness; yet hyperactive.
- **Mood, attitude and behavior.** Moodiness, often depressed, mood swings (tyrannical); anxious; irritable; critical; intolerant of others; low self-esteem; feels out of control; hopeless; rigid, highly controlled behavior; does not reveal feelings; perfectionist behavior; believe that weight loss can cause or prevent some life event (prevent parental divorce, attract romance); denies hunger; denies problem of weight loss (sees self as fat); denies eating disorder; distorted body image, overestimates body size and shape, "feels fat" despite emaciated appearance; ritualistic habits.
- **Mental ability.** Unable to concentrate, decreased alertness; has difficulty with reading comprehension, diminished capacity to think; memory loss; decline in ambition; narrowed interests.
- **Social.** Isolates self from family and friends, becomes increasingly aloof and withdrawn; lonely; feelings easily hurt; avoided by peers; family relationships decline.
- **Weight.** Preoccupied with body; frequently monitors body changes (may check with scale and/or mirror many times per day); compares size and shape to others, envies thinner persons; feels in control of body.
- **Food, eating and hunger.** Ignores hunger; fears food and gaining weight; eats alone; may secretly binge; dieting and weight increasingly important focus; has unusual food-related behaviors (makes rules for specific foods, placement on plate, time of eating, size of bites, number of chews per bite); progressively preoccupied with food and eating (may begin to cook and control family eating); need to vicariously enjoy food (may collect recipes, dream of food, hoard food, enjoy

watching others eat, pursue food-related careers — as dietitians, chefs, caterers).
- **Other.** Hypersensitive to cold and heat, hypersensitive to noise and light; insomnia.

Bulimia nervosa

The person with bulimia nervosa is often normal weight and may not experience the effects of starvation. However, if she has nutrition deficiencies due to purging, she may have starvation symptoms. When a patient with anorexia becomes bulimic, she or he experiences symptoms characteristic of both eating disorders.

Typically, these mental and emotional symptoms may be associated with bulimia nervosa:
- **Mood/attitude/behavior.** Anxiety, depression; mood swings; low self-esteem, self-deprecating thoughts; embarrassment, shame related to behavior; persistent remorse; paranoid feelings; unreasonable resentments; makes excuses to go to restroom after meals; may buy large amounts of food, which suddenly disappears; impulsive as compared to anorexics who are overcontrolled.
- **Mental ability.** Loss of ordinary willpower, poor impulse control, self-indulgent behavior; recognizes abnormal eating behavior.
- **Social.** Depends on others for approval; feels isolated; unable to discuss problem; distances self from friends and family; fears going out in public; family, work and money problems.
- **Weight.** Feels that self worth is dependent on low weight; constant concern with weight and body image.
- **Food, eating and hunger.** Eats alone; eats when not hungry; preoccupied with eating and food; fears binges and eating out of control; increased dependency on bingeing; feels out of control, cannot stop eating.
- **Purging.** Feels need to rid body of calories consumed during binge (through vomiting, laxatives, diuretics, enemas, fasting or excessive exercise); experiments with vomiting, laxatives and diuretics often leads to regular abuse.
- **Binge/purge cycle.** Spends much time planning, carrying out, cleaning up after bulimic episode; eliminates normal activities; complex lifestyle may develop with episodes occurring several times a day; worsening of symptoms during times of emotional stress; feels soothed and comforted by binge/purge cycle — it may serve to relieve frustration, anxiety, anger, fear, remorse, boredom, loneliness.
- **Other.** Dishonesty, lying; stealing food or money; drug and alcohol abuse; suicidal tendencies or attempts.

Physical complications

Anorexia nervosa

- **Electrolytes.** May be low in potassium, sodium, chloride, calcium, magnesium, and high or low biarbonate. Electrolyte imbalance more likely when there is dehydration and/or purging.
- **Gastrointestinal.** Constipation is likely, may promote laxative use. Commonly there is vomiting, feelings of fullness and bloating, and abdominal discomfort. There may be ulcers, and pancreatic dysfunction. Excessive laxatives over time may result in gastrointestinal bleeding and impairment of colon functioning.
- **Cardiovascular.** Commonly present are chest pain, arrhythmias, hypotension, edema and mitral valve prolapse. Electrocardiogram (EKG) changes. Heart rates lower than 40 beats per minute are common and as low as 25 reported in severe starvation. Prolonged QT intervals can lead to sudden death syndrome.
- **Metabolic.** Abnormal temperature regulation and cold intolerance are common. Abnormal glucose tolerance, fasting hypoglycemia, high B-hydroxybutyric acid, high free fatty acids, hypercholesterolemia, hypercarotenemia are common. Diabetic patients with an eating disorder may have fluctuating blood glucose levels leading to serious long-term consequences.
- **Bones.** Decreased bone mineral density may lead to fractures, growth retardation, short stature and osteoporosis.
- **Renal.** Elevated blood urea nitrogen, changes in urinary concentration capacity, and decreased glomerular filtration rate are common.
- **Endocrine.** Amenorrhea is 100 percent, by definition, although many anorexia nervosa patients begin to menstruate over time. Amenorrhea related to weight loss but may precede weight loss (in one-third); may cause delayed puberty, contributes to osteoporosis, breast atrophy, infertility. Hypometabolic state resulting in cold intolerance, dry skin and hair, bradycardia, constipation, fatigue, slowed reflexes. High plasma cortisol, decreased cortixol response to insulin.
- **Hematologic.** Anemia, leukopenia, bone marrow hypocellularity, common; these effects are usually mild, but can include bleeding tendency.
- **Neurological.** EEG and sleep changes are common; epileptic seizures affect up to 10 percent.
- **Musculocutaneous.** Muscle weakening, muscle cramps. Hair loss, brittle hair and nails, lanugo hair, dry skin and cold extremities are common.

Bulimia nervosa

- **Electrolytes.** Low potassium, low chloride, dehydration and metabolic alkalosis are common. May lead to cardiac arrest, renal failure. Dehydration is common along with hypotension, dizziness, weakness, muscle cramps. Cardiac arrhythmias affect 20 percent; unpredictable, may require emergency treatment. Hypochloremia is common; limits kidney's ability to excrete bicarbonate.
- **Gastrointestinal.** Constipation and increased amylase common. Rarely gastric and duodenal ulcer, acute gastric dilation and rupture. Frequent abdominal pain. Severe abdominal pain may lead to rigid abdomen and shock which may result in death. Abuses of laxatives may lead to iron deficiency anemia, rectal bleeding and cathartic colon.
- **Pulmonary.** Aspiration pneumonia possible from aspiration of vomitus.
- **Cardiovascular.** Peripheral edema is common along with EKG changes and QT changes, which can lead to serious arrhythmias and congestive heart failure. Uncommon is sudden cardiac death. Ipecac syrup abuse may lead to death through cardiomyopathy, myocarditis.
- **Metabolic.** High B-hydroxybutyric acid, free fatty acids. Less common edema, abnormal temperature regulation and cold intolerance.
- **Renal.** Possible changes.
- **Endocrine.** Menstrual irregularities with low body weight, dexamethasone nonsuppression common.
- **Hematologic.** May be anemic with nutrition deficiency.
- **Neurological.** EEG changes common. May have epileptic seizures with malnutrition and electrolyte imbalance.
- **Musculocutaneous.** Calluses on dorsum of dominant hand are common from inducing gag reflex. Muscle weakening with ipecac abuse.
- **Dental.** Enamel erosions with vomiting.

CHAPTER 5

Weights continue to rise

■

What's alarming is that rates of overweight were fairly stable during the 1960s and 1970s. But since the early 1980s, both children and adults have gained consider- able weight. ... Prevention is an urgent concern throughout the world.

When is a woman overweight? What causes it? How serious are her risks? And what can we do about it? These are old questions and yet ones so new that before 1980, many believed obesity to be simply a problem of too many calories. As a result, the solutions offered by experts were often simplistic and ineffective.

Faced with the failure of the old approaches, researchers are asking some new questions: What are the hallmarks of obesity? Does it start in childhood through excess fat cell development, or even in the womb? What happens during pregnancy? Breast-feeding? Menopause? How powerful are genetic factors? And if heredity is the important determin- ing factor, why are we seeing such steep increases in obesity in just the past decade?

While there have been advances, much about obesity remains un- known and the subject of intense debate. The bottom line is that more and more researchers and health professionals now recognize obesity as a complex condition that resists intervention. The fact is, there is much we don't know about obesity — or what to do about it. "Obesity continues to humble the scientific community by eluding effective under-standing and intervention in many important respects," says Shiriki Kumanyika, professor of nutrition epidemiology at Pennsylvania State University.[1]

Weight increases

While researchers and health professionals ponder the causes and outcomes of overweight or obesity, one thing is clear. The prevalence of overweight in the United States increased sharply in the last decade for both adults and children. Not only are more people overweight, but they are more severely overweight than ever before.

The landmark study that reveals this striking new evidence is the Third National Health and Nutrition Examination Study (NHANES III), which gathered measured data on representative samples of Americans across the country between 1988 and 1994.

This study found the woman at the median, or midpoint, is now 5-foot-4 ½ inches tall and weighs 144 pounds. This is an increase of a half-inch taller and six pounds heavier since 1980. She has a body mass index (BMI) of 25, up from 24. The *average* woman is a little heavier, but since this statistic can be a distortion it is used less often.[2] (The median man is 5-foot-10, weighs 176 pounds, and has a BMI of 26, an inch taller and six pounds heavier than in 1980.)

For practical purposes, the terms overweight and obesity are often used interchangeably, as they are in this book, to denote any degree of excess weight or fat.

However, the new NHLBI (National Heart, Lung, and Blood Insti-tute) Guidelines on obesity have defined two official levels: *overweight* is a BMI of 25 to 29.9, and *obesity* is a BMI of 30 or more. *(For BMI chart, see appendix.)* This distinction is controversial because it sug-gests the health risks of excess fat begin at levels much lower than supported by research. Most risks are found with severe obesity, not at these lower weight levels. In addition, new studies show these risks may have as much or more to do with lack of exercise than weight.[3]

These definitions put 55 percent of American adults, 97 million people, into the two categories. It increases the number of overweight people to from 30 to 32 percent and the number of obese people from 13 to 22 percent. Under these standards, 25 percent of women are overweight and 25 percent are obese. The categories define 39 percent of men as overweight and 20 percent as obese *(figure 1)*.

Minority people tend to have higher rates of obesity under these standards, with the highest rates among African American and Mexican American women.[4]

American Indian populations have particularly high rates of obesity, and it is often related to high rates of type 2 diabetes. In the Navajo Health and Nutrition Survey, 1991-1992, 35 percent of men and 62 percent of women were overweight with BMIs at about 27 or more.[5]

What's alarming is that rates of overweight were fairly stable during the 1960s and 1970s. But since the early 1980s, both children and adults have gained considerable weight, particularly at the upper end. In other words, heavier men and women became heavier.

World prevalence

The same increases in obesity are seen worldwide. There is every reason to expect that obesity and its associated health risks will extend globally into the future as developing countries modernize. Thus, prevention is an urgent concern throughout the world.

Some of the highest rates of obesity in the world are found in Polynesian populations. About 77 percent of women in American Samoa and 63 percent of native Hawaiian women have a BMI of 27.3 or more. One study in Hawaii found an average BMI of 31 for both men and women.

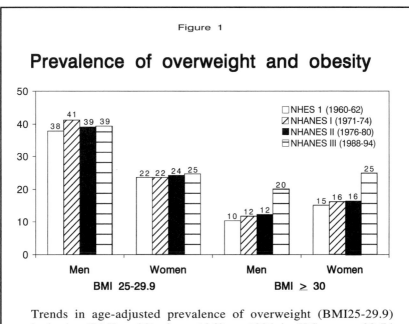

Figure 1

Prevalence of overweight and obesity

□ NHES 1 (1960-62)
☑ NHANES I (1971-74)
■ NHANES II (1976-80)
目 NHANES III (1988-94)

Trends in age-adjusted prevalence of overweight (BMI25-29.9) and obesity (BMI ≥ 30), from 1960 to 1994 in U.S., ages 20-74 years. CDC/NCHS.[1]

NHLBI CLINICAL GUIDELINES ON OVERWEIGHT AND OBESITY 1998/ WOMEN AFRAID TO EAT 2000

Obesity is less common in Africa and Asia. However, obesity is more prevalent in urban areas and is growing as people move from their rural villages to the cities. In Asian cities, there is growing concern for escalating rates of both obesity and eating disorders. It should be noted that for most countries statistics are still incomplete, and not based on representative samples.[6]

Health risks

Research shows that being obese can put you at a higher risk for a number of health problems, including hypertension, diabetes, heart disease, stroke, gallstones, osteoarthritis, sleep apnea, breast cancer after menopause, dieting and even death.[7]

Some researchers claim that these health problems and their association with obesity cause 300,000 deaths a year in the United States. That assertion is highly controversial since causes have not been established and the researchers have not taken into account the protections extra weight afford some people, such as women from osteoporosis and breast cancer before menopause.

An authoritative statement from the editors of the New England Journal of Medicine said in 1998, "The data linking overweight and death are limited, fragmentary, and often ambiguous ... Although some claim that every year 300,000 deaths in the U.S. are caused by obesity, that figure ... is derived from weak or incomplete data."[8]

Glenn Gaesser, PhD, associate professor of exercise physiology at the University of Virginia, makes a strong case for a lack of connections between obesity and risks such as high blood pressure, and challenges the assertion that thinner is healthier in his book, *Big Fat Lies: The truth about your weight and your health.*[9] Gaesser cites research that suggests obesity may be neutral in matters of health.

The NHLBI Clinical Guidelines on obesity define the range of "normal weight" at a BMI of 18.5 to 24.9 and anything over that as being at risk *(figure 2)*. However, the Guidelines themselves do not make a strong case for risks below 30, and actually show the point of least risk at around 25 for most people. For ethnic minorities and older people it appears to be considerably higher.

A recent four-year study of women age 50 and over found their lowest mortality rates at a BMI of around 34. Risks were in a broad U-shaped relationship between BMI and mortality, suggesting that a broad range of weight is well tolerated by women at midlife. High risk at lower weights did not appear to be explained by smoking.[10]

New studies are challenging some of the risks traditionally blamed on obesity. These risks may have more to do with lack of exercise than with weight. Most active healthy people probably do not have weight-related risks, even when moderately obese. Weight loss will not improve their health. And as they grow older, weight is even less of a factor in their good health. (Also, some of the risks are so slight, they mean only a difference of a few days or weeks in life span.) Even at higher weights, where risks appear to be stronger, they often disappear after initiating a moderate physical activity program. In fact, the NHLBI Guidelines report that weight loss without increased physical activity fails to improve cardio-respiratory fitness.[11]

Laura Fraser, author of *Losing It*, makes the case that even though Americans are gaining weight, we're suffering from fewer of the diseases traditionally associated with obesity.[12]

Related risks of obesity

Some people suffer from a cluster of metabolic abnormalities, often termed Syndrome X, which has been linked to obesity. The problems include the "big four": glucose tolerance, insulin resistance, plasma lipids and hypertension, which are associated with diabetes, cardiovascular disease and stroke. However, it is not yet clear whether obesity is causal to Syndrome X, or if a third factor causes both, possibly high

---

Figure 2

Classification of overweight and obesity

Disease risk relative to normal weight and waist circumference

	BMI	Obesity class	Men ≤102cm (≤40 in) / Women ≤88cm (≤35 in)	>102cm (>40 in) / >88cm (>35 in)
Underweight	<18.5		—	—
Normal**	18.5-24.9		—	—
Overweight	25.0-29.9		Increased	High
Obesity	30.0-34.9	I	High	Very high
	35.0-39.9	II	Very high	Very high
Extreme Obesity	≥40	III	Extremely high	Extremely high

* Disease risk for type 2 diabetes, hypertension, and CVD.

** Increased waist circumference can also be a marker for increased risk even in persons of normal weight.

Classification of overweight and obesity by body mass index (BMI), waist circumference and association of disease risks.[2]

NHLBI CLINICAL GUIDELINES OF OVERWEIGHT AND OBESITY 1998/
WOMEN AFRAID TO EAT 2000

stress or inactivity.[13]

Fat patterning

Your health risks associated with being overweight or obese may depend on where the fat is located on your body. People with upper body obesity, or an apple shape (also called abdominal or centralized obesity), are more likely to have risk factors related to heart disease and diabetes. Upper body obesity is often regarded as a male pattern, but many women are built this way, too. People with lower body obesity, or a pear shape, have more rounded shoulders and wider hips.[14]

African American, Mexican American and Native American children tend to have more upper body fat than white children, and this increases with age, particularly for boys. Women in these minority groups tend to have higher rates of obesity.[15]

Another critical factor in determining health risks from obesity is whether your excess abdominal fat is internal (visceral) or located just under the skin. People who put on weight internally or viscerally tend to have a higher risk for obesity-related health problems, such as heart disease. Health professionals measure visceral fat through a scanning technique or measuring the sagittal diameter, or height of the abdomen while lying down.[16]

As people grow older, their fat shifts around somewhat so they have more visceral fat. With aging, both women and men increase their percent of body fat as they lose lean body mass.[17]

One way you can determine your potential for health risks related to obesity is by finding your waist-to-hip ratio. The waist-to-hip ratio can be calculated by dividing your waist measurement by your hip circumference. Ratio of lowest risk is .95 or under for men, 0.8 for women. A simpler method is offered by the National Institutes of Health, which uses only the waist circumference. The NHLBI Guidelines suggest that health risks increase with a waist measurement of 35 inches or more for women and 40 inches for men.[18] Again, these last numbers are controversial.

The mystery of obesity

What causes obesity? And why did obesity rates jump across the board for young and old, male and female, and for every ethnic and racial group, during that last decade of the 1980s and early 1990s?

The nature of obesity is not well understood, but it is far more complex than once thought. The causes of obesity are complex, and the interplay of factors likely differs for individuals. Sedentary lifestyles, high-fat and high-calorie foods, disruption of normal eating habits, smoking cessation, high stress, higher weight gains in pregnancy, and genetic vulnerability probably all play a part. Also, we have an older population.

Genetic factors

Your family makes a difference when it comes to weight. A child of two overweight parents has an 80 percent chance of becoming overweight, compared with 14 percent for the child of two normal-weight parents, in one analysis.[19]

Studies of rats and mice with different genetic backgrounds show clearly how genes influence the ability to store fat. In one study of seven strains of rats fed a high-fat diet, one strain did not become obese, while the others did. In another study of nine mouse strains fed a high-fat diet, there was a continuous range of increasing obesity; some strains showed no weight gain response at all. Similarly, certain breeds of dogs are especially susceptible to obesity, while greyhounds and other slim breeds seldom grow fat.[20]

About 25 to 40 percent of obesity is probably genetic, perhaps coming from a number of genes, says Claude Bouchard, PhD, a professor of exercise physiology at Laval University, Quebec. He has done extensive research comparing identical twins, reared apart and together, adoptees and their two sets of families, and nine types of relatives.[21]

The tendency to gain excessive fat varies from one person to another, even in the same family and even when food intake and physical activity appear to be the same, Bouchard has found. It's quite clear that genetic factors do affect metabolism, thermogenesis, and how fast one's "inner clock" is set. Our genes appear to have some control over when we feel hungry and when we feel full. They also appear to control how our bodies burn or store fat and when our bodies protect or burn those fat stores.

African Americans, American Indians and some other populations seem to have a special vulnerability to obesity under modern conditions of sedentary living and abundant high-fat food. The *thrifty genes* theory explains why. It holds that under harsh conditions, only people who stored fat easily survived to pass on those genes. This was helpful in primitive times, but today people with efficient genes are more prone to obesity and related diseases, especially diabetes.[22]

Still, Bouchard cautions against putting too much blame for obesity on genetics. Many factors are involved, and there's "a lot of chaos in the body system we're working with," he says. "We are probably overemphasizing the importance of genetics in obesity. ... We are seeing big increases in obesity worldwide. This has to be the result of environmental factors."

Physical inactivity

Americans are less active today than they have ever been. Most are not very active in their work, travel, recreation or at home. Women are less active than men, African American and Hispanics are less active than whites, and everyone seems to get less active from childhood on. Half of women rarely or never engage in exercise vigorous enough to work up a sweat, according to NHANES III statistics. Only about one-fifth of adults are regularly active during their leisure time (5 times a week for at least 30 minutes).[23]

Less smoking

While smoking cessation efforts have succeeded in lowering national smoking rates, they have in turn contributed somewhat to obesity rates. Smoking dropped from 40 percent of U.S. adults in 1965 to 26 percent in 1991, with a slower decline for women than men. Smokers tend to have lower weights than nonsmokers do and people who quit smoking appear to "catch up" with the weight they kept off through smoking. This averages about six pounds for men and eight pounds for women.[24]

Is fat intake to blame?

Eating fat was thought to be a major culprit in obesity and its rising rates. But maybe not. Many scientists, pediatricians, and nutritionists are rethinking lowfat advice.

At first it seemed simple, back when those first studies came in showing rats and mice gained more weight and more fat when fed high-fat diets.

Americans responded by dropping their dietary fat intake from a high of about 44 percent of total calories in 1965 to 33 percent in 1996 — and health gurus urged a still lower drop to 30 or 20 percent.

On average, women reduced their fat intake from about 83 grams per day in 1965 to 62 in 1989. Men dropped their fat consumption even more — from 139 to 96 grams between 1965 and 1989, with a slight increase to about 100 grams since.[25, 26]

Now we have the dangerous situation in which college women strive to eat no fat at all. Some of their diets have been analyzed at only 4 percent fat. Health-anxious, thin-obsessed parents wean their babies on skim milk, stunting the growth of some. Many teenage girls, already the most poorly nourished of any group in America, no longer drink milk or eat meat in their extreme fear of consuming fat.[27]

At the same time, obesity rates have skyrocketed. The same thing happened in Europe and Australia, where obesity went up as fat intake dropped.

Was it because of the advice to eat less fat? Or in spite of it? Either way, there is a growing realization that decreasing the amount of fat one eats is not the answer that had been hoped for.

"Diets high in fat are not the primary cause of the high prevalence of excess body fat in our society, nor are reductions in dietary fat a solution," concludes Walter Willett, Department of Nutrition, Harvard School of Public Health.[28]

Without question, high-fat diets promote the development of obesity in several species of lab animals, although there are numerous individual differences. Usually, but not always, overeating is stimulated by a high-fat diet.

But studies in humans are less convincing.

In the Women's Health Trial, a breast cancer study, women reduced their fat intake from 38 percent to 20 percent. At first the women lost weight on the lowfat diet, but then regained even though compliance was excellent. By the end of two years, they weighed almost the same as the control group that had maintained the original fat levels.[29]

Yet it is clear that fat is stored easily in the body, and is not regulated in the same way as protein or carbohydrates. Dietary fat is considered especially fat producing because of its high caloric density, metabolic efficiency, and palatability — it makes food taste good, so people often overeat.

The problem with fat is that the body doesn't burn more fat when more is available, as it does with carbohydrates and protein, said Andrew Prentice, of the MRC Dunn Clinical Nutrition Centre, Cambridge, England. He cites a study in which volunteers were overfed and underfed on carbohydrates for seven days while the level of fat in their diets was held constant. Then they were overfed and underfed fat while carbohydrates were held constant. As the amount of carbohydrates they ate changed, their bodies made almost an identical adjustment in how it burned carbohydrates. Their calorie intake and output stayed in balance. But when their fat intake varied, there was almost no response by their bodies. The system seemed blind to differences in fat intake. Any excess was simply stored.

In his own research, Prentice finds that people do not compensate by eating less when their diets are high in fat. They may eat the same volume of food whether food is 20 percent or 60 percent fat, and therefore eat more calories with the higher-fat diet. However, not all studies agree.

Yet Prentice says that humans seldom eat pure sources of fat, and in mixed meals there do not seem to be big differences as long as people are not overeating.

If we don't eat to excess, he explains that there appears to be little difference in total calories used whether meals are high or low in fat, even with as wide a variation as 10 to 80 percent fat. The differences arise only when people eat too much. Then more of the excess calories are stored as fat in the high-fat diets. And the fat we store probably comes directly from the fat we eat, which is stored with an estimated efficiency of 96 percent.

Fat is also less satisfying in most studies, and especially for obese persons and restrained eaters. These people may eat many more calories when given high-fat foods.

Prentice believes there is a strong case for implicating high-fat diets in the cause of obesity, along with other factors. But he warns that reverting to a lowfat diet will not resolve the obesity problems of affluent nations. First, a high-fat diet is only one of many factors promoting over-consumption, including inactivity and aggressive corporate food marketing. Second, once obesity has occurred there appear to be powerful forces defending it.[30]

Another problem with lowfat diets is that they are not necessarily low in calories. Many lowfat processed foods are extremely high in sugar and calories, such as many of the fat-free cookies, cakes, chips, and candies that now crowd supermarket shelves.

In general, high-fat foods have more calories. But not necessarily. For example, adding three tablespoons of fat-free chocolate syrup to a glass of whole milk doubles the calories (from 320 to 640 per pound) but cuts the percent fat from 50 percent to 25 percent of calories. Now it is a lowfat food, but high in calories.

Thus, a lowfat diet works only if it reduces calorie density.[31]

Food intake

Whether people eating more calories is part of the equation is a matter of dispute. Americans may have increased their calorie intake slightly in recent years, according to NHANES III. It's clear that over-eating is being promoted in our culture today — in all-you-can eat buffets, extra large servings, jumbo sizes, and in advertising. Customers expect larger portion sizes today, and restaurants are responding by giving them more food. People are eating more meals outside the home.[32]

Still, the average intake of women age 19 to 50 is slightly below 1,800 calories, considerably less than the recommended 2,200 calories per day. Men average about 2,700 calories, somewhat less than the 2,900 calories recommended.[33]

In one large study, African American and white girls ages 9 and 10 kept food diaries for three days. The African American girls tended to be heavier, and ate more calories and fat than the white girls. They ate less meat, milk and cheese and snacked more on high-fat foods. They also watched more hours of television and videos per week — and it was this factor that seemed most directly related to overweight. For white girls, eating high-fat foods and watching TV were both associated with overweight.[34]

Medications can promote weight gain

Some needed drugs promote weight gain. And, unfortunately, some women regard this gain, as with certain anti-depression drugs, as worse than being ill or depressed. Given that depression is often associated with under-nutrition, this may make the condition worse as well as interfering with treatment.

"I hate the fact that my patient and I have to discuss which is worse: depression or 10 extra pounds," says Valerie Davis Raskin, MD, a psychiatrist at MacNeal HealthCare Center in Oak Park, Illinois. In some cases, she says, a different medication or altered dosage can reduce these effects.

One study suggests the reason for weight gain with anti-depressants may be a metabolic slow-down, not an increase in appetite or food intake. Patients have complained that the medication caused them to have "carbohydrate cravings," for sweet, high-fat foods. The researchers did find cravings for these foods in one third of depressed patients, but it was in the pre-medication period, before anti-depressants were prescribed.[35]

Depression can add fat

Although much concern focuses on weight loss from depression, it may also have the opposite effect for some people. More than one third of patients gained weight in a University of Pennsylvania study. The more overweight the person was initially, the greater the weight gain.[36]

Alcohol adds fat

Alcohol is often forgotten when we talk about protein, carbohydrate, and fat. This beverage accounts for about 6 percent of calories in the average American diet and can be as much of 10 percent of the calories for regular drinkers. This overlooked nutrient weighs in at 7 calories per gram, nearly as high as fat at 9 calories, and nearly double the 4 calories of protein or carbohydrate. Alcohol also may promote fat storage in a special way.

Alcohol acts more like a fat in the body, since it can be used as fuel instead of fat. The body burns the alcohol and spares fat, making it available to be stored, says J.P. Flatt, PhD, of the University of Massachusetts Medical School.[37] This means alcohol should probably be considered as a fat when figuring diet composition, says Flatt. For example in a diet that is 30 percent fat and 10 percent alcohol, the effect is similar to a diet of 40 percent fat.

Alcohol also promotes abdominal obesity and visceral obesity — so the term "beer belly" is probably to the point.

Paradoxically, alcohol seems to affect heavy drinkers differently. Long-term heavy drinking depresses the appetite and reduces food intake even to the point of emaciation and malnutrition. Alcoholics may consume more than 50 percent of their calories in alcohol, which has harmful effects on the liver and the body.

Despite the effect of alcohol on fat stores, it is still controversial whether alcohol intake and higher body weight are related. Some studies show they are for men, but not for women, for whom social issues may intervene to confuse the picture.

Does dieting make people fatter?

Doctors and patients have often observed that the more weight one loses, the more weight one gains. Instead just yo-yoing down-and-up, the weight of a chronic dieter often ratchets up higher and higher each time.

Sally Smith, former executive director of the National Association to Advance Fat Acceptance, says there are many 450-pound women in NAAFA who were once 250-pound women. But because of the hundreds of pounds lost and even more regained in trying to reach 150 pounds, through an endless series of diet programs, their weight climbed that extra 200 pounds. They are convinced that dieting and weight loss therapy is to blame.

Many scientists believe weight cycling makes a difference in ease of weight gain, even though no mechanism for this has been found.

Some authors have compared weight cycling to the efficiency of weight storage in hibernating animals that build up large fat stores in spring, summer and fall, and then slow down all body processes to live off it through winter.

"Repeated dieting may result in a higher setpoint, as the body adjusts to this modern form of 'famine' by storing more fat," warns Esther Rothblum in *Feminist Perspectives on Eating Disorders.*[38]

"People who experience periodic famine or endure long periods of inconsistent or inadequate food supply may unconsciously overeat and maintain a higher body weight in order to build fat stores in anticipation of a future period of limited availability of food," say William Bennett and Joel Gurin in *The Dieter's Dilemma.*[39]

Women experience natural weight cycling in pregnancy.

Weight gain in pregnancy

Just being a woman seems to put you at risk for gaining weight. Biologically, pregnancy sets women up to gain a lot of weight over several months in order to ensure a healthy baby. For some reason, however, the medical and health communities continue to ignore the weight-cycling realities of pregnancy and its effects on the female body.

On average, women gain about a pound with every child, but there is great variation. The Stockholm Pregnancy and Weight Development Study of 1,423 women found that a year after giving birth, some women had gained as many as 57 pounds from their pre-pregnancy. Others lost as much as 26 pounds. Women who gained most were more likely to:

- Gain more weight in pregnancy
- Gain more weight early, in the first trimester
- Gain rather than lose after giving birth
- Stop smoking
- Have irregular eating habits: skipping breakfast, and often snacking

Of these, the two most critical factors were higher weight gain in pregnancy and smoking cessation.[40] Lifestyle changes during pregnancy, such as a drop in physical activity and changes in eating habits and meal patterns had an effect.

Earlier, the Swedish researchers found weight gain during pregnancy was an important factor for obese women. They recalled gaining about 13 to 18 pounds with each pregnancy, and the more children they had, the more they weighed.[41] Another study in Sweden showed that 73 percent of obese women had retained 22 pounds from a single pregnancy.[42]

McGill University researchers found women retained 86 percent of the weight they gained in the first 20 weeks of pregnancy. They suggested that since fetal growth is minimal this early, the mother's surplus calories were accumulated as long-term fat reserves. It this study, a pregnancy gain of more than 27 pounds was more likely to result in lasting weight gain.[43]

Some studies show the more children a woman has, the more she weighs. Excessive weight gain in pregnancy is a special problem that needs to be studied in ethnic and racial groups that have high obesity rates for women. Research suggests that it is normal for African-American women to gain less in pregnancy and have smaller babies than white women. Small babies, who grow faster in their early years, are common in Africa, say experts.[44]

American Indian babies, too, were known to be smaller in earlier times and childbirth was easier, possibly a survival trait.

But since 1989, U.S. Public Health directives have called on women to produce larger babies (6.6 to 8.8 pounds, averaging about 8 pounds), by gaining more weight in pregnancy, in a move to reduce the number of small, premature babies.

I have considered this a mistake that potentially harms mothers. Gaining more weight in pregnancy clearly increases their obesity risk, and there is evidence that larger babies may be more prone to obesity. A national analysis shows birth weight influences later growth. Heavy babies are four times as likely to become heavy 5-year-olds.[45]

At the time, I urged decision-makers in the Public Health Service to investigate possible detrimental effects for mothers before establishing new directives. But my arguments fell on deaf ears.

"Bigger babies thrive better," one proponent told me. "If a baby is too big, the mother can have a Cesarean. If she gains too much weight, she can always lose it later."

It's time to examine this seemingly flippant advice. The effects of unnecessary weight gain in pregnancy on women need to be taken seriously by the health community.

The aim is primarily to cut down on the tiny premature babies born to so many young growing girls, many of them already malnourished from dieting. A worthy goal, but I doubt that urging women who are older, wiser, more experienced, and who in any case, would be good mothers, to have 8-pound babies will accomplish this. Low infant weights are influenced by many factors other than mother's weight gain: smoking and substance abuse, and mothers who are very young, of low socioeconomic level, with low pre-pregnancy weight. Smoking alone is blamed for an estimated 29 to 42 percent of low birth weight for babies.

High birth weight (over 8.8 pounds) increased from 10 percent of all babies in 1970 to 12 percent in the 1980s, and from 4.7 percent to 5.2 percent for African Americans. During the same time, the average pregnant woman reportedly gained 8 to 10 pounds more weight.[46]

More than half of mothers do not lose all the weight they gain during pregnancy, and nearly one-third of these retain over 11 pounds, according to Swedish research.

Whether a woman breast feeds her babies or not apparently makes little difference in how much fat she retains. The overall effect of breast-feeding on mother's weight was minimal in both the McGill and Stockholm studies.

We need research to determine the optimal weight gain in pregnancy for the long-term health of both mother and child. Women need help now in maintaining that weight during pregnancy and in losing the excess after childbirth.

The 1991 report *Nutrition During Pregnancy* by the Food and Nutrition Board of the National Academy of Sciences advises most women to gain 25 to 35 pounds during pregnancy. Thinner women are urged to gain a little more (28 to 40 pounds), and larger women a little less (15 to 25 pounds).[47]

This advice urges women to gain more weight than in the past: 15 pounds in 1932; 20 to 25 pounds in 1961; and 22 to 27 pounds in 1974.

Roy Pitkin, MD, chair of the committee that published the report, acknowledges, "It will contribute to the long-term obesity problem, particularly if it's followed by a succession of pregnancies."

I think it is important for women to try not to gain too much during pregnancy.

Women gain at midlife

Another weight gain comes for many women after their childbearing years. Most women gain 10 or 15 pounds or more during their 40s or 50s.

A University of Pittsburgh study of 485 pre-menopausal women, ages 42 to 50, found they averaged a 5-pound gain in the next three years.

In this study it made little difference whether the women had moved through menopause, or took hormone therapy, or not; weight gains were similar. Neither did it make much difference whether they were initially thin or large.

Physical activity did make a difference. Women who gained least were most active. If they changed exercise patterns, those who became more active gained less; those who became less active gained more.

Unfortunately, this study was too short and the women still too young to define a clear pattern of weight changes during menopausal years.[48]

Though many women blame this weight gain on estrogen replacement hormone therapy, it may not make much difference whether they take hormone therapy or not. A University of California study of 700 medical records of post-menopausal women, found those who took estrogen either continuously or intermittently gained no more weight over 15 years than women who never went on hormone replacement therapy.[49]

There is no evidence a moderate gain at midlife will harm normal healthy women. On the contrary, heavier women have stronger bones and are much less likely to have osteoporosis, one of the most severe and disabling diseases that hit older women, especially thinner women.

Being slightly heavier than average may even protect older women and men from chronic disease. The Longitudinal Study of Aging, a national sample of 7,397 men and women studied from 1984 when they were age 70 or over through 1990, found the lowest risk of death was at weights much higher than expected. The healthiest weight proved to be in a broad range from about 168 to 192 pounds for a five-foot-five woman (BMI 24-36) and 191 to 221 pounds for a six-foot man (BMI 24-32). Pre-existing disease did not make a difference. In fact, a higher weight seemed to protect against a number of diseases, including, surprisingly, diabetes, stroke and heart disease. The researchers concluded it seems unwise to encourage weight loss for older persons.[50] However, they said that over one-fifth of women are still trying to lose weight after age 70.

A Cornell University review of long-term studies found most of them showed that weight made almost no difference in death rates for women.

Another surprise is that Americans live longer after reaching age 80 than do elderly folks in Japan, France, Sweden, and England, even though life expectancy at birth is slightly higher in most of these countries.[51] Could one reason be that Americans are heavier at this age?

How ironic if someday the doctor's first line of advice at menopause, instead of prescribing pills, is "drink milk, lift weights, and put on a little weight."

Is obesity contagious?

Can obesity, or some part of it, be caused by a virus? Don't rule it out.

University of Wisconsin scientists have come up with an intriguing finding: a virus that fattens birds. They found that this virus, called the avian adenovirus, fattens chickens. Another virus of this type causes them to develop an unusual amount of visceral fat deposit. In screening human adenoviruses that cause respiratory infections, the researchers found one type that can cause obesity when injected into chickens and mice. When they tested 154 obese and 45 average-weight men and women, they found that 15 percent of the obese subjects carried antibodies for this virus, while none of the normal-weight controls did. They advise skeptics to keep in mind the analogy with stomach ulcers, which were blamed on infection only in 1983, drastically changing treatment.[52]

CHAPTER 6

Prejudice punishes
large women

■

"I think it's a miracle that I laugh every day and walk through my life with pride, because our culture is unrelenting when it comes to large people. I don't understand. We hurt nobody. We're just fat people."
— *Camryn Manheim*

Beauty, health, and strength come in all sizes. When can women join together to confirm this truth? When can we encourage the public to shift from an emphasis on thinness to health at any size, to appreciating people, not for appearance, but for themselves, their humanity, character and talents?

Life is difficult today for women who don't fit the cultural ideal. It is particularly hard for large women who too often bear the brunt of society's disapproval.

Her first experience in public humiliation came when she was a 185-pound sophomore in high school, recalls Terry Nicholetti Garrison, author of *Fed Up!*, when she heard one of a group of school jocks call out "Hey, fat ass!" as she walked down the hall. Hoots of laughter followed.

"I turned, my face flaming ... I shrunk with shame and slinked to the cafeteria, where I nursed my pain with a lonely lunch. I was sure that Billy was right. I should feel ashamed of my body. I was fat and bottom-heavy."

For 15 years her weight fluctuated between 135 and 205 pounds. At a low point in her weight, she met and married her husband. "I loved to dance. But I was so worried about how I looked that I rarely did. My husband told me that the first time we danced after I gained 30 pounds, he tried to keep us positioned with his back to the tables so people wouldn't notice my large hips. While he didn't say the words at the time, I'm sure I got the message."

Society's disapproval can be cruel

A woman who responded to an Internet listserv request on health care problems that large people encounter, for a special issue I was doing for *Healthy Weight Journal*, sent in her experience with a doctor's scornful treatment: "I was suffering from intense pain in my left knee. I put it off as long as I could but finally I had to go to the walk-in clinic. I sat up on the table and after the nurse took vitals, the doctor came in. He stood across the room from me and asked me what was wrong. I explained the problem to him and told him about the pain. His reply was 'Well, I can't see any swelling.' This man was standing 10 feet away! He said there was no way he'd be able to tell what was wrong because I was too fat. He handed me a prescription for an anti-inflammatory and said 'Take this with food, which shouldn't be a problem for you, and if it bothers your stomach just don't take it.' and he walked out."[1]

Fat prejudice is sexism in action, write psychologists Laura Brown, PhD, and Esther Rothblum, PhD. "Fat oppression is hatred and discrimination against fat people, primarily fat women ... (it is) the stigmatization of being fat, the terror of fat, the rationale for a thousand diets and an equal number of compulsive exercise programs. It is the equation of fat with being out-of-control, with laziness, with deeply-rooted pathology, with ugliness ... a catalyst for energy-draining self-hatred. It leads us to starve ourselves, to life-threatening surgeries such as stomach stapling and liposuction; it places women at high risk for the development of chronic and intransigent eating disorders ... Empirical data tell us that all the self-starvation done in the name of health and beauty leads women to feel like failures, while damaging their health in the process."[2]

Charisse Goodman describes a day in the life of a large woman in *The Invisible Woman*[3] that begins when she picks up the morning newspaper and reads ads and articles glorifying the slender figure and relegating her own body type to the weight-loss ads. "The message: lose weight. You're not a real woman unless you're thin. While taking public transportation to work, she may have to cope with seats designed for much thinner people, some of whom will clearly resent her presence should they have to share a seat with her. Once at work, she must listen to other women discuss at painful length their diets, their own perceived weight problems, and their anxiety and self-reproach at not being more disciplined. She winces as they express to one another, or her, their disgust and contempt for fatness as a general concept ... Eating in a lunchroom results in criticism or comments about her appetite and choice of foods. Perhaps she is even the object of coarse jokes made right to her face."

Goodman follows this woman through a visit to the hairdresser, a clothes shopping trip, a movie, and watching a series of television commercials, all of which portray thin women as attractive, lovable, successful, and glamorous, while portraying her and others like her as unattractive, unlovable, unsuccessful, and decidedly unglamorous. In fact, she is portrayed as loud, aggressive, oafish, alienated. If she dares to exercise in public she needs a great deal of courage and self-confidence to risk the snickers, pitying or contemptuous looks, or jeering from complete strangers who feel they have every right to comment on her size. At home she may have to face a companion or family members who hound her about her weight.

"What kind of life is this? How much energy do fat women waste just trying to move freely through a world which derides them with impunity purely because of their size?" asks Goodman. "Clearly, our thinness obsessed society expends a considerable amount of energy to ensure that fat women must struggle just to hold up their heads. Moreover, the human misery caused by weight bigotry is expediently attributed to the failures of the fat person, when in fact it stands as an appalling indictment both of modern social values and the American character."

In a letter to the editor published in the *Portland Oregonian*, Theresa Reed objected to offensive anti-fat comics. "Imagine living in a world where every time you walk out of the door of your house, you run the strong risk of public ridicule," she wrote.

In 1993, Leslie Lampert, an editor of the *Ladies' Home Journal*, had a "fat suit" made that made her look as if she weighed 250 pounds, and wore it for a week to see what life would be like. She was laughed at by a cab driver as she struggled to get out of the taxi, people peered disapprovingly in her grocery cart, two boys puffed out their cheeks at her and giggled, she was ridiculed in a fast-food restaurant, and kids talked loudly about the "fat lady." Afterward, she wrote an article about the openly contemptuous behavior she had encountered and how it had surprised her. The journal received over 900 letters from people who said she had written the story of their lives.[4]

Camryn Manheim is a larger actress who plays a straight-shooting attorney on *The Practice*, an ABC television drama. Her rise to stardom has not been easy. Manheim says, "Our culture really hates fat people ... There are billion-dollar industries invested in me hating my body: the fashion industry, the diet industry, the nutrition industry, and the cosmetic surgery industry are all invested in my hating my body. If women of my size were to actually enjoy being their size, those industries would collapse ... I think it's a miracle that I laugh every day and walk through my life with pride, because our culture is unrelenting when it comes to large people. I don't understand. We hurt nobody. We're just fat people."[5]

Size bigotry knows no national barriers.

It's not easy to be fat in Spain today, reports size activist Carmen Banuelos. In Spain, "fat people are often valued less highly as human beings than thin people. They get less of the good things in life and more of the bad. Men and women of average weight tend to disparage fat people: they despise them, feel superior to them, pay them less, penalize them, and laugh at them. Fat people are often objects of scorn and abuse due to their weight and thin people consider that this approach is fair, that fat people deserve this treatment. Such abuse is even seen as a humanitarian gesture, since supposedly the inflicted humiliation might drive them to lose weight. The shame of fatness is so intense and pervasive that sometimes fat people themselves come to believe that they deserve such treatment."

America is the great role model for German fashion, whether its a rock band, quirky clothing, or the thinness mania, says Barbara Bahr of Kassel, Germany. Discrimination there is extremely blatant, she reports. The diet industry cashes in, and the prevalence of eating disorders and body image problems is very high.

In New Zealand, discrimination exists in medical treatment, in accommodations like airline and theater seats, and "fat jokes" are seldom challenged, according to Pat Rosier, an activist in that country.

Discrimination in the workplace

In their work and careers, large women frequently meet size prejudice in hiring, in advancement, in salary. Sometimes they are the first to be fired.

In an example that size activists say is typical, one woman thought she had landed a job after three telephone interviews and a faxed resume to the publisher of a magazine ad department.

The publisher was enthusiastic. "We'll set up an interview as a formality — I can't wait to meet you," he told her.

But his face closed over when she walked into his office, and he brushed her off with a clumsy excuse that he had more candidates to interview.

Research confirms the truth of such complaints. One day I had a request from the director of the Employment Discrimination Project of the Legal Assistance Foundation of Chicago, which documents discriminatory hiring practices, looking for large women to serve as undercover agents to investigate size-discrimination in the work place. I put her in touch with a size-activist group. This is what they found, reported Lee Ann Lodder, project manager:

"One of our test teams was made up of two large-size women, one black and one white. We found they were treated markedly different by a number of the employment agencies we sent them to in Chicago. They would be kept sitting in the waiting room for an hour or more before anyone offered to help them. Their applications were lost. In one case, they had to go back and fill them out twice. They would arrive for a scheduled appointment and be told that the person that they had the appointment with was not there or was unable to see them."[6]

One highly-qualified woman was fired as a receptionist for a computer sales company because she didn't "present the kind of image" they wanted at the front desk. Several weeks later she stopped by the office and met her replacement, a thin blonde woman who had difficulty using the copier and no computer knowledge.[7]

Job discrimination is a major issue for large people, says Sally Smith, former executive director of the National Association to Advance Fat Acceptance. Smith divides the problems into two categories. First, the difficulty of getting hired, with the large woman often told over the phone that she has all the skills needed for the job, and when she arrives for the interview being told the position is filled. Second, is harassment on the job, which includes being singled out for torment by a supervisor or co-workers, even "people pasting cartoons that disparage fat people on their lockers."

Unfortunately, these are not isolated cases, but are all too common experiences for large women. A recent study shows that American women in the top five percent of weight earn nearly $7,000 a year less than women of average weight.

It's difficult to get legal recourse for job discrimination. Civil rights for large people have not yet caught up with other anti-discrimination laws. Only one state, Michigan, has laws against size discrimination.

Maureen Arrigo-Ward, a law professor, explains, "I think obesity discrimination today is where gay discrimination was maybe 20 years ago: Of course you discriminate. You can't take seriously a homosexual, that he should be able to be front and center? Of course not, these people shouldn't even exist, and, if they do, they should keep themselves under wraps. That's how it is for obese people today."

Prejudice in health care

But ironically, it is in health care that large women seem to suffer most. Health professionals are often seen as part of the problem.

"Fat people learn when they visit a doctor that getting quality, un-prejudiced health care is not something we can take for granted. Many of us feel that our health care is held hostage by doctors, used as a carrot to get us to lose weight," charges Lynn McAfee, Director of the Council on Size & Weight Discrimination.

Worse, she says, is the amount of sheer, inexcusable cruelty that large women endure at the hands of health professionals.

In a guest editorial on medical discrimination in *Healthy Weight Journal,* McAfee wrote that large people are forced to suffer severe verbal abuse from angry and contemptuous physicians who seem to blame every condition on obesity. Fat patients often receive no intelligible diagnosis — the diagnosis is that the patient is fat. While she agrees that many diseases are associated with obesity, naming obesity as a cause without offering a successful, affordable cure puts the blame squarely on the victim.

"We are given a diet as a first line of treatment. We are told not to come back until we lose weight, although we all know that weight loss and maintenance is a nearly unattainable task. If we can't lose weight, we are viewed as weak-willed or, worse, defiant. This is the kind of attitude that makes the 80-year-old woman afraid to see her doctor when her hypertension worsens. It causes a woman to die from uterine cancer because her doctor told her he wouldn't operate on her 225-pound body until she lost weight. Serious complaints, sometimes indicative of potential cancers, are dismissed under the mistaken impression that every fat woman should have menstrual problems. As a result, important testing is not done. Supersize women are particularly victimized by this treatment."

McAfee insists that health care needs to help large people be as healthy as possible now. Each health care interaction should make them empowered, more determined to take care of their bodies. "Studies show clearly that isn't happening. Physicians have been counseling people to lose weight for decades now, and the result has been that we are fatter, not thinner."[8]

What large people need from health providers is not a change in diet advice, but a change in attitude. They need to examine their own prejudices against large patients and understand how social discrimination affects the care they give them.

Some of the most poignant stories come from women who are pregnant, or trying to get pregnant.

One woman recalls that she was feeling pretty confident when she went to a specialist to find why she was having trouble conceiving. "This 'specialist' told me having a baby at my size would be irresponsible, that I was far too big to safely carry a baby and that I should use birth control until I lost at least a hundred pounds. The next sentence was that I couldn't possible ovulate at this size and would need to lose weight before I could get pregnant (contradicting himself). I left in tears. Later I found the courage to find a wonderful, caring fertility specialist who has been upfront about exactly how my size impacts both my fertility and ability to carry a child, while assuring me that all choices about my health care and life are mine to make — he is an advisor. I feel robbed of the year of fear and shame I can never have back of my childbearing years."

Another woman was humiliated during a pelvic exam. "I married, got pregnant, miscarried and put on almost 200 lbs. I developed Wolffe-Parkinson-White Syndrome. I knew I was fat, yet I still wanted a baby desperately. I went to an ob-gyn who told me there was no way he'd manage a fat morbidly obese woman. As he was giving me a pelvic and attempting to do the internal exam with one finger inserted and one palpitating the abdomen, he kept pushing down so hard, and I said, 'This is really uncomfortable.' He snarled back, 'Well if you weren't so damn fat this wouldn't hurt. This is your problem not mine!' I was humiliated. He told me I would hurt an unborn baby being fat, and would bring a baby with defects into the world being as fat as I was, and that if I had a baby while fat (he kept saying fat over and over) there would be a good chance I couldn't run after my toddler and care for him or her properly. Needless to say, I left in tears. He sent me home with condoms, foam, and a prescription for birth control pills. I stopped trying to have a baby then."

Another young woman, 26 and weighing 346 pounds, says she has been the target of more doctor-perpetrated fat jokes and insults than she cares to remember. "Here are some of the highlights: 'All fat women get toxemia when they're pregnant. You should never get pregnant because you'll die from toxemia. No fat woman can ever have a healthy pregnancy. Besides, if you did get pregnant, I'd tell you to have an abortion. But that's a moot point anyway, because you're too fat to get pregnant.' (I am now almost five months pregnant with absolutely no sign of difficulty or problems.)"

It's no wonder doctors fear the pregnancy of a large patient, says

Boyd Cooper, MD, an obstetrician and gynecologist at Women's Medical Group at Hollywood Presbyterian Hospital. "Consider what doctors are taught. The textbooks warn us about large-size women having a high risk of complications during pregnancy, such as pre-eclampsia, diabetes, hypertension, C-sections, poor wound healing. But in my own experience, large-size women do just fine as patients. Extremely large patients can encounter minor difficulties. It might take longer to hear the heartbeat, or tell how the fetus is lying, but an abdominal UltraSound will give us that information. Actually, most of the problems of larger women's pregnancies have solved themselves through technology."

For some women, it is the accumulation of years of abuse from health professionals that contributes to their shame.

At 360 pounds, Jennifer, 37, berates herself for feeling ashamed. "I am one of those women who avoids health care because of the fear of 'the weight lecture.' I'm not a stupid woman ... I have college degrees. It seems that whatever I'm going to the doctor for, my weight becomes an issue. I've gone to doctors because of an infected cut and been lectured about my weight ... I've gone to the doctor for a sprained wrist and been lectured. I postpone and postpone my yearly Pap smears for the same reason. I often feel ashamed that I let it get to me. I am allowing my fears to compromise my health."[9]

Felicia is haunted by her childhood experiences, and dreads going to a doctor for the first time in 10 years, required because of the restructuring of her health care insurance. "I'm scared out of my mind, and the whole experience makes me suicidal. I always left the doctor's office depressed and hurt, and wanting to crawl into a hole where I could never be seen again. All my pediatrician did was scream at me because of my weight. I remember the last time I went to her, she said 'You're too fat, if you don't lose weight I'm going to put you in the hospital.' I would rather have died right then and there, than to ever see another doctor."[10]

Many women fear seeing a doctor even for a virus, certain they will get the lecture on losing weight. One woman said, "When you go to a doctor, you feel so intimidated. You don't feel well, you're waiting for the 'lose weight' speech and sometimes you just don't have the energy to advocate for yourself. If doctors could be a little more compassionate and try to understand how much courage it took for a fat person to get to the doctor, maybe they would be able to treat the fat patient with a little more dignity and respect. As a fat person, I don't mind being told when my weight has an adverse effect on me, but don't blame every ache and pain on my weight."[11]

One woman sent this email message. "I dread going to the doctor.

I have not had a regular physical since I was a teenager. I have not had a Pap smear since my daughter was born five years ago (before getting pregnant I had not had one in 10 years). It's just the general dread of hearing the lecture about my weight, and the feelings of worthlessness and shame it invokes; even when I know my weight has nothing to do with the reason I am there! For example, the last time I saw a doctor was in 1994 when I had strep throat. The comment he made was 'When are you going to do something about your weight?' I mumbled something incoherent like 'not today' and he told me I was a walking time bomb, and did I want my daughter to grow up without a mother? Now, last time I checked, strep throat had nothing to do with one's weight ..."[12]

Lower quality care

A recent study that investigated cancer prevention testing reveals that size activists are telling the truth when they say large women often get second-rate health care. The study looked at data on 6,981 women from a cancer supplement to the 1992 National Health Interview Survey from the National Center for Health Statistics. The study adjusted for age, race, income, education, smoking and health insurance status.

It found that the higher the weight of women, the less likely they had had either a clinical breast exam, a gynecologic exam, or a Pap smear in the previous three years, even though they had as many or more doctor contacts. These three exams are critical for the early detection of cancer, and are especially important in this higher-risk population, since the effect of obesity on cervical, ovarian, endometrial and breast cancer is well documented. If detected early, many of these cancers can be successfully treated.

The only cancer screening exam that was being performed equally on these larger women was a mammography. The researchers wondered if this was because the physician could simply send the patient on to mammography, without direct physical contact. They warned that the lower level of preventive care large women are getting may account for some of the increased health risks found with obesity.[13]

A Connecticut study of 1,316 physicians showed they were more reluctant to perform pelvic exams on very obese patients. Seventeen percent stated specific reluctance to examining obese patients. In the same research, it was found that higher weight for 291 women was related to negative attitudes about their appearance, which in turn was related to lower frequency of pelvic exams.[14]

Another study suggests that physicians may be dissuaded from testing for cervical cancer by the technical difficulties associated with performing pelvic examinations on obese women.[15]

Large women who work in health care understand what's going on. They've heard it all, and it cannot be reassuring for their own treatment.

A veteran nurse confided her fears over an upcoming surgery to her daughter-in-law, "She reluctantly told me she was afraid the operating room doctors and nurses would not take as good care of her as they would a thin person, because she is not as worthwhile an individual because she is fat. She said that if something went wrong while on the operating room table, she did not think the doctors or nurses would work as hard at saving her life as they would a thin person. I could not understand how she could think that a whole operating room full of professionals would let something like that happen, even if one doctor discriminated against fat people. ... She started crying and said that she was sure they would let her die. I felt just awful that a medical professional degraded her so much that she could feel this way. The scariest thing about this is that my mother-in-law is a retired registered nurse who worked in a hospital for years. It makes me wonder what kind of treatment of fat people she witnessed over the years."[16]

From South Australia, Kathy Sandow, an Adelaide social worker, reports that she hears many health professionals express a personal dislike of fatness. "Some are repulsed by a fat body and do not want to touch. I have often heard accounts of fat women being refused treatment by doctors because they are fat, being told to come back when they have lost weight.

"Of course we never return ... unless our self-esteem is so battered that we actually think we deserve this treatment. Most large people have had some kind of negative experience with a doctor," writes Sandow.[17]

Sandow describes three recent visits she made to different doctors. During the first, for an immunization, she was weighed, blood pressure taken, and cardiovascular risk factors assessed, and even though all signs were good, and her risk low, was advised to lose weight. She visited the second doctor with flu-like symptoms and again was weighed, scolded for "eating at least twice as much food as my body needs," and told she would probably die young. Finally, the third doctor conducted blood tests for the same symptoms, as would likely be done for other patients, and found she was anemic. This time she was not weighed. Her weight was not mentioned.

"For the first time I felt I was getting the health care I am entitled to. He saw me as a whole person who just happens to be fat," says Sandow. "I dislike being weighed at every visit regardless of the problem. I feel like the only thing noticed is my fat."

A study of female health-care workers showed that 32 percent of the women with a BMI of over 27 (slightly over average weight) delayed or canceled physician appointments because they knew they would be weighed. The study concluded, "We will fail to meet our goals of health maintenance if a significant percentage of obese patients delay seeking medical care."[18]

Smith recalls growing up as a large child and being put on an endless series of weight loss programs. She says she has spent 20 years dieting her way up to 325 pounds, regaining more than she lost each time. "When I was 7, I was sent to a dietitian for my first diet. There were weekly weigh-ins, food charts, exchanges and servings, rare praise and more often, scoldings. When I was 9 and alone with my pediatrician in the examining room, he told me to take off my gown, get off the table, stand up and bend down and touch my toes, 'so I can see how fat you are.' There I was, a naked 9-year-old, being degraded and humiliated by my doctor. I remember public weighings where the nurse would make derogatory comments about my weight, and the doctor scolding me.

"When I was 16, my doctor told me that I was so fat I'd never live to see my 18th birthday. When I was 20, another doctor told me I'd never live to see 21. When I was 26, a different doctor told me I'd drop dead if I didn't buy the liquid diet program she was selling and lose weight immediately. This was the same doctor who had me on a high blood pressure medication unnecessarily for three years. It was a new doctor who used the proper blood pressure cuff and said, 'What are you doing on medication? Your blood pressure is low!'"

Inevitably, Smith's weight was always a doctor's focus, even though she was generally healthy. She describes a visit to a dermatologist for bumps on her forehead. "This woman was so fatphobic that she didn't want to get near me. She literally had her back against the door when she asked me what was wrong. I told her about the bumps and, peering at me from across the room, she said, 'Well, the first thing you need to do is to lose weight.' I asked if thin people ever got bumps on their foreheads, and she had to admit that, yes, they did. I said to her, 'Well, then, why don't you tell me what you usually tell them?'"[19]

A 30-year-old woman has not seen a doctor for 12 years, since she was 18 and taking a college medical examination. "My doctor weighed me, clicked his tongue, and said: 'I don't want to see you back here next year unless you've lost 50 lbs.' I was 5' 5' and 170 lbs, my health was good, with slightly low blood pressure but no problems whatsoever. The experience mortified me, filled me with shame.

"Well, I didn't lose and in fact, I gained, and continued gaining, until now I weigh 265. The idea of exposing myself to what will undoubtedly be a much worse experience now (considering how much heavier I am) is anathema to me, and so I remain nearly phobic about going to visit a physician. Fortunately, I have had no severe health problems."[20]

Size prejudice in health care is not new, according to some correspondents. One woman remembers that her large-bodied grandmother would fast the day before going to her doctor and drink a bottle of citrate of magnesium to lose weight. "She had a heart condition and went every other week. How unhealthy this must have been for her, and how sad that she felt she had to do this."[21]

Young children called lazy, stupid

Prejudice begins young: even small children feel the stigma and fear being a target. In one study children as young as six described silhouettes of an overweight child as "lazy, dirty, stupid, ugly, cheats and lies."

When shown drawings of a normal weight child, an overweight child, and children with various handicaps, including missing hands and facial disfigurement, children rated the overweight child as the least likable. Sadly, this bias even afflicted the larger children who expressed the same prejudices.[22]

Charisse Goodman recounts the unfairness of her childhood experiences — she was always "the fat kid," a stereotype.[23]

"I wasn't me. I wasn't a name or a person, just an object described by an adjective. If I was naturally shy, I became doubly so. I learned that no matter what anyone says, it really doesn't count if you're smart, kind, funny, sweet, generous, or caring because if you also happen to be heavy, you may find yourself on the receiving end of more cruelty than you even knew existed.

"I learned that keeping to myself and minding my own business didn't help because people would seek me out to ridicule and humiliate me. I learned that 'ignoring it,' as I was nonchalantly advised to do by my emotionally disengaged parents, usually just made me a greater challenge to bullies, so that I inevitably became 'the one to get.' I learned that adults are often indifferent to the suffering of a fat child, perhaps because on some level they agree with her tormentors, or maybe it's just convenient for them to believe that an abused child will somehow emerge unscathed into adulthood, magically free of emotional scars.

"I discovered that anytime I moved my body, people would laugh at me, and that even if I sat still and quietly read a book they would point and laugh. I learned that if they saw me cry or show any weakness, they would laugh at me even more. And so I learned to cry alone, and laugh alone, and live alone inside my head. I learned that the word 'pretty' never included me.

"Now I am a grown woman. I know without a doubt that in every town and every city, in every state in America, countless other fat children are learning the same heartbreaking, soul-destroying lessons that I was forced to learn. My pain and the pain of others like me has been conveniently invisible to thin people for far too long. They have been too comfortable with the price that we have paid for their imaginary superiority.

"At long last, I am angry."

Oppression against large children can be a form of persecution. They are teased on the playground, called names and chosen last to play on teams. Harassment of any kind is no longer allowed in many schools and should be reported.

It is at puberty when the problems of obesity become most painful. Despite the discrimination against them, studies show that when they are younger, large children's sense of self-worth is similar to that of average-weight children. But in adolescence, the powerful social messages become internalized and a lifelong negative self-image can develop, according to William Dietz and Nevin Scrimshaw, in *Social Aspects of Obesity*.[24]

Gaining a strong sense of self-worth is especially difficult for large teenagers in industrially developed countries, where both feminine and masculine ideals have become very thin. Male stars of movies, television, sports and pop music are not only lean, but appear muscular and fit.

"All this results in a distressing position for an obese adolescent who has to face up to the negative attitudes of colleagues at school or even in the family. Clumsiness, unattractiveness to the opposite sex, are serious problems at this age," note Dietz and Scrimshaw.

One study shows that large people who were obese as teens were more likely to develop negative body image and low self-worth, than those who gained their excess weight later.

Because of their youthful experiences, some women have a great deal of unresolved anger and rage. Jean Rubel, 36, in the book *Full Lives*, describes how she turned this anger against herself.

"Under my loneliness simmered a lake of molten rage. Sometimes I turned it loose when I felt ignored, criticized, misunderstood, or unloved. Most of the time, though, I held it in the pit of my stomach, where it became the only defense I could find against my belief that I was flawed in some critical way that kept me from joining the human race. Unfortunately, I too often turned this hateful energy against myself in storms of self-criticism and loathing. I began to blame my body for all my problems. If I weren't so ugly, so big, so soft and flabby, I would be happy and popular ... I wanted to be thin, admired, and loved. Instead I felt awkward, shy, fat, defective and extremely lonely."[25]

Obesity is the last socially acceptable form of prejudice, charge Albert Stunkard and Jeffery Sobal, in *Eating Disorders and Obesity*: "Obese persons remain perhaps the only group toward whom social derogation can be directed with impunity."[26]

Teachers reinforce prejudice

Discrimination has been shown in the way teachers evaluate and interact with larger students. Acceptance into prestigious colleges is lower in one study for large women, even when they do not differ in academic qualifications, school performance or application rates to colleges.[27]

In 1994 the National Education Association reported in its investigation of size prejudice in schools: "From nursery school through college, fat students experience ostracism, discouragement, and sometimes violence. Often ridiculed by their peers and discouraged by even well-meaning education employees, fat students develop low self-esteem and have limited horizons. They are deprived of places on honor rolls, sports teams, and cheerleading squads and are denied letters of recommendation."[28]

Effects of this stigma carry over into adulthood, especially for women.

Women who are overweight as adolescents or young adults earn less, are less likely to marry, complete fewer years of school, and have higher rates of poverty than their normal weight peers. Fewer of these effects occur for overweight males.[29]

A double standard criticizes obesity in women while overlooking it in men. In one study 16 percent of employers said they would not hire obese women under any conditions; another 44 percent said they would not hire them in certain situations.

The larger the woman, the more severe the discrimination in all areas. Supersize women and men may have serious work- and recreation-related disabilities, more health problems, and they must deal daily with a constraining physical environment that limits mobility and subjects them to humiliation. Many cannot fit through subway turnstiles, or sit in theater seats or waiting room chairs. In almost every aspect of living they are made to feel different and as if they don't fit in.

Invisiblity of large women

Goodman contends that large women in America are in many respects invisible in today's thinness-obsessed culture. Regardless of her unique personal qualities, a large woman is often not seen as an individual, but as a stereotype, portrayed as having physical and emotional problems, as being unattractive, compulsive, self-indulgent, even anti-social. Thus, often she is not treated as a normal human being with normal needs, desires, virtues and vices, but rather as a failure, an example of what not to be, not to become. She may be discreetly or unconsciously excluded from office or extracurricular social interaction. She may be automatically passed over for promotions, even paid less than thinner people for equal work.

On the other hand, says Goodman, she becomes all too visible when someone is looking for a scapegoat. Then she's an easy target for the neighborhood bully, the insecure person in need of a cheap ego boost, and for the weight loss industry.

"It takes a powerful character not to vanish beneath this avalanche of stereotypes, which is all that American society sees when it looks at a fat woman," she concludes.

Myths stigmatize

Along with the stereotypes, society abuses large people with myths. "All large people overeat ... are unhealthy ... have personality problems ... if they wanted to, they could lose weight."

Some of these myths:

• *Romance is not important to large women.* Certainly, a large woman like any other longs for romance, love, admiration and appreciation. This is important and desired. Fortunately, 5 to 10 percent of the population prefer large-size partners, according to the National Association to Advance Fat Acceptance. Yet it sometimes takes courage for men to date large women, even when they want to, fearing stigmatization and disapproval from their peers.

• *Large people have unhealthy lifestyle habits.* Many large people are extremely fit and maintain healthy lifestyle habits. Others may be sedentary, as are other people of all sizes. Some critics have the erroneous notion that if large people would just adopt healthier habits and live more actively, they would automatically lose weight. This is not necessarily true, as normal weight is defended. But developing an active and healthy lifestyle has many benefits for people of all sizes.

• *Large people overeat.* This is still controversial, but the latest official word is that there's little or no correlation between weight and calorie intake. Calorie intake fails to predict weight, and vice versa. This comes from the Healthy Eating Index, the nation's newest "report card" on how Americans are eating. It pulls together extensive recall data based on national intake studies, compiled by the Center for Nutrition Policy and Promotion, CDC.

Statistics in the Healthy Eating Index show that men and women with a body mass index of 20 or less and those with a BMI greater than 30 have a similar range of calorie intakes, as do the two categories between. Weight factors were omitted entirely from the final statistics in the Healthy Eating Index, because researchers could find no relationship between weight and calorie intake or percent fat in the diet.[30]

Various studies have attempted to compare how people of different sizes eat, with mixed results. Some studies indicate that people's eating may be regulated by the amount of their lean body mass.

Another theory is that people who are in a dynamic state of weight gain eat more, at any size. One study found that obese women who were gaining weight ate about 480 more calories a day than either women of normal or stable obese weight. At the same time, there were no differences in intake between women of normal weight and those of stable obese weight.[31]

What does seem clear is that there is great variation in how much people eat. Some large people eat more calories than average, and others don't. Some small people eat and burn a great many calories, and others don't.

The severely obese people publicized in the tabloids as eating insatiably and consuming great amounts often have a condition called Prader-Willi syndrome. Prader-Willi affects about one in 15,000, both sexes and all races, and may relate to a chromosome abnormality. It is characterized by compulsive eating, obsession with food, abnormal growth, characteristic facial traits, cognitive limitations, obesity and balance problems.[32]

• *Large people are unhealthy.* Often the health issue serves as a smoke screen to justify denying large people their civil rights. The assumption that they must be unhealthy is used to defend discrimination in employment, education, housing and adoption.

However, there is, in fact, very little or no added risk for most moderately obese people. Granted, the health risk is statistically increased with obesity, but this is most significant for public health policy, when considering populations. Individuals should not take statistics too personally. It is possible for one ill person to double the risk for everyone, in a statistical sense.

Furthermore, if people are physically active, research shows there is little difference in longevity between the different weight categories. Active people are much more likely to live long lives than inactive people of any size.[33]

It is true that with severe obesity, health risks are more likely to be serious. However, no research has investigated the damage done by a lifetime of hazardous weight loss attempts. None has assessed the harm from racheting one's weight upward through repeated weight loss and gain cycles. None has counted the costs of lower access to preventive health care.

• *Rapid weight loss is healthy for large people.* One of the most harmful myths among health professionals, which has caused much injury and death, is the myth that obese persons are at such severe health risk that radical weight loss methods are justified. The thinking here is that high-risk people must lose weight at any health cost to reduce their risk. Does this make sense to you?

This myth is widely promoted by the weight loss industry, yet any doctor who has practiced a few years and has the interests of his or her patients at heart should spot the fallacy in this thinking at once. The severely obese patient who has high-risk factors is not well served by the severe shock to the body that comes with large, rapid losses. Rather, it is even more critical that this person be treated conservatively and that weight loss be gradual and lasting.

Yet hundreds of thousands of large women underwent radical very low calorie diets of 800 or less calories, usually liquid diets, suddenly losing great amounts of weight, and at the same time losing proportionate amounts from heart muscle and all other organs, causing great disruption of body processes, and then just as rapidly regained the weight, causing a wild swing in risk factors. Many died. Others suffered many subsequent health problems. Some of these women have written me long, impassioned letters about recurring health problems that followed. Even their immune system seemed compromised.

One day a woman called me, frantic after a visit to her doctor, asking my opinion of a liquid diet rapid weight loss program. "I weigh 300 pounds. The doctor says I have to lose weight right now or I might die!" I tried to calm her down, found she had no actual risk factors, and suggested she consider carefully before putting herself at even greater risk with the program she mentioned, which was almost guaranteed to weight cycle her right back to 300 pounds, or higher.

• *Large people have psychological disturbances that prevent weight loss.* There are still traditional psychotherapists who take a Freudian view, following theories such as that fear of sexuality, suppressed rage, aggression, oral fixation, or Oedipal impulses are involved in maintaining excess weight. They may believe that the conscious wish to be thin is sabotaged by the unconscious desire to be fat.

However, research finds no common patterns to explain obesity is a result of personality factors, emotional conflicts, faulty training in self-care, or dysfunctional family systems. Judy Rodin of Yale University reviewed studies and concluded, "There are virtually no data showing a causal relationship between emotional disturbance and obesity ... Even evidence supporting a correlation is, at best, weak. Nor is there any evidence that certain personality types are more likely to become obese than others."

Albert Stunkard also looked at the evidence and reported, "The old view that obese persons have a specific personality profile is no longer held, and population studies of obese people show that they differ little, if at all, from non-obese people in overall levels of psychopathology." He further suggests that psychosis may be present in people of any weight, but is being blamed on weight only for obese persons.[34]

After reading all this you might wonder that any large woman is able to live her life with a smile on her face, but upcoming chapters will show how they do it every day. It's not always easy, but it is possible.

This information might make you sad, it might make you angry, it might leave you feeling overwhelmed. But knowledge is power. Knowing what the research says can help us all to move ahead.

Research tells us that large women are no different than thin women. Each is an individual and deserves to be regarded this way and treated with respect.

CHAPTER 7

Living in starvation mode

■

"I fell in love with a girl ... but see her only occasionally now. It's almost too much trouble to see her even when she visits me. It requires effort to hold her hand ... If we see a show, the most interesting part is scenes where people are eating."
— *Volunteer in Minnesota study*

The other day, a New York radio talk show host named Brian called me to talk about why women are so obsessed with their bodies.

"When I hang out with chicks, sometimes all they want to talk about is how they should take fat off their thighs or waist, they shouldn't eat this or that, and gotta lose some weight. They look just fine to me."

It's boring, he said.

"And when you take them out to dinner they just pick at their food, right?" I countered.

He was astonished that I could guess what went on during his dinner dates. "That's right! And afterward I pay this huge bill, and nearly all the food is left on their plates."

The sad thing is that half a continent away, I know all too much about Brian's girlfriends and what's uppermost on their minds — their weight, body image, and how they can avoid eating in spite of gnawing hunger. It's how undernourished women act. This is living in a starvation mode.

Well-nourished women can't be stereotyped. They develop the many fascinating facets of their personalities, expand their interests, reach out to others. I couldn't guess. But malnourished women are far too much alike, and the hungrier they are, the more they are alike. In a sense their personality is reduced to the lowest common denominator.

A recent United Nations UNICEF report notes the disappearance of personality for starving people: "Personalities slip away ... A person grows confused and disoriented and is easily irritated. Many exhibit self-centered behavior."[1]

Listen to your body's opinion

How do you discover your natural, healthy weight? The weight at which you can maintain a high quality of life, keep well nourished, feel a sense of well-being, and be at your personal best?

Most people call it the setpoint. Or, as Mohey Mowafy, PhD, a nutritionist at Northern Michigan University, has dubbed it, the "settling point."

It's the weight our bodies "want" to be at this time in our lives. What you and I weigh right now, when fully nourished and not dieting. It's the result of genetics, family and eating and activity patterns up to this point.

"The body has an opinion about what it should weigh," says Richard E. Keesey, PhD, a setpoint researcher and professor at the University of Wisconsin, Madison.

Indeed it does, whether we like it or not. It's misguided to choose a number on a chart and say this is our ideal weight. It's even worse to encourage others to devote their lives to reaching this number.

Keesey points out that most people maintain a stable weight, despite wide variations in calorie intake. This is because the body makes its own adjustments to match food intake. With overeating or undereating, the adjustments are made. Metabolism speeds up or slows down, temperature rises or drops, heart rate adjusts to try to balance calorie intake.[2]

Unfortunately for the woman who loses weight, all this combines to defeat her best efforts. Her setpoint remains the same but her body shuts down, metabolism drops, along with other calorie-burning processes, and continues to be abnormally depressed. At the same time, she feels a very normal increasing desire to eat. After a time of dieting and deprivation, she probably "breaks" the diet with a binge, and weight returns to her normal setpoint.

In one study that illustrates this principle, obese people dropped their calorie needs by 28 percent through weight loss. After they lost weight, they still weighed 60 percent more than a control group, but even though they weighed more, their calorie requirements were much less. And this did not change in four to six years for the three people who kept off their weight that long.[3]

In mice and rat experiments, Keesey reports that weight loss is countered by both lower energy expenditure and higher calorie intake as soon as the animals can eat freely. These act together to bring their weight back to normal.

Weight returns to setpoint

Why don't weight loss programs work?

Because, of course, the setpoint theory is true. The secret is out. The diet industry has tried to bury the idea of a setpoint, to pretend it's not true. But there's a great body of convincing evidence that says it is true, and none that I am aware of against it.

We each do have a setpoint weight. Without effort our bodies regulate body temperature, salt in the bloodstream and many other conditions — so why wouldn't they also regulate body weight? Researchers are looking for the signal that tells the body it is back to setpoint weight. If they could find this signal, maybe they could change its message.

Our setpoint is not fated at birth, but is the result of both genetic and environmental factors up to this time in our lives. It's the weight our bodies want to weigh now.

If we lose weight, there are many regulatory processes in our bodies working to shut down the furnaces, burn fewer calories, and at the same time increase the drive to eat. So we gain back all the weight we lost, usually just as quickly as we lost it.

Certainly there are some successes, people who lose weight and keep it off in a healthy way, apparently lowering their setpoint.

But we are also haunted by other so-called "successes" — gaunt, hollow-eyed shadows of women and girls, who are keeping their weight low by eating less food than their bodies need. They experience a body shutdown to some degree that affects them physically, intellectually, emotionally, socially and spiritually.

Anyone who works with eating disorders knows the symptoms all too well. With weight kept below setpoint, a woman lives in a starvation mode, or what might be called the *starvation syndrome.*

Evidence of a setpoint

One of the most convincing arguments for a setpoint concerns the remarkable stability of weight. Many people vary only two or three pounds in weight throughout most of a lifetime.

Twenty years ago Albert Stunkard, PhD, a pioneer obesity researcher, calculated that a person eating 3,000 calories a day consumes a million calories a year. An error of only 300 calories either way from an exact daily balance of food to physical activity, would add or subtract 30 pounds in a year. Obviously, this does not happen. Weight rarely varies more than a couple of pounds a year, if that. Stunkard reported that when a person's weight does go up or down through diet or various life events, it soon returns almost precisely to its previous level.[4]

One writer reports that for 24 years he has weighed within two pounds of high school graduation size. Assuming he ate about 24 million calories, the two-pound gain represents .8 calories a day, or about equal to one carrot stick. To come this close in balancing calories with activity would be virtually impossible had he counted, which he didn't.[5]

One German nutritionist who did count early in the century found a remarkable wasting of calories when he overate. For one year he kept a stable weight while consuming 1,766 calories daily. The second year he increased to 2,199 calories, and the third year to 2,403, carefully weighing and analyzing all his food. He calculated that his excess eating should have added 40 pounds the second year and another 60 the third, if 4,000 extra calories equals a pound (theoretically 3,500 to 4,000). Yet he gained only a few pounds over the three-year period. He concluded that his body adapted to overfeeding by somehow wasting the extra calories.[6] We now know this calorie wasting comes in part from increased metabolism and body heat.

The almost inevitable regain after weight loss also furnishes strong evidence for a setpoint. For over 16 years I have evaluated virtually every type of weight loss treatment worldwide, as praised in news reports, conferences, and the scientific press by major obesity experts. Many were hailed at the time as the miracle people were waiting for.

However, the sum result of this 16-year full-time effort by the biggest guns in the business is that, no matter how hard they try, none can show long-term success past one year. Even on the strongest programs maximum weight loss comes at about six months, followed by inevitable regain until nearly all participants have gained back what they lost. This takes a few months to as long as two to five years.

For example, in one carefully controlled Danish study, 57 patients, averaging 264 pounds, were randomly assigned to very low calorie diet or gastric surgery. They lost an average of about 50 pounds. If they could keep off 22 pounds they were categorized as successful. By the end of three years, only 23 percent of those on the diet and 47 percent of surgical patients were deemed successful. (They still weighed an average of 242 pounds.) At the end of five years, this had deteriorated to 3 percent of the dieters and 16 percent of surgery patients who were defined as successful. Even though surgery gave somewhat better weight loss, the researchers advised the hospital to stop the surgery because its complications were so numerous and severe.[7]

A Pennsylvania study that compared three programs and showed excellent one-year weight loss results was widely praised as a shining example of success. But the researchers took another look in three years and found that only 13 percent of participants were "successful maintainers." Worse, all of these so-called successes had been on several intervening weight loss programs during that time. The researchers wisely asked themselves: If the original program was so successful, why did these people join other weight loss programs? And what if, even now, they were only caught in the down swing of another weight cycle?[8]

Metabolism drops with weight loss

Many studies confirm a drop in resting metabolic rate and total energy expenditure with weight loss, in humans as well as lab animals.[9]

Keesey says a 5 percent drop in weight ordinarily results in a 15 percent drop in metabolism. Sustaining a lower weight at this level does not lower setpoint and requires a lifelong commitment. He warns this may be too great a price to pay for the modest weight losses most obese individuals would be able to achieve and sustain.[10]

Metabolic rate is markedly reduced for dieters, says David Garner, PhD, Director of the Toledo Center for Eating Disorders,, showing "the body's extraordinary ability to adapt to low caloric intake by reducing its need for energy."

The starvation syndrome chart on page 145 describes what happens when the body adapts to defend its weight against calorie deficit and loss of fat and lean body mass. The physical effects as well as mental, emotional and social effects can be profound.

Survival traits

Can some of the abnormal effects of dieting be explained as survival traits that kept our ancestors alive through periods of famine and starvation? I believe they can.

During weight loss or starvation three things happen. First, the body shuts down, slowing metabolism and other processes, and burns fewer calories. Second, the drive to eat increases. Third, there's evidence that fat may be selectively routed to storage instead of being burned as usual, so that half-empty fat cells are replenished quickly.

This complex set of factors appear to come together to defend weight and retain fat stores. It's a precise system of monitoring and readjustment, as if aimed at keeping consistent body weight as a natural protection against death by starvation.

So what happens when women ignore their setpoint and go on a severe diet to lose weight? They do lose weight rapidly at first as cells release water, and may lose fat and muscle rapidly for a time. Then the defenses kick in. Six months is the longest period of weight loss that obesity treatments can show. After that, the body rebounds to its setpoint weight, usually as fast as the weight was lost.

It may be that the setpoint can be lowered in healthy ways, which we'll talk about later, but probably not through dieting, especially rigorous dieting.

The reality of setpoint is all too real to women who repeatedly lose weight, then inevitably regain every pound. It is all too real to women who maintain a lower weight than natural. To go against setpoint means a continual struggle to which many women dedicate their lives.

Garner warns that people who override the body's regulating mechanisms and stay at an unnaturally thin weight do so "at great personal sacrifice, in the face of constant biological pressure to return to higher body weight levels."[11]

Sadly, many women are not content to work with their setpoint, but instead choose to live in a chronic state of suppressed weight or continued weight-cycling.

What happens during starvation?

Our bodies are well prepared to defend against starvation. Looking at the long history of the human race, our ancestors' biggest threat was not enemy tribes or large predators, but starvation.

So what traits would most ensure survival of the human race? Clearly, the ability to go into a protective "starvation mode," shut down the body, bank the fires, endure privation, and at the same time sharpen the drive to search for food.

In fact, this is just what happens. The evidence is plain: the woman experiencing starvation or even a calorie deficit, shuts down physically and mentally. She burns far fewer calories than normal. To her dismay, her body reacts defensively just as it would to famine.

"This makes complete evolutionary sense," explains Garner. "Over hundreds of thousands of years of human evolution, a major threat to survival of the organism was starvation. If weight had not been carefully modulated and controlled internally, early humans most certainly would simply have died when food was scarce or when their interest was captured by countless other aspects of living."[12]

The drive for food is an important facet of this defense. Our ancestors did not just lie around, listlessly waiting to die, when starving. Their intense craving for food drove them out in search of it. Hunger is a survival trait we all have.

Ironically, in well-fed nations throughout the world, thousands — probably millions — of women and men are living this way by choice, existing in an undernourished state that keeps their bodies in a defensive starvation mode, in order to keep off a few pounds. Thousands more are driven unwittingly into the starvation mode by unproven weight loss programs that either ignore or fail to realize the harm they do.

At what point does the starvation syndrome begin? This is unclear. It appears to vary for individuals, and may depend on such factors as initial weight, body fat, genetics, health and mental stamina.

One man developed major personality disturbances after just 10 weeks in the Minnesota wartime experiment in human starvation. He had lost only 10 pounds, 7 percent of his weight, and his diet of 1,570 calories was much higher than that of many weight loss regimens. Yet mentally and emotionally he was well into the starvation mode.[13]

It is not known what triggers the starvation syndrome. It could be loss of weight, loss of muscle mass, fat cell depletion, calorie deficit, diet composition, or nutrient deficiency. Several writers view reduced weight or reduced fat cells, rather than diet, as the determining factor.[14]

How does living in the starvation state affect girls and women? How does it alter their lives? How does it shrivel relationships, impact friends and families? What is the potential harm to the fabric of our culture? Is it worth the price they pay?

Let's take a look at the evidence.

Starving in Minnesota

The classic study on what it's like to live in a starvation state was done in 1944 and 1945 at the University of Minnesota, aimed at finding how best to help the starving people of Europe after the war. Thirty-six men were selected from 100 volunteer conscientious objectors. Of these, 32 finished the 12-month program, and their lives were changed forever. For six months they received half rations (about 1,570 calories a day).

The Minnesota Starvation Study, as it is commonly called, conducted by Ancel Keys and colleagues, shows clearly how weight is defended by internal adjustments, and how setpoint weight is restored when food is again available.

In even more profound and heartbreaking ways, it reveals what happens to people who are deprived of food, to their personalities, thought pathways, and social intercourse.[15]

They make the "great personal sacrifice" that Garner warns of. So do their families.

Personality changes

Starvation causes high stress. There is no peace for starving people. They crave food and focus on this one overriding need.

Men in the Minnesota study tested healthy and strong both mentally and physically during the initial three-month control period. The researchers said, "The psychobiological stamina of the subjects was unquestionably superior to that likely to be found in any random or more generally representative sample of the population."

The young men were noted for being friendly, idealistic and good-humored. They were well-educated; over half were college graduates, and all others had completed at least one year of college. Many were members of the pacificist Brethern Church. They opposed war, and expressed a deep desire to heal the war's devastation.

But during six months of semistarvation, their idealism evaporated. As these friendly and dedicated young men lost one-fourth of their weight, profound changes occurred. They became highly nervous, restless, and anxious. Apathy, fatigue, moodiness, and depression increased. Many experienced profound mood swings, elation to "low periods."

When the men tried to continue their cultural interests and studies, they felt distracted and could not concentrate. Interests narrowed and they lost their ambition. They felt ineffective and frustrated by the discrepancy between what they wanted to do and could actually accomplish. Intellectual pursuits, self-discipline, mental alertness, comprehension, and concentration declined.

The men's general apathy extended to appearance and they often neglected to shave, brush their teeth, or comb their hair. They continued bathing as one source of pleasure, because in their chilled condition they enjoyed the warm water and soothing of aches, pain and fatigue.

Most of the men experienced severe emotional distress at times, and nearly 20 percent an extreme emotional deterioration that markedly interfered with their functioning. Personality tests revealed significant increases on the depression, hysteria, and hypochondriasis scales, confirming what the researchers were noticing. Before the study was over, personality profiles measured an average rise toward the neurotic end. Six men reacted with severe character neurosis. Two developed psychotic disturbances that included violence and hysteria.

One man was so depressed he cut off three fingers so he could be released from the program. First, he jacked up his car and dropped it on his fingers, without success. Two weeks later he smashed off the fingers by slamming his car trunk on them.

Eating disorder specialists often see the same personality traits in women and girls who are undernourished through self-starvation. Many exhibit self-injurious behavior including higher tolerance for pain and discomfort. They feel the same obsessive concerns, the same irritability, distrust and intolerance.

Food preoccupation

One of the most striking changes in starving people is how intensely they are occupied with food, while other interests decline. Food became the central topic of conversation for the men in the Minnesota study. Food was constantly on their minds. It was the major topic of their conversation, their reading, and their daydreams.[16]

They talked of little else but hunger, food and their weight loss. Even though some were annoyed by this in others, they could not resist doing it themselves. They fantasized about food, planned how to stretch out their foods, collected recipes, studied cookbooks and menus.

They would dawdle up to two hours over a meal, and developed bizarre eating rituals, toying with their food, cutting it in small pieces, adding spices, sometimes in distasteful ways, trying to make it seem like more and of more variety. For some an inner conflict seemed to rage as to whether to ravenously gulp their food, or stall out eating. They smuggled out bits of food from their plates, hoarded food, and spent much time planning, preparing and eating food saved from meals. They demanded that food and beverages be hot. They ate their allotted food to the last crumb, and, yes, they licked their plates.

The men reported feeling pleasure from watching other people eat, but grew angry if they saw anyone wasting food. They drank more tea and coffee, and chewed more gum — one man chewed as much as 40 packs a day. They increased their smoking, and some nonsmokers took up the habit. They often chewed their fingernails.

In anthropologist Colin Turnbull's vivid account of the Ik, a starving tribe in east Africa,, the same thing happened. Turnbull relates in *The Mountain People* how every person focused single-mindedly on food.[17]

Food is one of our five basic needs. Lacking any of these — air, food, water, sleep, shelter — the body goes into an emergency state and strives to serve that one need. If you're missing sleep, for example, you crave sleep and grow anxious, irritable, unable to concentrate. When you finally sleep, you may drop off for a long time. Similarly, people wandering the desert without water can think of little else but the taste of water — cool, clear water.

Deprived of air, we have no need more desperate. Kathy Kator, an eating disorder therapist in Minneapolis, asks sixth graders to breathe through a straw in their mouths to make this point. She instructs them to hold their noses while breathing entirely through the straw. She teases them that they might look better if they would cut back on oxygen so their faces would be bluer: Surely they can cut back, it will be worth it to have the "right look." When they drop out and gasp for air, she chides them, "Have you no will-power? What's wrong with you?"

Kator discusses the consequences of being deprived of one of the five basic needs, the difficulty in concentrating on anything else, the powerful cravings for it, the irritable and self-centered feelings that arise, and when finally available, needing much more than normal. When she asks them to predict what would happen if they were deprived of food, they correctly list the symptoms of dieting women.[18]

Social interests deteriorate

Social and family relationships suffer when a person is living in a state of semistarvation. The friendly young men in the Minnesota study became loners, each looking out only for himself.

In volunteering for starvation research, the men had hoped to make a contribution to humanity. Many asked to serve overseas in hunger relief, and they planned evening training classes. Sadly, their intentions dried up during the six-month starvation period. Plans for careers in foreign relief work quietly collapsed, and instead many said they wanted to be chefs or cooks. They no longer enjoyed group activities, complaining that dealing with other people was too much trouble, even though earlier they had taken an active interest in making group decisions.

Social devastation for the starving African Ik people was much more severe. They lost all sense of caring about one another, all sense of love and compassion. Again, these are familiar eating disorder traits, known to professionals who work with anorexia and malnutrition, and sadly, to their families.

Starving tribesmen reject love

As Turnbull's eloquent and moving account reveals, people may lose all sense of humanity as starvation advances.

He describes the dehumanization of the Ik tribe as its culture deteriorated through a period of drought and starvation in the mid-1960s. Forbidden by the Uganda government to hunt game in the newly established Kidepo National Park, their traditional hunting ground, the Ik tried with little success to farm and forage for food in the barren mountains adjoining the park.

Starvation made them a strange and heartless people, distrustful, their days occupied with constant competition in the search for food. They seldom spoke. Cruelty took the place of love as their culture broke down. Men and women went out alone to forage for food, eating quickly and in secret, hiding any surplus bits of food and returning empty-handed to avoid sharing with crying children, weakened parents or spouse.

These people would be kind, generous and friendly if they were well nourished, Turnbull writes. But as starvation progressed during the two years he spent with them, basic human survival instincts took over. Reduced to desperate hunger, they became as "unfriendly, uncharitable, inhospitable and generally mean as people can be."

"The lack of any sense of moral responsibility toward each other, the lack of any sense of belonging to, needing or wanting each other, showed up daily and most clearly in what otherwise would have passed for family relationships," he says.

One day a baby left on the ground was carried off by a leopard. Turnbull describes the mother as delighted: she was rid of the child and it also meant the big cat would be sleeping nearby and an easy kill.

"The men set off and found the leopard, which had consumed all of the child except part of the skull. They killed the leopard and cooked it and ate it, child and all," he reported.

On another day, an old blind woman tripped, fell, and rolled a distance down the mountain. "There she lay on her back, her legs and arms thrashing feebly, while a little crowd standing on the edge above looked down at her and laughed at the spectacle," Turnbull observed.

When Turnbull gave her food and water, she suddenly began to cry, explaining that all of a sudden he had reminded her of a time when her people had been kind and good, and had helped each other.

As starvation wore on for the Ik, there was less and less that could be called social life. Turnbull says there was simply no community of interest, family or economic, social or spiritual. Spiritually, they lost their religion, and all sense of moral obligation. They no longer practiced any religious rituals after the three old priests died of starvation.

Turnbull says he searched for evidence of love almost from the beginning. He did not believe people could behave this way, especially in Africa where he had previously seen much evidence of loving families and strong tribal bonds. "But love implies mutuality, a willingness to sacrifice the self. The Ik are without love."

I wondered whether women might survive longer in a malnourished situation. Women have that extra layer of fat, we're told, so they can survive longer in famine and care for children.

So I asked a United Nations official who works with starving people in central Africa, "Who lives longest? Is it the women?"

He was silent for a time. Then he sighed, "No, it's the men. They are stronger and can better find food and get to the relief centers to save themselves."

They save themselves and maybe they don't return to their families with food. It's what starving people do.

Sexuality all dried up

Turnbull observed that men and women had lost all sexual interest, and did not flirt with each other, a missing factor that deprived them of a major drive toward sociability. Men told him they had better uses for their energy than to waste it on sex. Each person was simply alone, solitary, living in isolation, seldom speaking. It was this apathy and sense of isolation that made love almost impossible, he explains.

This same decline in sexual interest and libido was observed in the Minnesota starvation study. At first the men had girl friends or were looking for women. But they soon stopped seeing or writing to their girl friends — they didn't flirt, they didn't care. They had lost interest. They took down photos of girls and put up food pictures.

One man wrote in his diary, "I fell in love with a girl (in the control period) ... but see her only occasionally now. It's almost too much trouble to see her even when she visits me in the lab. It requires effort to hold her hand ... If we see a show, the most interesting part is scenes where people are eating."

A physical shutdown

The outcome of six months of semistarvation in the Minnesota study was documented by extensive medical tests, as the men's weight dropped an average of 24 percent.

Resting metabolism fell by almost 40 percent, an adaptive savings of 600 calories per day. Heart volume shrunk by about 20 percent and heart work output per minute dropped by half. The men's pulses slowed and their body temperatures fell. They felt cold. With muscle loss, their arms and thighs shrunk and their strength dropped by half.

The men complained of aching eyes, an inability to focus and seeing spots. Their hearing sharpened to the point where ordinary sounds were disturbing, and some had sensations of ringing in the head. Their skin grew pale, cold, dry, thin, scaly, rough, inelastic and marked with brownish pigmentation. Skin ulcers and sores were common. Their hair thinned, dried and fell out. Sexual function and testes size were reduced.

Over the weeks, the men lost their endurance and capacity to work, especially lifting, pushing, carrying loads, climbing, walking long distances, and standing for long periods. They slept poorly, and needed less sleep. Giddiness and momentary blackouts upon rising were common, and the men often felt dizzy. They had stomach pains and headaches. Their muscles frequently cramped, felt sore and extremities "went to sleep" or had tingling or prickling sensations. Tendon reflexes became sluggish. Urination was frequent. The men appeared and behaved as if they were much older, and often said they felt old, but there were no physical indications of accelerated aging.

On the rebound

It is instructive to read Turnbull's disappointed tale of recovery, which he observed a year later when he returned to find the drought eased and relief efforts underway. Relief brought food to the Ik, but failed to restore their spirit. Everyone still ate alone. They still laughed cruelly at others' misfortunes.

"If they had been mean and greedy and selfish before ... now that they had something, they really excelled themselves in what would be an insult to animals to call bestiality," he reports.

The Ik were no longer starving. The old and infirm had already died and younger survivors were doing well. They kept many of their dead on relief roles, so they could benefit from double rations. Often those who traveled to relief centers were given food for hungry people at home, but Turnbull says they did not bring it to them.

"So those who were in no real need got the relief intended for themselves as well as that intended for all their truly needy kin."

Turnbull does not blame individuals, but rather the conditions of starvation that made them this way. "There is no goodness left for the Ik. They have made of a world that was alive a world that is dead, a cold, dispassionate world that is without ugliness because it is without beauty, without hate because it is without love."

Men in the Minnesota study fared better in recovery.

Yet, surprisingly, the refeeding period, with a gradual calorie increase after the diet ended, did not immediately revive their spirits. Morale slumped even lower, and many of the men grew more depressed and irritable for about six weeks than they had been before.

They became even more argumentive and questioned the value of the experiment, their role as "guinea pigs," the competence of the researchers, and said they felt "let down." Not until the 15th week of refeeding did social behavior at meals improve. Slowly humor, enthusiasm and sociability returned, and the men began looking forward to their plans for the future. Not until the 20th week, nearly five months after the study ended, did the men all say they felt nearly normal and less preoccupied with food.

Rebound appetites insatiable

Bingeing began as soon as the men were allowed to eat more. Their appetites grew insatiable. They ate voraciously. All wanted more food than they were allowed and most found it hard to stop eating even when physically full and "stuffed to bursting." Table manners and eating habits had deteriorated and now during refeeding became worse. These highly educated young men continued to lick their plates at the meal's end.

During the 13th week after the starvation period ended, when food restrictions were lifted, the men consumed a daily average of 5,218 calories. On weekends they sometimes ate 8,000 to 10,000 calories.

They ate nearly continuously, as many as three consecutive lunches, and spent most of their time eating and sleeping. By the 15th week, table manners improved to normal for most, yet over one-fourth still gobbled their food, and had the desire to lick their knives and plates. Four of the 14 men being tested at the laboratory were still overeating eight months after the test period ended. One ate 25 percent more than initially and gained so much weight he tried to reduce, but grew so ravenous he couldn't stand it, and returned to excessive eating.

The evidence of binge eating being experimentally produced in the Minnesota study should temper the speculation of some specialists that psychological disturbances are the cause of binge eating in patients with eating disorders, says Garner.

As they binged, the men rapidly gained fat tissue, and soon overshot their original fat levels by 10 percent. A "soft roundness" became their dominant characteristic. Lean tissue recovered more slowly. Over the next two or three months the men gained back their baseline weight plus an average of about 10 percent. Then, as their eating normalized, weight gradually dropped back, until by about nine months after refeeding began, all except two were near their initial weight.

Metabolism speeded up as the men ate more calories, and there was a sharp increase in the energy burned through metabolic processes. The men who consumed larger amounts of food had the largest rise in basal metabolic rate.[19]

A study of 45 male bodybuilders also showed binge eating. While dropping 15 pounds in trying to get rid of subcutaneous body fat, 81 percent reported being preoccupied with food often, sometimes, or always. Nearly half described distress, anxiety, short temper and anger, and half reported bingeing after the contest.[20]

Weight gain not easy

The thin person who overeats to gain weight is fighting a similar but opposite battle. Increasing your weight above the setpoint and keeping it there is almost as difficult as losing weight. When weight is elevated, appetite is diminished so calorie intake drops; at the same time, calories are burned faster until weight is brought back down to its usual level.

Researcher Ethan Sims tested this with inmates at Vermont State Prison who volunteered for overeating studies. The men tried to gain 20 to 30 pounds. Eventually 20 did reach that goal, but almost all found it extremely difficult. One 132-pound man ate great amounts of food and reduced his activity to less than half its former level, but could not get his weight above 144 pounds, a gain of only 12 pounds. One who gained more easily increased his weight from 110 to 138 pounds, but had to eat 7,000 calories a day to do so. As the men gained weight, they became lethargic, apathetic, and neglectful of their duties.[21]

When the overfeeding period ended, most of the prisoners dropped quickly and naturally back to their original weight. Only the two men who had gained more easily stabilized slightly above their starting weight. Investigation showed they had a family history of obesity or diabetes.

"Essentially all of the subjects to date have lost weight readily, with the same alacrity, in fact, as that with which most of our obese patients return to their usual and customary weight after weight loss." said Sims.

He concluded that the men had some biochemical means for burning off or "wasting" excess calories, so they could not be stored as fat. Weight at setpoint is optimal for activity and mood, Simms suggests, and people become apathetic if weight goes much above or below.

In the same way, the person who eats a huge holiday dinner or celebrates on New Years Day by eating all day long, does not usually gain weight. Rather, it seems that most calories are wasted, and the person eats less the next day.

Over the six-week holiday season that begins with Thanksgiving and extends through Christmas and New Year's Day, many women gain 5 to 7 pounds. Most would probably lose it naturally, but they are afraid to wait. They launch their annual New Years diet, during which they "successfully" lose that extra weight and keep it off. But if they try to lose an extra 10, it doesn't happen — or they lose and regain it so they stabilize about at the same weight as before the holidays began.

Not everyone keeps a stable weight through life. Many experience an upward drift of setpoint, gaining perhaps a half to one pound a year.

Setpoint theory revisited

The Minnesota study challenges the popular belief that if people will just show a little initiative and will power, they can easily lose weight and keep it off.

As Garner points out, it demonstrates that the body is not simply "reprogrammed" at a lower setpoint once weight loss is achieved.

The setpoint theory is well accepted by health professionals — even though it is still regarded as a theory. Introduced in the 1970s, the term was popular in the media for a time, then disappeared.

The setpoint suggests that our bodies have finely tuned ways to monitor weight and fat, and make accurate adjustments during disturbances. We don't question other adjustments made by the human body: body temperature is kept at the same point whether a person works in sweltering summer heat or chilly winter blizzard; fluid volume keeps steady in the body; salt levels in the blood stream, and dozens of similar readjustments are made that require close monitoring to maintain homeostasis.

There is no reason to suppose that weight is any less regulated.

Industry renounces setpoint

When setpoint research burst on the scene in the 1970s, it brought a flash of insight to dieters: So that's it! That's why I can't keep off lost weight. It's not my fault.

Doctors said: No wonder my patients can't lose weight. Maybe we can't blame them after all.

Suddenly it all made sense. But after a brief spin in the public eye — a few research articles, a few textbook chapters, presentations by Richard Keesey, a rash of news stories — came silence. That's how science makes unacceptable truths go away, with silence.

The notion of setpoint was dropped like a hot potato.

It was a hot potato.

If the idea of setpoint weight were established as true, it would rip a hole in existing weight loss services and the new advertising campaigns hovering on the horizon. The heavy promotions for very low calorie liquid diets couldn't have happened. This was going to make no money for anyone. It was going to cause big problems for commercial diet companies and the psychologists and clinicians who treat obesity.

Setpoint explains why weight loss programs don't work. It explains why they seem to work at first, as we lose weight, then ultimately fail as our bodies readjust to restore lost weight. Needless to say, this was unpopular with the diet industry.

A set of arguments emerged against the idea, and eventually they prevailed. Ostensibly, the reasoning went that if setpoint were preordained at birth, then why was this other research showing that lifestyle matters? Why was there an increase in obesity in populations that had the same gene pool as an earlier, slimmer generation? Not that setpoint researchers had ever suggested setpoint was set at birth, but now it seemed that they had.

It was thought that the public should not be discouraged from losing

The starvation syndrome
A defense of body weight

Cutting calories, dieting and losing weight results in a
body slow-down or defense that includes decreased
metabolism, heart rate and temperature, and increased drive
to eat. This can lead to the following effects:

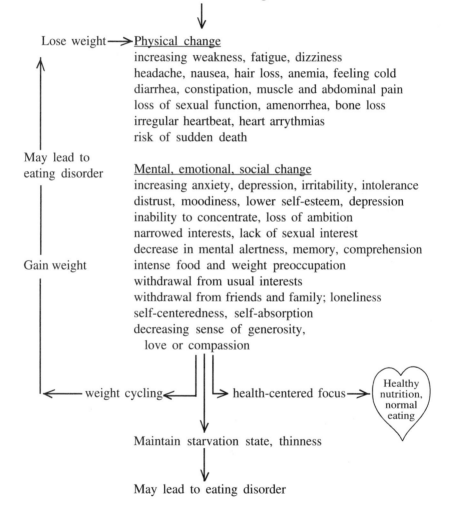

Lose weight → Physical change
increasing weakness, fatigue, dizziness
headache, nausea, hair loss, anemia, feeling cold
diarrhea, constipation, muscle and abdominal pain
loss of sexual function, amenorrhea, bone loss
irregular heartbeat, heart arrythmias
risk of sudden death

May lead to
eating disorder

Mental, emotional, social change
increasing anxiety, depression, irritability, intolerance
distrust, moodiness, lower self-esteem, depression
inability to concentrate, loss of ambition
narrowed interests, lack of sexual interest
decrease in mental alertness, memory, comprehension
Gain weight   intense food and weight preoccupation
withdrawal from usual interests
withdrawal from friends and family; loneliness
self-centeredness, self-absorption
decreasing sense of generosity,
    love or compassion

← weight cycling ← | | → health-centered focus → Healthy nutrition, normal eating

Maintain starvation state, thinness

May lead to eating disorder

weight. Experts came to believe that, in the interests of health, consumers need to keep trying. So Americans turned away from the uneasy setpoint notion and returned their trust to diet gurus.

Setpoint talk was quiet for years, but now the idea is being accepted again. The ascendency of drugs has altered the thinking: Diets don't work, so it will take drugs to lower the setpoint.

Yet, this talk is guarded because for current drugs to show important weight loss, the patient needs to go on a diet at the same time, and this means only temporary loss — and back to setpoint. If expensive drugs without diet can offer only a small reduction in setpoint, an average of about 5 to 8 pounds, will people want to take them on a long-term basis and possibly suffer harmful side effects?

Open the dialogue

As a responsible and caring society, we need a wider understanding of the setpoint and the starvation syndrome so we can begin to find solutions that make a real difference.

Why do women sacrifice their intellect and energy and humanity for the sake of thinness? Why are we so desperate for any gimmick or drug or diet that will help us lose weight that we risk our health?

Why have we allowed our national health leaders to ignore the effects of the setpoint and starvation syndrome as they press one weight loss program after another on us, squander our tax money on hundreds of virtually identical studies which measure only short-term weight loss, when the harmful effects have been known for over 50 years?

The alarming information on the starvation syndrome needs to be investigated. Unless we can fully understand its effects, how can weight reduction programs succeed in a way that ensures health and well-being?

Scientists who worked on the Minnesota study ventured the astounding opinion that many of the so-called American characteristics — abounding energy, generosity, friendliness and optimism — may be understood as the expected behavior of a well-fed people. These are not characteristic traits of people who live within the starvation syndrome.[22]

In anguish, Turnbull asks: Is love a luxury permitted only to the well fed?

While the effects are not as severe for most dieting women, they risk some of the same changes.

We can do better than this. Women can live their lives, if they will, as strong, capable, loving, generous individuals who live up to their rich potential.

CHAPTER 8

The risks of losing weight

■

"Until we have better data about the risks of being overweight and the benefits and risks of trying to lose weight, we should remember that the cure for obesity may be worse than the condition."

— *Marcia Angell, MD*
and Jerome Kassirer, MD

Is the cure for obesity worse than the condition? Yes, in many cases, it is.

In 16 years of reporting worldwide weight and eating research, I've watched a stream of miracle cures come and go. At best, these would-be miracles only weight cycle people. The best statistics any program can show is weight loss up to six months, then a steady regain back to setpoint weight.

Most popular plans make about a four-year swing: two years ascending (driven by heavy advertising), two years at peak frenzy, then a sudden decline, after which absolutely no one wants to have anything to do with that disaster again.

The fallout is tragic. I get heartbreaking calls from victims and their families. A man from California whose 38-year-old wife died in her sleep from drinking herbal weight loss tea. The distressed husband of a woman whose stomach stapling surgery went awry. "It breaks my heart," he said. "That surgeon should not be allowed to practice, but he keeps right on."

Even the wedding is a dangerous event, as each member of the bridal party tries to fit into the smallest dress possible for the wedding pictures. I know of two brides who died on the eve of their weddings. One was losing weight at a commercial diet center, the other on fen-phen pills.

I've been told by physicians of two patients who died on the very low calorie liquid diet not far from my home. One was a young woman in her early 20s, an only child, who died suddenly. When her mother was called with the terrible news, she turned to her husband and said, "Mary's dead." In that moment, the father clutched his heart and died. Their family doctor told me sadly, "It was the only time I've known this to happen in my practice, when a person gets a fatal heart attack from bad news. And now the mother is left alone."

I was there when John Garren introduced his Garren-Edwards stomach balloon to an enthusiastic crowd of admiring physicians — and a few years later at a Harvard meeting as he stood alone by his posters, forlorn and rejected, his hastily-granted FDA approval withdrawn.

But by then enthusiasm had moved on to the very low calorie diets, known as VLCDs — 300 to 800 calories — with their "amazing, miracle" results. Large patients lost one-third of their size in months — and gained it back just as fast, with sometimes terrible side effects, like sudden death. I knew Peter Lindner, MD, famed diet doctor of the 1980s, who co-authored with George Blackburn, MD, of Harvard, one of the early VLCD studies that "proved" success. Their study was referenced, quoted and followed up by hundreds, probably thousands, of nearly identical studies attesting to the success of VLCDs, most no longer than 3 to 6 months. Lindner's friend told me he later made a five-year check of former patients, and not one of them — not one — kept off for five years any of the weight they lost so successfully.

Then came Slim Fast and its imitators filling grocery aisles for a couple of years. There were surgeries, intestinal bypass, stomach stapling, liposuction, jaw wiring. And thigh cream. Fen-phen and Redux became wildly popular, and about 6 million people reportedly took these diet pills, before they were abruptly withdrawn. New prescription drugs were soon approved, and others are in the pipeline, awaiting approval. And these are just the legal, medically-sanctioned cures. People have been subjected to a steady stream of quackery as well. In the journal we've reported on over 200 fraudulent or questionable products, almost guaranteed to weight cycle their victims.

Everything works short-term

The irony is that everything works short-term, and nothing works long-term. And this plays into the hands of promoters. They can boast their short-term success, and shift blame back to the dieter for her inevitable regain. How wonderful that *their* method worked so well and you lost weight so easily — too bad *you* failed to keep it off. And if, unfortunately, a large patient dies, it conveniently can be blamed on obesity, pre-existing factors, or a supposed "unhealthy lifestyle."

If even one method worked, we'd have no need for the others. Yet we spend $30 to $50 billion annually on these services, not including smoking for weight control, that unacknowledged but highly lucrative windfall for the tobacco industry.

Yes, a National Weight Control Registry has been pulled together over recent years that documents weight loss success for 629 women and 155 men, most of whom maintained a 30-pound loss for five years. It is great these people have succeeded. But looking at it in another way, that's a pitifully small number out of the millions who make the attempt, considering that the call went out nation-wide in the health community and the media for names. Half these people came in on their own, and the other half were referred as their very best examples over many years by hundreds of obesity specialists and weight loss centers.[1]

In truth, we have no safe and effective methods of losing weight. Yet more people are trying to lose weight than ever before. About half of American women and girls and one fourth of men and boys are trying to lose weight at any one time.

Weight loss boosts death rates

Worse than being ineffective, most large, long-term studies show that losing weight is a risk factor for earlier death.

The NIH conference on Methods for Voluntary Weight Loss and Control first compiled this evidence in 1992. It showed that weight loss is associated with increased risk of death, rather than the other way around, as had been assumed.[2]

During 18 years of follow-up in the Framingham Heart Study, both men and women who lost weight through 10 years had the highest death rates. For younger men, death rates were lowest in the weight stable group, and for older men lowest in the group that gained weight. In younger women, mortality rates were lowest in the group that gained weight, except for the first six years, when mortality rates were similar at all weights. In older women, mortality rates were lowest in the weight stable and weight gain groups.

Similar findings were reported from a number of long-term comprehensive studies including MRFIT, the Harvard Alumni Study, CARDIA (Coronary Artery Risk Development in Young Adults), a follow-up of the NHANES I study, and a 10-study review by Reubin Andres, MD, clinical director of the National Institute on Aging. All showed higher mortality with weight loss. Most controlled for age, smoking, race, early deaths (such as from a pre-existing disease), and other possible confounding factors. Andres concluded, "For the general population, the results of the 10 studies do not support the idea that losing weight will increase longevity ... (but) the opposite."

The question is why? Why, if short-term studies show benefits with weight loss, do long-term studies show higher death rates?

Some have thought it was bone loss, and the increased risk of fragile bones that comes with weight loss.[3]

But it may be more than this. A new study analyzing data separately from two large longitudinal studies shows the problem may be that people lose too much lean body mass (including muscle, bone and organ) when they lose weight. Results were remarkably similar in both samples: weight loss was associated with higher death rates, but fat loss with lower death rates.

In the Framingham Heart Study, weight loss of 1 standard deviation resulted in a 39 percent *increase* in mortality risk, and fat loss of 1 standard deviation resulted in a 17 percent *decrease* in mortality risk. In the Tecumseh Community Health Study, comparable figures were a 29 percent increase in risk with weight loss, and 15 percent decrease with fat loss. Results showed that on average the harmful effects of losing weight outweighed the benefits. While loss of fat appears to be healthy, loss of muscle, organ and bone is not.[4]

When the researchers used different analyses, and controlled for smoking, age, gender, initial weight and fat, they basically arrived at the same outcome and confirmed these results.

David Allison, PhD, of the Obesity Research Center in New York the lead author says, "Past research has shown people who lose weight don't live as long, on the average. This suggests they may be losing an undesirable ratio of fat to lean."

The body powerfully defends its fat, says David Garner, PhD, director of the Toledo Center for Eating Disorders, citing studies that show a defense of fat at the expense of lean muscle and vital organs. Autopsies of emaciated patients show a shrinkage of vital organs, including heart, liver, kidneys and spleen, equal to the percent of weight loss.[5]

Weight cycling may compound the problem. After weight loss, regain of fat appears to outstrip regain of lean body mass.[6]

These facts prompt disturbing questions. Are people compromising their health by trying to lose weight? Even short-term, are the methods they are sold safe and effective? If not, why are they not being told this? Why is the cult of thinness being promoted so vigorously in the health community?

For the first time, in January 1998, a major scientific journal questioned weight loss treatment in a realistic way. Marcia Angell, MD, and Jerome Kassirer, MD, editors of the *New England Journal of Medicine*, wrote in their famous New Years Day editorial that the $30 to 50 billion dollars being spent on weight loss is wasted. Their editorial said bluntly that weight loss is not effective, it involves serious health risks, and it is untrue that the risks of obesity are so high this kind of treatment is justified. They concluded, "Until we have better data about the risks of being overweight and the benefits and risks of trying to lose weight, we should remember that the cure for obesity may be worse than the condition."[7]

Today's dieting craze has changed eating habits for millions of people. While the term dysfunctional eating may be new, disturbed behaviors on the eating continuum are familiar to most of us — from simply counting calories to the extremes of anorexia and bulimia.

There is a whole other world of treatments and gimmicks that claim to help people lose weight. Some are a waste of money. Others are deadly. The most notable of these seen during my years at *Healthy Weight Journal*, are outlined here.

Drugs for weight loss

We can list many drugs that claim to help people lose weight. They include prescription drugs, over-the-counter diet pills, fraudulent pills, laxatives, diuretics, herbal weight loss tea, gum, appetite sprays and, of course, nicotine. These don't claim to be drugs, merely food supplements that reduce your appetite, increase your metabolism, block digestion, or "flush out fat." Most of these are illegal claims.[8]

Prescription pills

Weight loss is modest for prescription diet drugs: an average of less than 5.5 pounds greater than placebo at the end of one year for fenfluramine,[9] 7 to 11 pounds for sibutramine (Meridia, by Knoll Pharmaceutical),[10] and 8 pounds for orlistat (Xenical, by Hoffman-La Roche)[11] Most studies show maximum weight loss at about 20 weeks, and weight regain when the drug is discontinued. This is about the same effect as smoking.

Sibutramine/Meridia. Sibutramine, sold under the brand name Meridia, was approved by the Food and Drug Administration (FDA) in November 1997. Meridia works on brain chemicals to suppress appetite.

But it tends to raise blood pressure, speed up heart rate, and is advised only for seriously obese patients — but not if they suffer from poorly controlled hypertension, heart disease, or irregular heartbeat, or if they have survived a stroke, according to the FDA.

During one-year tests, Meridia helped patients shed 7 to 11 pounds more than control groups but that weight was regained when the pills were stopped.[12] Only one-year studies of safety and effectiveness of this drug are available, which means it's not wise to take sibutramine for more than one year. Yet paradoxically, this drug, like all others, must be taken long-term to keep off lost weight. But this is not assured, either. In the past, when companies have provided only one-year data, it frequently meant weight was being regained by the year's end.

Orlistat/Xenical. Orlistat, sold as Xenical, acts on the intestine instead of the brain, blocking up to 30 percent of the fat absorbed into the intestines. Orlistat has been criticized for the side effect of causing soft stools and oily leakages as it sends undigested fat out of the body. Promoters say this helps train the user to eat less fat.[13] Others point out similarities between this purging effect and eating disorder behaviors.

Fen-phen/Redux. About 6 million people took the diet pills fenfluramine and dexfenfluramine alone and in combination with phentermine (fen-phen/ Redux), which were withdrawn from the market in September 1997. The FDA says up to one-third may have developed leaky heart valves, and reported a study confirmed by five investigators at five medical centers showing that 25 to 30 percent of patients taking the drugs who were evaluated had abnormal echocardiograms even though they had no symptoms.[14]

At the time the pills were banned, FDA had reports of more than 100 patients who had heart valve disease, and three deaths from it. In addition, FDA reported 16 cases of the disease with fenfluramine alone, dexfenfluramine alone, or dexfenfluramine in combination with phentermine. There were also 55 confirmed reports of primary pulmonary hypertension related to fen-phen, nine of them fatal. Primary pulmonary hypertension, a rare disease that is fatal within four years for nearly half its victims, had long been linked to the fenfluramine drugs.

Who died? Most were young healthy women. FDA says the injuries and deaths are almost exclusively of women. With about 6 million treated, the number of young American women injured by the fen-phen/Redux tragedy staggers the imagination. Some used the pills less than a month.

For instance, FDA reported the death of a 29-year-old Boston woman who took fen-phen for only 23 days and died of pulmonary hypertension eight months later. A healthy nonsmoker with no family history of the disease, she weighed 193 pounds at 5-foot-5 and had a body mass index of 32. She stopped taking the drug when she experienced increased heart rate and shortness of breath with moderate exercise. She was hospitalized five months later for fever, shortness of breath and chest pain. Released from the hospital, readmitted and again released, she died two days later in sudden cardiac arrest.[15]

Of the first 28 heart valve cases, all were women, median age 45, who had taken the diet drugs for an average of 10 months. Six underwent valve-replacement surgery; one died. The condition did not resolve in any of the patients after stopping the drug; in two there was progression from a new heart murmur to valve replacement surgery within a year and a half.[16]

Patients' heart valves were coated with a glistening, white, waxy substance that kept them from closing fully. Blood leaked back into their hearts, forcing them to pump harder. Symptoms were fatigue, shortness of breath, and lower extremity swelling.

In addition to potential heart and lung damage, evidence suggested these pills may cause brain damage. This was documented in more than 80 animal studies, including research with monkeys.[17] Brain disturbances from the pills in humans have shown up in sleep problems, depression and psychotic reactions.

As fenfluramine and Redux were pulled off the market, some doctors turned to phen-pro, a phentermine and Prozac combination. Prozac acts on brain serotonin, is approved for treating depression and bulimia, and reduces appetite in 9 percent of users, while phentermine has often been used to jump start a diet. Like fen-phen, this combination is "off label," unapproved by the FDA and prescribed at the physician's discretion. Experts say the combination could be risky.[18]

Nonprescription diet pills

You don't need a prescription for diet pills sitting on drugstore and grocery shelves. Pills containing PPA (phenylpropanolamine) are readily available under such names as Dexatrim, Accutrim, Control, Dex-A-Diet, Diadex, Prolamine, Propagest, Rhinecon and Unitrol. Many teenage girls confess they shoplift these pills and swallow them by the boxfull.

PPA and benzocaine (seldom used, but said to numb the tongue) are the only two weight loss drugs approved for nonprescription sales. With the efficacy and safety of both under question, they are now "on review" by FDA — a move that effectively sidetracks action and keeps the popular PPA on the shelves. More than $40 million dollars are spent annually by drug companies to advertise PPA diet products. Sales go virtually unregulated.

Abuse is widespread. In the 1990 congressional hearings on the weight loss industry, there were numerous pleas to take PPA diet pills off the shelves and restrict sales.

A bereaved father testified against their easy availability. "The lights went out in our lives on July 12, 1989, when our beautiful, fun-loving, and soon-to-be-married daughter, Noelle, died of cardiac arrest. These stores have no more business selling these drugs to children than they do liquor to a minor."[19]

A Michigan State University study of 1,368 female and 1,062 male college students found that nearly half the women and 6 percent of the men had taken a PPA diet drug — 27 percent of the women within the past 12 months, and 3 percent in the past 24 hours. Although most women didn't start using them until age 16, one fifth did begin much earlier, as young as 12. Even 9 percent of those who perceived themselves as slightly underweight had used PPA diet pills in the last 12 months. None had ever consulted a physician about their use, even though labels advise this for users under age 18. Many took more than the recommended daily limit of 75 mg of PPA. About one-fourth of the women using diet pills had also double-dosed with other PPA-containing medicines at the same time. One woman with a severe cold had taken a total of 675 mg. within 24 hours of the interview — a diet pill and four nonprescription decongestant products containing PPA.[20]

Nearly 7 percent of adolescent girls in the U.S. are currently using diet pills, and many more have used them, according to the Youth Risk Behavior survey.[21] In a study of 1,269 Cleveland high school students, 23 percent of the white girls and 16 percent of African American girls had used diet pills. They were also used by 6 percent of white boys.[22]

PPA leads all other major nonprescription drugs in the number of adverse drug reactions and in number of contacts with Poison Control Centers. Nearly 47,000 in 1989, the subcommittee was told. These included documented cases of fatal strokes, dangerously high blood pressure, heart rhythm abnormalities, heart and kidney damage, hallucinations, seizures, psychosis, headaches, nervousness and insomnia from PPA use. Other risks noted are cerebral hemorrhage, increased intercerebral pressure, nausea, vomiting, anxiety, palpitations, reversible renal failure, disorientation, and death. Further, expert witnesses said, PPA is regarded by most users as ineffective and no data contradicts this.[23]

Fraudulent weight loss pills

Quackery flourishes in the diet pill market. In the past 15 years, *Healthy Weight Journal* has reported on more than 200 questionable and fraudulent weight loss products, including herbal and "natural" pills, herbal teas, bee pollen, chromium picolinate, mushroom tea, starch blockers, and body detoxifying programs, as well as many other gadgets and gimmicks that claim weight loss success.

Weight loss quackery relies heavily on the exploitation of herbs and "natural" products that are sold as food or dietary supplements. This works because Congress allows herbal products to be sold as foods, as long as no drug claims are made. (Drug claims are claims that the product can alter body functions such as suppressing appetite, speeding up metabolism, reducing fat, or blocking out calories, fat or sugar.) These illegal claims are often made in advertising but not on the product label, which lists only ingredients to avoid FDA seizure. A red flag of likely fraud is when you find only ingredients listed on the label of a weight loss product, with no directions given on how or when to use it. By contrast, check an aspirin bottle for appropriate information.

Ephedrine, often sold as Ma huang, a Chinese herb, or ephedra, has proven to be one of the most deadly of quack pills.[24] The FDA warned consumers not to use Nature's Nutrition Formula One products that contain both Ma huang and kola nut, cautioning that overdosing with ephedrine can cause heart palpations and death. Yet overdosing is common with diet pills. In the past two years, FDA reported over 800 adverse reactions to ephedrine-containing products, including at least 17 deaths. Reactions included life-threatening conditions including irregular heartbeat, heart attack, angina, stroke, seizures, hepatitis and psychosis. Temporary conditions such as dizziness, headache, memory loss, and gastrointestinal distress were also reported.[25]

Bee pollen, too, has caused fatal allergic reactions. FDA warns that bee pollen holds hazards for anyone with allergies, asthma or hay fever — although promoters claim it is "naturally safe" and "safe for any dieter."[26]

False claims for chromium picolinate, the main ingredient in many weight loss products and muscle-building pills, have often been exposed. But it seems to bounce back with more outrageous claims that it burns fat, causes weight loss, increases muscle mass, and provides health benefits. All these claims are false and misleading and must cease, the FTC finally ruled in 1997, after a long and profitable run for marketers of chromium picolinate.

In 1985 FDA documented more than 100 cases of adverse reactions to Herbalife weight loss products, including nausea, headaches, diarrhea, constipation and vomiting and investigated several fatalities. The company says ingredients like mandrake and pokeroot, which posed a potential danger in some Herbalife products, are no longer being used.

The weight loss product Quickly was found to contain the prescription drug furosemide in amounts that could be dangerous. Excessive doses can lead to profound depletion of water and electrolytes, blood volume reduction, dangerously low blood pressure, heart complications, nausea, diarrhea, vomiting, hearing loss, dizziness, headache and rash, said FDA.[27]

Drinking herbal weight loss tea can be fatal, too. Of particular concern were reports to FDA of at least four recent deaths of women who drank Laci Le Beau Super Dieter's Tea. All died suddenly, and three of the four had cardiac effects. They had used the tea several times a week.

Similar teas under FDA scrutiny are Trim-Maxx, 24-Hour Diet Tea, and Ultra Slim Tea. Adverse effects from these teas ranged from diarrhea, cramps, fainting and permanent loss of bowel function, to death due to chronic diarrhea and electrolyte loss, warns FDA. Many teas for weight loss contain large doses of stimulant laxatives such as senna, cascara, castor oil, buckthorn, aloe and rhubarb root. Since the teas are not regulated, they contain unknown amounts of laxatives. Potency varies widely with growing season, amount used, and steeping time.

Scam artists imply that because herbs are natural they are safe. This is untrue. Many plants are poisonous and contain potent drugs. Furthermore, herbs vary greatly in strength, since there is no regulation or standard dosages. Unfortunately, federal agencies take action against herbals only on a case-by-case basis, and usually only after injury complaints.

When heavily advertised, fraudulent products can pull in enormous profits. Slim America netted $9.5 million with its Super-Formula in one year, between the time full-page advertisements ran in major newspapers across the country and the Federal Trade Commission froze company assets. By then most of the money had disappeared, an FTC spokesman said.[28]

Weight loss fraud works because people want to believe in weight loss miracles. Con artists exploit this with a mixture of mysticism, pseudoscience and sensationalism. Selling on the internet makes weight loss marketing easier, more targeted and cheaper than ever before.[29]

Amphetamines

Amphetamines are no longer recommended because they can be addictive, but they are still being prescribed for weight loss by some doctors. In their youth, many large people took amphetamines prescribed by their doctors and struggled with addictions.

Gloria, now 43, tells of taking her first amphetamines at age 12. In the book *Real Women Don't Diet*, she explains, "They weren't called 'yellow jackets' or 'uppers' back then. They were just some little yellow pills given to a healthy 12-year-old to lose weight ... Withdrawing from years of diet pills, which meant having vivid hallucinations and periods of extreme paranoia and finally becoming bulimic, were the most dangerous, physically damaging aspects of my war with my body, but the psychological damage and pain have been far more lasting."[30]

Laxatives and diuretics

Taking laxatives or diuretics is a dangerous and ineffective way to lose weight, yet they are used by many young women today. In the Cleveland high school study 18 percent of African American girls used laxatives and 11 percent used diuretics in attempts to lose weight, more than other girls. About half took them at least every month.[31] Laxatives cause weight loss through dehydration due to a large volume of watery diarrhea. Calorie absorption is not really affected, but nutrients may be poorly absorbed.

Laxative abuse can cause both acute and chronic lower gastrointestinal complications, including abdominal cramping, bloating, pain, nausea, constipation and diarrhea.[32] It may also cause malabsorption of fat, protein and calcium, and loss of electrolytes, including potassium, essential for heart function.[33] Chronic abuse can cause nerve damage resulting in sluggish bowel that can become so severe a colectomy is required. The body develops a tolerance to laxatives over time, so abusers sometimes increase to 60 or more tablets daily.[34]

Diuretics or "water pills" are used less, but their abuse is even more dangerous. The big concern is rapid and dramatic potassium loss causing heart arrhythmia and kidney damage. Using several purging techniques together intensifies the overall effects.

Smoking for weight loss

Whether we acknowledge it or not, the fact is that nicotine is the most popular diet drug in use today. Its effects are similar to prescription diet pills in that smoking keeps off an average of about 7 to 10 pounds, which is regained upon stopping smoking. Women and teen girls are well aware of this effect, and many depend on it. (The health risks of smoking probably would not show up if we looked at only one-year studies, as is being done with diet pills.)[35]

Smoking rates are up for young women. And they begin early. For the first time ever in the 1995 Youth Risk Behavior Survey, white high school girls are smoking more than boys in their desperate attempts to control weight. Forty percent of white girls smoke occasionally (defined as at least one cigarette a month), compared with 37 percent of white boys, 35 percent of Hispanic boys. Twenty-one percent smoke frequently (at least 20 cigarettes a month), compared with 18 percent of white boys, 11 percent of Hispanic boys, 9 percent of Hispanic girls, 8 percent of African American boys, and 1 percent of African American girls.[36]

Tobacco has its own powerful industry promoting smoking for weight control. Smoking ads in magazines targeted to women do this in a subliminal way, with thin models and "slim" copy — making it clear that tobacco companies are in the weight loss business. There are Virginia Slims, Capri Superslims, and even "slim price," which seems ridiculous, and always the supremely thin models. The industry does not admit this, of course, and seems happy with the current health policy that pretends smoking has nothing to do with weight, just as long as teenage girls know the truth.[37]

A valuable area for investigation might be searching those 39,000 secret tobacco documents, that the tobacco industry turned over to the Minnesota Supreme Court, for mentions of weight loss, how to influence women's smoking through advertising, and the encouragement of thin female ideals in the health community and media.

The jump in women smoking and a 500 percent rise in lung cancer for women smokers began during his tenure in the late 1970s, confesses Joseph Califano, Jr., former secretary of Health, Education and Welfare. The thinness obsession is a great boon to tobacco companies and they play shrewdly on the fear of weight gain, he says. Califano now wishes he had done something about the fear of weight gain early in the fight against smoking.[38] Tobacco is responsible for more than one of every six deaths in the U.S. While there is a decline in smoking, the decline has been slower among women than men. Fewer women dare to quit smoking, it seems.[39]

If you smoke, you may know that smoking eventually drags down the face with deep vertical wrinkles, muddies the complexion, and makes people look older than they are. As for improving those wrinkles, plastic surgeons say it's difficult to work with a smoker's unresponsive skin.

Quitting smoking can bring on a miraculous reversal. You may regain those 7 to 10 pounds, but would that be the worst possible outcome? It's doubtful anyone you know would even notice. (If you are a smoker who cannot or does not want to quit at this time, just move on and don't allow this to block other healthful changes you'd like to make.)

A Healthy People objective for the year 2000 was to reduce regular smoking by 20-year-olds to no more than 15 percent. It seems this goal was sabotaged by the same officials who tried to promote it, by their pursuit of thinness.

The irony is that it is not considered politically correct to mention that smoking affects weight, because the health community refuses to acknowledge it. So instead, its campaign to curb youth smoking persists in focusing rather foolishly on the influence of Joe Camel. Acknowledging that a desire for thinness is a major reason for female smoking is the only way to deal with the problem of more girls smoking. That it isn't being done suggests this would expose the hypocrisy of the current health policy.

Even former Surgeon General C. Everett Koop has aligned himself with the commercial weight loss industry in a well-financed anti-obesity campaign. Perhaps he is unaware of the irony: that a man long identified with the fight against smoking is now so pressuring teenage girls to be thin that they are turning to smoking as never before.

Very low calorie diets[40]

There are many kinds of diets and ways of restricting food including flexible and rigid diets, faddish food-combinations, fasting, "detoxifying" the body and vomiting to eject food before it can be digested. A diet limits calories and/or fat. It can specify certain foods or food combinations, or replace meals with liquid formulas or pre-packaged food. Low and moderately low calorie diets provide about 1,000 to 1,500 calories daily.

But most devastating to physical and mental health are the very low calorie diets (VLCDs) of 300 to 800 calories per day, usually liquid, which were extremely popular in the late 1980s and early 1990s. They carry severe health risks, even when medically monitored and administered by medical teams. They are now considered ineffective, and are disavowed even in the NHLBI Guidelines.

Yet despite poor results, these diets have often been prescribed for high-risk large patients, and still are, with the rationale that they need to lose weight quickly to reduce their risk factors. This is twisted thinking — that their risks from obesity are so high any high-risk treatment is warranted. Large patients do lose weight rapidly on these diets; unfortunately, they regain that weight just as rapidly, and many have suffered injury or death as a result.

While there is much less support for VLCDs today amid the wreckage of their heyday — when talk show host Oprah Winfrey publicly lost and regained 67 pounds on Optifast — many specialists still promote them.

These diets hold special appeal because people lose weight rapidly. Moreover, they lose their appetite for awhile, so they don't even feel hungry. It seems like a miracle that will last forever. But reality hits when they taste real food or with the first binge. After that, there's no stopping the hunger and rapid regain.

Even some of its most prominent medical promoters admitted early, "After the first time, the magic is gone. VLCD doesn't work the second time around." (Well, it didn't work the first time either, then, did it?)

In Britain, the 1987 COMA Report of the United Kingdom Department of Health recommended that VLCDs provide at least 400 calories and be limited to four weeks because of the high risk. There are no such standards in the United States, where VLCDs are usually prescribed for 12 to 16 weeks and often much longer, even over a year.

Weight losses can be huge. An Oregon man lost over 300 pounds in one year, dropping from 506 pounds to 205. A 500-pound woman in Cape Town lost 288 pounds in 18 months. Most losses range from 40 to 80 pounds.[41]

The modern VLCD is an outgrowth of the zero calorie diet of the 1950s, the Metrecal craze of the early 1960s and the liquid protein diets of the 1970s and early 1980s. Deaths associated with VLCDs have been reported for more than 30 years.

The VLCD has one of highest risks for sudden death syndrome during weight loss, warn researchers at the NIH Obesity Research Center in New York. Fatal cardiac arrhythmias with these large, rapid losses may be related to loss of heart volume, they report.

The dieter's risk for gallbladder disease is greatly increased with VLCDs. University of Alabama nutrition researchers found new gallstones developed in 10 to 26 percent of persons on VLCDs, often within the first four weeks.[42]

In 1989 at the height of its popularity, the Michigan Health Council Task Force, which had documented seven deaths in Michigan, warned of potential risks from VLCDs.[43] The task force identified the following risks: cardiac arrhythmias that can occur suddenly without warning and are potentially fatal; loss of muscle and organ tissue; potentially fatal dehydration; ketosis, hypoglycemia with related headaches, fatigue, inability to concentrate, sleepiness and cardiac arrhythmias; low levels of potassium in the blood, which may lead to cardiac arrhythmias; gallstones; excess uric acid levels related to gouty arthritis or uric acid kidney stones; an abnormal increase in fibrous connective tissue in the organs; anemia, characterized by fatigue, lassitude, weakness, pallor, reduced resistance to infection, lowered exercise tolerance and decreased attention span; re-feeding edema; and other documented side effects such as constipation or diarrhea, headaches, nausea, dry skin, hair loss, muscle cramps, bad breath, fatigue, cold intolerance, menstrual irregularities, and transient skin rash.

In addition, the task force warned of emotional changes, of withdrawal, depression, anxiety, irritability, and the discouragement and diminished self-esteem likely to follow the probable weight regain.

In the early 1990s, the Federal Trade Commission investigated and charged the makers of these six VLCD programs with false and misleading advertising about their safety and effectiveness: Optifast (Sandoz), Ultrafast (National Center for Nutrition), Medifast (Jason Pharmaceuticals), HMR Fasting Program (Health Management Resources), UWCC Permanence Program (United Weight Control Corporation), and New Directions (Abbott).[44]

Dieting groups

Commercial diet centers and dieting groups can offer much social support and acceptance for regular participants, especially if they are actively losing weight. People may learn healthy lifestyle habits that are long lasting. However, in general, clients are merely weight-cycled, and dropout rates are high.

Laura Fraser, author of *Losing It,*[45] notes that commercial diet groups, now in a slump, need to keep adding gimmicky ways to compete. Aggressive marketing has always driven the weight loss market, she notes. "It's the fresher approaches — the gurus who market diets in the guise of not dieting, the doctors who sell gimmicky high-protein diet books or promote prescription diet pills — that are attracting attention. Those who devise commercial diet programs are learning that they have to adapt to the current consumer climate, in which monitoring grams of fat and minutes on the exercise machines have replaced counting calories, and come up with aggressive new marketing strategies to survive."

Dieting meetings have been compared to religious rituals by Natalie Allon, a pioneer in the social analysis of obesity and dieting. She sees the meeting as a religious ritual:

1. Entry from the profane outside world into the sacred dieting group.
2. The weekly paying of dues, or alms, as redemption for eating sins.
3. The weighing — an anxious procession to the scale, with the scale passing judgment on salvation and cleansing of cheating sins.
4. The procession back into the outside world of temptation

Group members represent four types of religious fervor, in Allon's view. They are: saints-in-the-making, women (usually) who accept the moral code of worshiping thinness and seeking deliverance from the fatness evil and are losing weight; theoretical saints-practical sinners, who accept the morality but don't lose weight; theoretical sinners-practical saints, who reject the moral code but are losing weight; and proud sinners-devil's advocates (or Doubting Thomases) who reject the ideology and do not lose weight.[46]

Fad diets and quackery

Unbalanced fad diets rely on gimmicks and food combinations such as the Zone diet, Sugar Busters, Protein Power, Scarsdale Medical Diet, Beverly Hills Diet, the Cabbage Diet, Fit for Life, Dr. Atkins' New Diet Revolution, and Dr. Cooper's Fabulous Fructose Diet. Coming up with a new gimmick is a way of recycling old diets with a new twist — and of course, a catchy new name. The gimmick might be to combine foods in a specific way, to ban foods claimed to have fat-producing effects, or to evoke a mystical state in which mind and body work at peak efficiency and weight disappears, as in the Zone. Fad diets often omit many important foods, creating nutrient deficiencies. Luckily, most people don't stay on these diets long enough to matter.

Detoxification. Detoxifying the body is part of an elaborate hoax spun by unscrupulous purveyors of alternative medicine and supplement dealers. It's a way to manipulate gullible consumers into buying often-expensive treatments and supplements for weight loss and a wide range of ills. The idea is that modern life so fills us with poisons from polluted air and food additives that our bodies (especially intestines, colon and blood stream) become lodged with undigested foods and need periodic cleaning. It's an irrational, unscientific concept that is gaining much ground today.

Detoxification involves fasting for several days, once or several times a year, while drinking only water with lemon juice or teas and taking various combinations of pills. It's a great way to jump start a diet, promoters believe.

For example, in the Inches Away Diet Center plan, the customer first detoxifies by eating no solid food for three days, drinks only water with lemon juice and honey, and takes three kinds of herbal capsules several times a day. This supposedly cleanses the digestive tract of accumulated waste and putrefied bacteria, cleans out the major organs and blood, and gives mental clarity because it stops the bombardment of the mind by chemicals and food additives. (Not true, of course.) After three days of detoxing, the client shifts to a combo of four diet pills to a maximum of 30 pills a day, and visits the diet center for daily simulated action on 10 passive exercise tables and weekly body wraps. Costs are about $400 a month.

Surgery

Surgery[47] for weight reduction reduces stomach size, and some procedures shorten, alter or bypass various digestive processes. Related surgery includes liposuction, tummy tucks, jaw wiring and the stomach balloon (gastric bubble).

About 15,000 "stomach stapling" surgeries are performed in the U.S. annually. Insurance usually pays the $25,000 to $30,000 cost, according to a spokesman for the American Society for Bariatric Surgery.

Improvement in related risk factors and lifestyle often follow this surgery and its accompanying weight loss. It can be very successful. Yet this is an elective surgery that carries a relatively high risk of complications and death. Mortality rate is up to 2.5 percent in published studies, according to the 1996 *Guidance for Treatment of Adult Obesity*.[48] Another estimate gives a mortality rate of 1 percent with a morbidity rate of 10 percent for the two most popular stomach-reduction surgeries, gastric bypass and vertical banded gastroplasty, according to a DATTA panel of 38 experts convened by the American Medical Association in 1989. The panel of surgery and gastroenterology specialists could not reach a consensus on either safety or effectiveness. About half agreed the two surgeries were safe, half disagreed.

A Norwegian study of 174 vertical banded gastroplasties found 25 complications during the first 30 days, including severe wound infections. After five years, a total of 60 late complications were registered in 48 patients. Twenty-six patients were re-operated, 24 with removal of the band, 13 because of gastric retention with unacceptable vomiting. Incisional hernia occurred in 15 patients, of whom six were operated. There were a total of four deaths, one clearly unrelated, one unknown.

The Norwegian study supports size acceptance activists' charges that the first two years are a favorable "honeymoon period," and then problems commonly develop. Five-year results may be very different than after the first two years. The Norwegian researchers report that many of their patients had late complications. Fewer than half maintained their weight within 30 percent of desirable for five years. The researchers said that their five year results changed "our early optimistic view to a more realistic one." They concluded that surgery is not a final solution to obesity.[49]

A Canadian report in *Surgery 1990* discussing three deaths in 201 patients, says one patient died of pulmonary embolism 30 days after surgery; another died of myocardial infarction 18 months after surgery, after losing 36 percent of initial weight; and the third, a 51-year-old woman, died of suicide 30 months after surgery.[50]

In reporting late mortality from two studies with a total of 490 patients, R. Armour Forse, MD, PhD, assistant professor of surgery at Harvard Medical School says the first study had four late deaths and the other three late deaths, with no deaths during the operation. Of these seven deaths, three were suicides; the others due to "obesity related" problems.[51]

The high suicide rate with gastric surgery has not been explained, but may be related to complications cited by size activists. Because of the severe adverse effects many of their members have suffered, both the Council on Size and Weight Discrimination and the National Association to Advance Fat Acceptance (NAAFA) call for an end to weight-reduction surgery. William Fabrey, founder of NAAFA, says, "Perhaps 10 percent of our members have had weight loss surgery at one time or another, have gained the weight back and suffered health problems as a result of the surgery. Unfortunately, two people I knew personally died after having this surgery."

A common complaint of patients who suffer complications is that they were not informed before hand what can happen: months of hospitalization, foul odors, adverse food reactions, nausea, infection and abesses, pain from the staples, skin eruptions and exema, profound body changes, depression, nutritient deficiencies, severe diarrhea and the need to stay close to a bathroom. Later, they are told by numerous physicians that their sometimes-permanently debilitating effects are common. Had they known of these potential complications beforehand, they would have been less likely to go ahead with surgery.

Surgery deaths are reported in inconsistent ways. Some surgeons report only immediate deaths. Others believe late deaths, including suicides, are very relevant to this type of surgery. This information is often lacking in reports. A National Institutes of Health Consensus Conference on Gastrointestinal Surgery for Severe Obesity held in 1991 called for better statistical reporting of surgical results, particularly long-term effects and survival. The conference report said lack of adequate studies make evaluation difficult: "The euphoria seen commonly in patients in the early postoperative period may be supplanted later by significant depression."[52]

When surgery is done at major surgery centers, mortality rates are relatively low, reports Forse.

Paul Ernsberger, PhD, assistant professor of medicine at Case Western Reserve University School of Medicine in Cleveland, charges that there is a lack of sufficient prior animal testing for this type of surgery. Another risk is that a surgeon may use less approved procedures or experiment with his own variations. For example, some use the biliopancreatic diversion operation, long discouraged in the U.S. because of higher complication risk, because its malabsorption of food results in greater weight loss. Ernsberger says the earlier 1987 NIH conference on weight-reduction surgery approved the intestinal bypass surgery at a time when that operation was already under fire for its numerous adverse effects and just before it was disavowed. Because of NIH endorsement, the operation was accepted for health insurance coverage. Its legacy, "is perhaps a hundred thousand patients worldwide, the majority of whom have suffered severe complications."[53]

Nutrient deficiencies are common after all types of weight reducing surgery. Iron deficiency anemia is a frequent long-term complication.

Other weight loss methods

Numerous other weight loss methods in use today include dehydration, withholding needed medications which may promote or appear to promote weight gain, and an array of fraudulent gadgets and creams being heavily advertised for losing weight.

Liposuction

Liposuction is the most popular of all cosmetic surgeries, with about 177,000 being performed a year in the U.S. Most procedures are done in private offices and not subject to hospital regulations, so there can be serious risks if the doctor is not well trained or pushes the margins of safety. Publicity on three liposuction deaths of women in California is being called just the tip of the iceberg. And one expert says for every death there are "at least 15 to 20 cases of severe injury.[54]

Dehydration

Dehydration is a dangerous way to lose weight. Three college wrestlers died in supervised athletic workouts during six weeks in the fall of 1997 as they tried to "make weight." All three were restricting food and fluids and promoting dehydration through perspiration by wearing vapor-impermeable suits under cotton warm-up suits and exercising vigorously in hot gyms, which resulted in hyperthermia and death.[55]

Vomiting

Many young women resort to vomiting to avoid digesting the food they eat. Anecdotal reports suggest this is so common in some college sororities and dorms today that it is no longer kept secret, and young women teach each other techniques. The Cleveland study found one in six white high school girls were vomiting to lose weight, half of them monthly or more.[56]

Repeated vomiting can cause upper gastrointestinal tract irritation, sore throat, difficulty in swallowing, indigestion, heartburn-like pain, and dehydration.[57] "Chipmunk" cheeks may develop, likely from repeated gland stimulation by the acid contents of the stomach. Forceful vomiting may also cause small tears in the mucosa of the gastrointestinal tract and break small blood vessels in the eyes. The esophagus can rupture after ingestion of a large meal and subsequent forceful vomiting. This is a medical emergency with very severe upper abdominal pain, worsened by swallowing and breathing. It has a high death rate if left untreated. Surgery is usually needed. Prolonged vomiting may cause loss of potassium, an electrolyte essential for muscle and heart functioning. Low levels can trigger cardiac arrhythmias.[58] Ipecac syrup, to induce vomiting, is extremely dangerous.[59]

Those who vomit three times a week or more will eventually cause erosion of their tooth enamel from acid vomitus. This erosion can take as little as six months. Teeth become sensitive to heat and cold, develop spaces between, lose fillings, and eventually deteriorate down to painful cores. The pulp may be exposed, teeth become thinner and sharper, and edges break off and wear away, reducing the tooth to half or one third its original height.[60]

Quack devices, gadgets and promotions

In the quackery genre are numerous gimmicks aimed to catch the attention of women desperate to lose weight. Creams, gels, toning lotions, thigh creams, and liquids touted to dissolve fat and move "cellulite" are always popular items in the quackery medicine show — so popular that many cosmetics companies have joined in the scam.

Appetite patches are to be placed like a band-aid on "accupressure" points at the wrist; accupressure earrings are clipped at similar points on the ear to suppress appetite; and rows of knobs on slimming insoles supposedly stimulate reflex zones that control digestion. There are appetite sprays, fiber cookies, body wraps, Chinese defatting soap, chewing gum, and even vacuum devices and heating gadgets that claim to disperse fat under the skin.

Other gadgets promote spot reduction and effortless exercise. Such gadgets as muscle stimulators, continuous passive motion tables, buzzing belts, and body shapers do not give exercise or weight loss benefits, says FTC. All claims that they do are false.

Traveling hypnosis seminars for weight loss are taken across the country by practitioners who book a motel room, buy glowing ads in local newspapers, gather a crowd, and charge $39.99 per customer for a two-hour pep talk. The fastest traveler in all this is Ronald Gorayeb, who claims the title of "Certified Hypnotherapist," and continues to operate despite FTC charges of false advertising and deceptive acts or practices.

There are even mystical ways to lose weight: "mind power" methods to search the subconscious for the source of hunger, to realign mental "energies" and "soul patterns," or to mobilize the mind and spirit to effect "weight release." Aromatherapy is said to help create weight loss atmosphere.

Needless to say, all these are worthless and many are potentially hazardous.

As national coordinator of the Task Force on Weight Loss Abuse for the National Council Against Health Fraud (NCAHF) I have a collection of these items that I've shown on national television talk shows. Hosts and audiences always have a good laugh at the foolishness of a "buzzing belt," vacuum pants, or slimming insoles, but seem to get the message about the widespread fraud that exists in the weight loss industry and how it dangerous it can be.

These are the kinds of products we spotlight in the Slim Chance Awards given each January during Healthy Weight Week to the "worst" weight loss products of the year, sponsored by *Healthy Weight Journal* and the NCAHF.[61]

CHAPTER 9

Food and activity choices intensify problems

■

One of the biggest barriers to making reasonable food choices is the confusion in the media over foods and health. Newspapers seemingly cannot resist bringing us the health scare of the day. ... Many people instantly stop eating that food, then learn the scare is of no consequence. Yet they are left a bit more shaken, more fearful.

The problem of unhealthy eating goes far beyond the dinner table. So do the problems of a sedentary lifestyle. Both these problems are interrelated with mental health and well-being.

In Canada, people are encouraged to enjoy eating well, to be active and to feel good about themselves — clearly the best way to prevent weight and eating problems.

But we in the United States don't get that message. The results are disturbing, even shocking. After many years of teaching about healthy living, I was appalled, but hardly surprised, by recent nation-wide reports that many American women and girls are severely undernourished. And I was alarmed that authors of these reports, federal policy makers, expressed no concern about female deficiencies.

What is the problem? Why are so many women undernourished, even starving in the midst of plenty?

Restricting food

The answers to these questions, I believe, are in a culture that encourages women to restrict their eating in unhealthy ways, to reshape their bodies to be thinner than is natural for them.

A recent national study showed the median calorie intake for women in the United States is reported at about 1,600 calories. This is considerably below the Recommended Dietary Allowance (RDA) of 2,200 calories for women in their childbearing years, as set by the Food and Nutrition Board, National Research Council.[1]

Why this low intake? The desire for thinness is a major factor in a woman's decision to withhold nourishment from herself. In addition, many women are extremely sedentary and may not feel hungry. Or they are too busy with sit-down work to take time either to eat or exercise. Poverty may be a factor for some women.

If sedentary women would increase activity, they would be more likely to feel hungry at appropriate times. In sync with body rhythms, their appetite mechanisms would work better; they'd feel hunger and fullness more readily, eat more and be better nourished. And their weight would stabilize at a natural point since what they eat would be balanced by activity.

When women have such low calorie intake as many do today it is difficult to get all the nutrients they need. When they are also inactive, their body regulators may not work as well.

If these women then snack and binge on cookies, candy, crackers and sweetened soft drinks, as many do today, they waste an important part of their limited calorie intake on high-calorie, non-nutritive foods. For example, it is estimated that in the 1970s Americans were eating over 40 percent of their calories in fat and 25 percent in sugars. This left only about 35 percent of calories for important, more nutritious foods in the five food groups.

If this were the case today, the average woman would be eating only about 560 calories of these needed foods. This may well be, because, while percent fat has dropped to 33 percent, a USDA assessment finds a 16 percent increase in calories from added sugars and sweeteners since the early 1980s. This marks a steep rise in high fructose corn syrup, more than offsetting a decline in refined sugar. It's an average of 32 teaspoons of added sugars and other sweeteners every day, for women more than two and a half times the 12 teaspoons suggested as an upper limit.[2]

It's no surprise, then, that the average woman in her child-bearing years is short on iron, calcium, magnesium and zinc, as well as the vitamins E and B_6. Except for iron deficiency, which can be related to menstrual blood losses, these shortages extend through older ages as well. The "hungry one-fourth" of women at the bottom end, are extremely deficient in these and other nutrients.

Teenage girls age 12 to 19 have the poorest diets of all Americans — the lowest in calories and nutrients — and are most at risk from nutrient deficiencies. Next come young women in the age 20 to 29 group who get 76 percent of recommended calories at the median, and only 60 percent at the 25th percentile, according to this intake data *(figure 1)*.

For young African American women, even more are at the very low end of food intake — and slightly more are at the higher end. Twenty-one percent report calorie intakes below 50 percent of RDA, compared with 13 percent of white women in this age group. At the higher end, 23 percent of young African American women are at or above the recommended level, compared with 18 percent of young white women. Very few women of either race have food intakes as high as 150 percent of RDA in these reports. (The statistics given here, except as noted, come from the US Department of Agriculture's Continuing Survey of Food Intakes by Individuals [CSFII], known as the *What We Eat in America Survey*.)[3]

It's more common that African American women have low nutrient

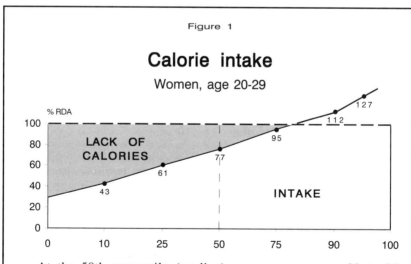

Figure 1

Calorie intake
Women, age 20-29

At the 50th percentile (median) young women age 20 to 29 consume 77 percent of the Recommended Dietary Allowance (RDA=2,200 calories). Women below this point have a much lower calorie intake than this.[1]

CONTINUING SURVEY OF FOOD INTAKES BY INDIVIDUALS 1998
WOMEN AFRAID TO EAT 2000

intake than that white women do. The percentages of young African American women who consume less than 50 percent of the RDA are: calories, 21 percent of women; calcium, 47 percent; iron, 24 percent; zinc 26 percent. Comparable figures for young white women are: calories, 13 percent of women; calcium, 24 percent; iron, 18 percent; zinc, 21 percent.

For older African American women, age 60 and over, calorie intake is lowest of any group. Over 24 percent of these older women have an intake that is below 50 percent of RDA and only 8 percent are at or above RDA. According to these intake studies, there is no evidence African American women are consuming more calories, even though they have much higher rates of obesity. There is evidence to suggest they may be eating a higher percent of their diet in fat, however.

At the other extreme from deficit calorie intake, we recognize that some women in every age and ethnic group are likely overeating and consuming excessive fat and sugars. Again, many are sedentary, and thus subject to the chronic disease risks related to inactivity and nutrition. Experts are now looking more seriously from a woman's health perspective at concerns like heart disease, breast cancer, diabetes, menopause, pregnancy, stroke and hypertension. Nutrition is one factor involved in these diseases and conditions.

The reference woman

For woman and teenage girls the recommended daily calorie intake is 2,200 calories from age 11 to 50, and 1,900 calories after age 50, assuming light-to-moderate activity. For very active women, this figure should be adjusted upward, according to the Food and Nutrition Board.[4]

This is based on needs for the reference woman, which is the young woman, age 19 to 30, at the midpoint of height and weight. (She is 5-foot-4 and weighs 133 pounds.)[5]

The CSFII *What we eat in America survey* collects food intake data for representative samples of individuals on two days (three to 10 days apart) during in-person interviews, using the dietary recall method. Evidence suggests there is considerable underreporting of food intake, especially at the upper end, and that this may stem from the tendency to give answers that seem socially desirable or an unconscious self-deception.[6] Many people also underestimate their portion sizes. It seems most appropriate to take these figures as estimates, recognizing that they may be somewhat low for some, and will vary by how individuals choose to report their food intake.

While RDAs provide a safety factor (except for calories), an intake below 75 percent is often considered to be at risk for deficiencies.

Calcium deficiency

Two of the most critical nutrients for health are iron and calcium, but according to these surveys most women and teenage girls in the U.S. consume less than two-thirds of what they need.

At the median, the 50th percentile, young women in their 20s report only 64 percent of the RDA for calcium *(see figure 2)*. This means half get less and may have major deficiencies. At the 25th percentile, young women get only 41 percent of their needs, and intake drops off painfully below this point. Calcium is extremely low for African American women; nearly half have an intake below 50 percent of RDA.

Today we are in what is being called a calcium crisis. RDAs for calcium for older adults over 50 were raised in 1997 to 1,200 mg a day, and for age 19 to 50 to 1,000 mg a day. Yet the average adult consumes only 500 to 700 mg. Women especially fall short.

Calcium is critical to maximize bone development, and is even more important for women. We build peak bone mass until about age 26. After this, bones begin to deteriorate. Women who don't drink enough milk, and especially if they are thin and often dieting, may be setting themselves up for a future of fragile bones, fractures and osteoporosis. Osteoporosis (literally, "porous bones") is painful and expensive. Women with severe cases can break their ribs sneezing, or break a hip by standing the wrong way. It can rob a woman of her independent and

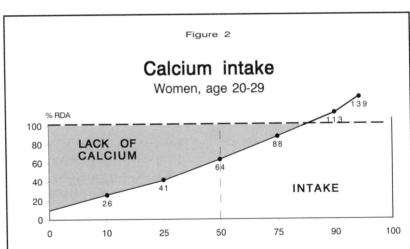

Figure 2

Calcium intake
Women, age 20-29

Women are getting much less calcium than recommended. At the 50th percentile (median) young women age 20 to 29 consume only 64 percent of the Recommended Dietary Allowance (RDA), and at the 25th percentile, 41 percent of RDA.[2]

Women Afraid to Eat 2000/CSFII 1998

active life. Normally a disease of older women, and some men, it is hitting at much at younger ages today. Experts fear an epidemic of osteoporosis when today's thin, dieting teenagers reach mid-life.[7]

Iron deficiency

That women often suffer from "iron-poor blood" should be no surprise. It takes a toll on feminine well-being. Menstrual losses, low iron intake, and lack of heme iron in the diet all contribute to the problem.

At the median, young women in the United States get only 77 percent of the RDA for iron, and at the 25th percentile, 55 percent (*figure 3*).

Some racial and ethnic data is provided in nationwide studies brought together in the Third Report on Nutrition Monitoring in the United States. While at the median American women ages 20 to 59 consume only about 72 percent of the iron they need, African American women are below this level. Mexican American women are in between, while white women get a little more.[8]

The NHANES III survey examined a large national sample and found 5 percent of women age 20 to 49 tested as having iron deficiency anemia (3.3 million women). Eleven percent were iron deficient (7.8

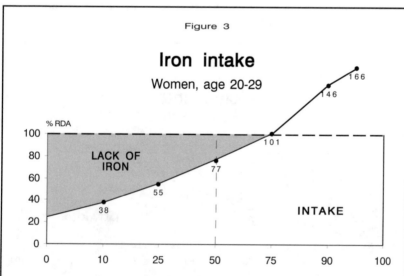

Figure 3

Iron intake
Women, age 20-29

Women fall short in their intake of iron. At the 50th percentile (median) young women age 20 to 29 consume only 77 percent of the Recommended Dietary Allowance (RDA), and at the 25th percentile, 55 percent of RDA.[3]

WOMEN AFRAID TO EAT 2000/CSFII 1998

million women and girls of childbearing age). Iron deficiency was defined as having an abnormal value for at least two out of three tests for iron status. Anemia was defined as iron deficiency plus low hemoglobin. Iron deficiency was twice as high or greater in minority women compared with white women. Other women with some degree of iron deficiency, or one abnormal value were not included in the totals.[9]

Iron is not easily absorbed by the body. If women are not getting heme iron, from animal sources, as much as 80 to 98 percent of the iron they consume may be wasted.

It is believed there may be some increased absorption when iron stores are low. Nevertheless, lack of iron is one of the most common nutrient deficiencies for women the world over. Some degree of iron deficiency appears to be a major reason why many women feel tired and get sick more often. Anemia is all too common in countries where meat is seldom available or where women eat last, and may contribute to the subjugation of women, and their treatment as second-class citizens in many parts of the world. Tests of blood hemoglobin concentrations find that on average the less meat a person eats, the lower her iron levels, even when iron intake would seem to be adequate.

Anemia or iron deficiency can cause fatigue, pallor, palpitation, impaired work performance, temperature abnormalities, and compromise the immune system. The heart may become dilated and "hemic" murmurs heard. Often the person has cold hands and feet and vague stomach complaints, such as diarrhea, gas, nausea and constipation.[10]

Zinc

Women with low iron stores usually have low zinc levels, as well. However its intake is even lower than iron. Zinc comes from the same rich animal sources. At the median, young women get 68 percent, and at the 25th percentile, 51 percent of RDA.

Low zinc is of most concern to the immune system. Research on animals finds all major branches of the immune system are compromised, even at relatively mild zinc-deficient levels. Low zinc is also related to decreased attention, difficulty in solving problems, and impaired short-term memory in tests of both animals and humans. Other risks are birth defects, retarded growth, and delayed sexual maturation.[11]

Hungry one-fourth

Calcium, iron and zinc are only three of many nutrients often deficient in the diets of the "hungry one-fourth" of women at the lower intake level. Their deficiencies can cause long-term or even permanent health problems related to growth and development, and mental prob-

Median daily intake
Percent of Recommended Dietary Allowances (RDAs)

Female

	12-15 years			16-19 years			20-59 years			≥60 years		
	NHW	NHB	MA	NHW	NHB	MA	NHW	NHB	MA	NHW	NHB	MA
Food energy	79	88	78	74	89	81	79	78	78	75	71	66
Protein	124	137	135	139	150	150	128	126	126	112	104	100
Vitamin A	63	64	59	73	60	54	75	52	66	104	63	60
Vitamin E	70	85	63	72	78	76	80	75	75	74	57	54
Vitamin C	106	180	144	102	140	127	110	97	110	143	135	102
Thiamin	108	120	107	105	118	107	112	111	112	121	106	95
Riboflavin	112	112	127	119	116	112	118	101	110	124	98	102
Niacin	97	115	100	100	112	96	118	111	103	129	109	90
Vitamin B_6	78	96	83	75	83	87	83	74	82	88	73	67
Folate	120	117	121	102	83	106	107	86	115	127	99	94
Vitamin B_{12}	169	145	170	170	154	148	156	146	150	140	116	114
Calcium	62	51	66	66	52	56	80	62	79	77	50	62
Phosphorus	87	81	94	88	87	90	130	113	134	116	96	102
Magnesium	64	70	74	62	58	66	85	66	85	83	67	65
Iron	67	65	68	63	69	68	74	66	72	103	96	84
Zinc	67	71	72	70	78	72	70	65	70	62	55	54
Copper	67	62	59	63	66	67	70	59	68	65	55	56
Sodium	108	124	106	103	129	106	110	111	106	96	83	76

NHW-nonHispanic white   NHB-nonHispanic black   MA-Mexican American

Shaded areas show median intakes that are below recommended amounts (except for sodium, which is above). Current public health issues that need attention are the low intakes of food energy (calories), calcium, iron and zinc. Considered to be potential public health issues for which further study is needed are vitamin A, vitamin C, vitamin B_6 and folate. Low intake of these nutrients for girls and women is a serious concern, especially for those below the median in each age and ethnic group. Values represent percentage of Recommended Dietary Allowances (RDAs); for food energy, values represent percentage of the Recommended Energy Intake (NRC, 1989a). *(For intake of men and boys, see appendix.)*[a]

Women Afraid to Eat 2000/NHANES III, 1988-1991

lems such as depression, confusion, hysteria and psychosis. Furthermore, this intake data does not reveal food quality, whether the protein they get is high-quality, or the iron is heme or nonheme.

Why don't these women drink milk? Many fear milk is fattening. Why don't they eat iron-rich meat and eggs? It's the same sad story. Many have a fear of fat. (Even though they could eat these foods with little or no fat).

How we've changed our eating

Dramatic changes have taken place in the past 35 years in how we eat.

Americans today have doubled their intake of foods like crackers, chips, bakery goods, pretzels and corn chips over the last few decades. We eat more desserts and candy.[12]

We have sharply increased our foods from the tip of the food pyramid: added sugars and sweeteners, soft drinks and alcohol. More fats and oils for some, though as a whole, we are eating less. These tip-of-the-pyramid items are not "bad" foods. They can fit into a healthy eating plan. But they are mostly "empty-calorie" foods, non-nutritive, with calories that add up quickly. They may be less satisfying, too, so we eat more.

What's missing? We're still not eating enough fruits and vegetables; we lack fiber. We're consuming less meat, eggs and milk. This is a significant departure from balancing the five groups in the food pyramid and eating them in variety.

Soft drinks make up about one-third of all refined sweeteners in the American diet, the single biggest source. Young adults have doubled and tripled their soft drink consumption since the 1970s. At the same time, they have cut milk by nearly half from three decades ago.[13]

Eating out more

Americans are eating out more. The percent of meals eaten away from home nearly doubled between 1995 and 1997 — an upward trend that will likely continue, experts say. We now eat one-third of our calories in meals eaten away from home (this figure includes take-out and ordered-in foods). These meals usually contain more fat and less iron, calcium and fiber than home-cooked meals, says a government survey. This would not be a problem if people ate out occasionally, as in the past, but when it happens every day or every other day, these food choices are critical in the overall diet.

And at home, more people are snacking or "grazing" — instead of eating regular meals — a practice that makes it less likely they are

following the healthy eating principles of balance, variety and moderation.[14]

Normal eating patterns have been disrupted with the increasingly
chaotic eating that is going on today, and many people have lost touch
with their normal signals of hunger and satiety. While many are reducing
their intake to a bare minimum, others are eating too much. They don't
know when they're full.

Some have even called ours a "toxic environment." That's stating
it a bit too strong, but it makes the point that many aspects of our
environment influence us to be less active and to eat more high-fat and
high-calorie foods more often.

Cutting fat too drastically

Americans have taken the anti-fat message to heart. Over the past
two decades, we have reduced fat intake to 33 percent of total calories.
For women this figure is 32 percent, and for younger women 31 percent,
bringing them close to the goal of 30 percent set by the Dietary Guidelines for Americans.[15]

Reducing fat from an estimated 40 percent in 1977-78 is a positive
change. High fat intake is a risk factor for chronic disease.

Fat can also contribute to obesity. Studies show that fat converts
easily to body fat, and it's where most of our body fat comes from. Not
so carbohydrate, for which one-fourth is used up in conversion, or
protein, of which almost none is stored as fat.

But the advice to cut fat has led to a deep fear of fat.

Some women have taken their fear of fat to the extreme, developing
fat phobias and striving for diets with "zero" fat, reducing their fat intake
dangerously low.

This is painfully apparent in working with young college women.
Cynthia DeTota, MA, RD, University Nutritionist at Syracuse University in New York, tells me college girls know fat as evil.

She has analyzed some of their diets at only 4 percent fat. "When
I give them the results, they are proud instead of concerned. They have
an intense fear of fat. They really think if they increase their fat intake,
they'll immediately gain weight. I encourage them to try a small change:
'If you could add one or two tablespoons of peanut butter on your
bagels at breakfast. Just try it for a week and see if it makes a difference in how you feel.' Some will do it, and they say they feel so much
better, are more alert, and don't fall asleep in class. But many are afraid
to try."

Excess fat and saturated fat should be avoided, like too much sugar,
salt or alcohol. However, fat is essential for good health. Unexpected

health problems related to low dietary fat are beginning to surface.

Lowfat diets were supposed to lower heart disease risks. But recently Ronald Krauss, head of the American Heart Association's nutrition committee, reported that one-third of people actually increase their risk of heart disease on a lowfat diet. One-third are unaffected, and another one-third benefit, he said. One study found 67 percent of men following a very lowfat diet had adverse changes to their blood lipids, which could put them at increased risk for heart disease.[16]

Lowfat diets lower the "good" HDL cholesterol, which is protective for heart disease. The effect is strongest when carbohydrates replace fat. Lowfat, high-carbohydrate diets also have been found to aggravate insulin resistance.[17]

And there are concerns that lowfat eating has increased deficiencies of essential fats and other nutrients. One study found more deficiencies in calcium and iron for women who went on lowfat diets.[18]

Older women, age 70 and over, have now reduced their fat intake more than other women, to 31 percent of calories. But they eat the fewest calories of any women (1,384), and are very low in zinc, magnesium and calcium. Sadly, many older people are malnourished. Many are taking to heart the popular advice to eat less fat, meat, eggs, and fewer of the nutrient-rich foods they have always enjoyed, and they fill up the void with supplements and herbals "guaranteed" to give them more energy.

Lowfat diets are not appropriate for everyone, especially the elderly or children, insists Alfred Harper, PhD, professor emeritus of biochemistry at the University of Wisconsin.

Harper says the idea that limiting fat intake will provide children with healthier lives as adults has not been validated by research. In Canada, health experts agree, and have not allowed this to happen. They find no evidence that lowering fat benefits children, lowers their cholesterol levels, or reduces illness in later life, but instead that it is more likely linked to deficiencies in energy, protein, calcium, iron, and other nutrients, and to shorter stature.

Harper also argues that blaming fat for the increase in chronic disease is a myth. He points out that the increase in these diseases is a natural consequence of a healthier aging population that has overcome acute infectious diseases with improved medicine. Most people no longer die young. They die in old age of chronic diseases, especially heart disease — and that's as it should be.

Neither has the drop in fat intake had a beneficial effect on obesity rates, as expected. Instead, they went up steeply as fat went down. There is a growing realization that lowering fat intake is not the answer.

In the U.S. it appears that calorie intake went up for adults in the past two decades, perhaps two or three hundred calories. But this is not true everywhere.

Studies rather consistently show people in most countries are heavier than 15 or 20 years ago and are eating less fat; some also find they are eating fewer calories.[19]

Two studies, in England and Finland, show percent of fat and calorie intake dropped at the same time obesity rates rose.[20]

All of these studies put the origins of obesity into question, and contradict the idea that lowering fat intake can stop the increase in obesity. The body appears to defend its fat stores and maintain a setpoint whether the diet is high or low in fat.

The debate goes on. Some researchers conclude that high fat in the diet makes little difference except with overeating: fat is not stored. But when total calorie intake is excessive, it is stored all too easily.[21]

Harper argues that lowfat foods may be making people fatter because they have lost the satiety cues formerly relied on. And perhaps they do not feel as satisfied with the processed and prepackaged eaten today, he says, as when eating home-cooked foods in family meals at home.

Adding to the confusion are emerging health effects of different kinds of fats. New findings about the potential benefits in cancer protection of conjugated linoleic acid (CLA) from animal fats, and harm from transfatty acids, as in vegetable oils made solid in shortening and margarine, and an overbalance of omega-6 polyunsaturated fats, complicate the once-simple advice to reduce fat and saturated fats.[22]

One result of the current fear of fat is that people are eating more lowfat foods that substitute double or triple the sugar for fat. Then there's the backlash of "low carbohydrate" diets pulling people to the other extreme of unbalanced eating.

At *Healthy Weight Journal*, we have long championed the advice to reduce fat in the diet. But in recent years I have backed off somewhat, appalled by the havoc wreaked by the growing fear of fat.

What today's consumers seem to need most is a break from the overemphasis on fat. It has diverted them from key health messages, such as the benefits of eating in balance, variety and moderation, and being active. As a people, we need to enjoy food again, all kinds of foods, reject the "good food, bad food" mentality, and stop feeling guilty about what we eat. A balance of fats, from a variety of sources and used in moderation, may be the smartest choice for most people.

Missing out on meat

Americans today are consuming less meat, eggs and milk than in the 1970s. Many women and teenage girls are turning away from animal-source foods entirely in their desperate fear of fat. This should be a concern when combined with dieting, but is being largely ignored in the current climate of media health scares, food fears, and confusion about healthful eating.

Women who cut out meat, poultry and fish because of a desire for thinness or because of guilt feelings, are often the same ones who restrict all foods severely. They fail to fill the nutritional void with baked beans, tofu, nuts and spinach, but instead snack on cookies, cake, pastries, bakery goods, chips and candy. They are more likely to feel tired, apathetic, unable to concentrate, are sick more often, more frequently depressed, and are the most likely to be malnourished. Menstrual irregularities and amenorrhea are more common with meatless diets.

We need to respect individual decisions on food choices, yet this can be a serious health issue.

Lean meat, poultry, fish and eggs are not "fattening," but are relatively low in calories. The nutrition is highly concentrated, and even a small amount can dramatically improve a poor diet. These foods are high in protein, and researchers have discovered that protein is not usually stored as fat in the body, unlike dietary fat, and carbohydrate when eaten in excess.[23]

People who do not eat meat need to balance their diets with alternates from that food group. But do chronic dieters eat one-third cup peanut butter, or a cup and a half of baked beans, as an alternate to a 3-ounce serving of meat, and multiply that by two to three servings a day? It seems doubtful.

It has become trendy and "politically correct" for some in the health community to denigrate the contribution of meat, and to call for diets low in meat. This is not supported by mainstream nutrition. These advisers are likely trying to reduce the overeating of high-fat meat, principally by men. Unfortunately, it seems that restricting women are the ones who keep getting the message loud and clear, and are most likely to cut down even more, just as they are with fat.

There appears to be no credible evidence that eating lean red meat is unhealthy, and volumes of scientific evidence that show meat is health-promoting, especially for women and growing children. But this trendy notion is having a profound impact.

Some earlier research seemed to link meat, or at least high-fat meat, to high cholesterol levels in men. Research today is much more refined, and finds the link too complex and tenuous to make this assertion. For example, even though their diets consist mainly of lean meat and animal products, reindeer herders in Siberia and cattle raising tribes of East Africa have very low cholesterol and triglyceride levels. They also have high activity levels.[24]

Instead, evidence continues to accumulate of the health benefits of meat in the context of a balanced diet. One study of older Americans found that high meat intake was linked to superior nutrition and not to any increase in heart disease, compared with people who ate little or no meat.[25]

The higher incidence of colon cancer in affluent societies was once attributed to high-fat diet, and especially the consumption of meat. But a long-term study of 120,852 middle-age men and women in the Netherlands contradicts this. Colon cancer was not related to intake of fresh meat, beef, pork, minced meat, chicken or fish.[26]

In Europe big-game hunters of 30,000 years ago were tall and strong with massive bones. They grew six inches taller than their descendants who settled down to farming, raised grains, vegetables and fruit, and seldom had animal foods to eat. And it took these descendants until the Industrial Revolution, when they again ate more meat, eggs and milk, to gain back that height.[27]

Meat and other animal-source foods are the building blocks of healthy growth that have made Americans among the strongest and healthiest people in the world. Worldwide, the striking difference between well-fed and ill-fed people is the greater consumption of animal products in the well-fed nations.[28]

Yet, from coast to coast, eating disorder experts tell me they are seeing alarming numbers of young women and children with stunted growth, fragile bones and stress fractures who have stopped eating meat and animal-source foods. When young people choose to give up meat, there is concern about how they are doing it and to what extremes they might go. Disturbing one important component in our diets such as meat can affect others in unexpected and detrimental ways.

In Glendale, Arizona, eating disorder specialist Monika Woolsey, MS, RD, says she consults with young people who are afraid to eat meat. "There is a sense that they have been traumatized by the message that animal rights people are taking into the schools. They are trying to eat perfectly, and they get this black and white sense of what is perfect: 'If I'm a nice person I'll be a vegetarian, and if I'm not a nice person, I'll eat meat."[29]

Woolsey says vegetarianism seems to be a politically correct way to have an eating disorder. Often giving up meat is one of the steps along the way to this pathology. She has developed a self-test to help people determine whether their choice is eating disordered or well-considered. *(For self-test, see appendix).*

William Jarvis, MD, long-time president of the National Council Against Health Fraud, suggests that vegetarianism often attracts young people who feel guilty. "And it seduces the unskeptical by causing guilt and instilling false guilt. Guilt leads to self-denial, even asceticism ... This is very dangerous for kids."[30]

Abstaining from animal foods is more of a problem for women than men. Women need more of certain nutrients, especially those abundant in meat, because their bodies prepare for pregnancy and bear children. They are more likely to suffer deficiencies, due to monthly blood losses. Yet they usually eat less.

But, ironically, it is women who are more likely to stop eating meat. Perhaps they are more susceptible to the guilt message.

As a Wisconsin mother told me, "You send your daughters to college, you know they're going to come home vegetarians." She seemed concerned about her daughter's many other food restrictions, as well.

Personal food choices need to be respected both within and outside the family. Yet when a severely dieting mother or daughter decides to stop eating meat, poultry and fish, it can be of great concern to others. They may notice many adverse physical and mental changes.

Vegetarians frequently express concern about their anemia, lack of energy, stomach pain, digestive problems, flatulence, and stunting of children's growth. Taking pleasure in eating and social meals is also a consideration for health and well-being. Paul Obis, founder of *Vegetarian Times* and a longtime advocate of vegetarianism, recently began eating meat again, according to *Newsweek*. He explained, "Twenty-two years of tofu is a lot of time."

Certainly vegetarianism can be healthy, particularly for people who choose this way of life for philosophical, religious, or cultural reasons and follow sound nutrition practices. For many people it is a natural part of their cultural traditions. They keep well nourished and enriched by their lifestyle choices. People of different cultures may also be adapted to different kinds of healthful diets, as some nutritionists suggest.

But unfortunately, as vegetarianism is being practiced by many young women in the United States today, it is often just one more self-abusing diet, unbalanced and severely deficient in nutrients.

Confusing the public

One of the biggest barriers to people making reasonable food choices at this time is the confusion in the media over foods and health.

The problem is, we get an overload of startling but insignificant information. Newspapers seemingly cannot resist bringing us the health scare of the day. Headlines warn of popcorn, peanuts, Mexican or Chinese food, mad cow disease, or alar treated apples. People instantly stop eating that food, then learn the scare is of no consequence. Yet they are left a bit more shaken, more fearful. It adds to the unfortunate confusion people already feel about healthy eating and food safety.

On a recent flight from Chicago, where I was a guest on the Oprah show, I sat next to a frequent flyer businessman.

He told me, "I was on a plane the morning when headlines in *USA Today* read, 'Coffee raises cholesterol.' No one drank coffee! On another flight the headline said coffee prevents suicide, and everyone was calling for coffee. Another time everyone drank orange juice because of a news story. We're crazy, aren't we?"

Right. And headlines sell newspapers. Nevertheless, the media needs to be more responsible in helping people put these bits of information into perspective.

Some sources they quote are barely credible. Others appear to be irresponsible, headline-grabbing "experts." They get lots of press. Scientists today are often embarrassed and chagrined by "health terrorist" messages beamed out by researchers who certainly know better.

The irony is that this national panic over food and health comes at a time when Americans are healthier and longer lived than ever before, and when our food supply is the best it's ever been, and without doubt one of the safest and healthiest in the world.

In actual fact, many of the headlined risks are negligible. If they made any difference at all, it might be three days of longevity for a few individuals in a particular subgroup.

Other studies are very preliminary, or represent one unorthodox view of an obscure controversy. These reports are better aimed at scientists talking to scientists, discussed in the laboratory and pursued with more research, rather than targeted to people on the street with little or no knowledge of the subject.

And some of this fearmongering about food may be a deliberate smoke screen laid over more serious health issues, as charged by Elizabeth Whelan, president of the American Council on Science and Health. She claims the nearly $6 billion spent yearly by the tobacco industry on advertising and promotion, plus the deep roots the tobacco industry has forged throughout corporate America, and the financial support it gives members of Congress "clearly buys silence and diversion" to hide the fact that half of all premature deaths before age 80, a half million each year, are directly and causally related to tobacco. She says nothing could make "this killer advertiser more content than having the word 'carcinogen' used so often it loses all its meaning. Remember: when everything is dangerous, then nothing is. The leading cause of death has enough clout to keep the legislative and publicity spotlights off the cigarette — and on the multitude of nonrisks around us."[31]

What we are hearing, too often, instead of clear health messages that put all this into context, is an endless parade of contradictions and confusion. The emphasis on "good foods/bad foods" adds fuel to the misguided notion that some foods are medicines that heal us, and others are dangerous health hazards that shorten our lives.

Instead, we need to restore confidence in the basic principle that good health depends on the total diet, not on a few special components. It's best to ignore scare headlines and advise journalists to report this kind of research in reasonable ways.

Are women physically active enough?

Today women have opportunities as never before to engage in an array of sports and activities. Many accept the fun and challenges. However, most women are not very active either in work, transportation, or during leisure time. They are less active than women have ever been.

Defining vigorous exercise as "enough to work up a sweat" (or raising heart rate to 60 percent of maximum for age), the latest NHANES III statistics find that half of women rarely or never engage in any vigorous exercise.

Only 19 percent of adult women are this active at least five times a week, while 13 percent are this active every day. Younger women age 20 to 29 are barely more active than women in their middle years.[32]

Even among youth, only about one-half between ages 12 to 21 regularly engage in vigorous physical activity. One-fourth report no vigorous physical activity at all. Most girls develop more sedentary lifestyles by age 15 or 16, and the older they get, the less active they become.

Inactivity increases with age and is more common among women than men, African American and Hispanics than whites, older than younger adults, and among those with lower income and less education than among those with higher income or education.

The 1996 Surgeon General's Report on Physical Activity and Health reported that:

• 15 percent of U.S. adults engage regularly in vigorous physical activity during leisure time (three times a week for at least 20 minutes).

• 22 percent of adults engage regularly in sustained physical activity of any intensity during leisure time (five times a week for at least 30 minutes).

• 25 percent of adults report no physical activity in their leisure time.[33]

What is clear, is that both children and adults live less active lives than their peers a few decades ago, not only in work and school, but also in recreation. (Consider that in much of Africa, a woman spends 30 to 150 minutes every day of her life just carrying water.)[34] Today we rely on ever more conveniences and remote controls, more TV channels, computer games, and videos, and hours spent at the computer and on the Internet. And the 21st century promises more, not less, of these kinds of sedentary recreation.

Inactivity links to obesity

Being active is important in long-term weight maintenance. Regular activity helps maintain muscle size and strength, builds lean body mass, and allows people to eat more so they can be well-nourished while keeping a stable weight.

Researchers find a relationship between the decrease in physical activity and the increasing prevalence of obesity, even though it has been difficult to measure both physical activity and its relation to obesity. Most studies suggest that keeping regularly active through life can prevent excessive weight gain and, conversely, that being physically inactive is a risk factor for obesity.

A 10-year follow-up study of 2,564 men and 2,695 women age 19 to 63 in three towns in Finland found the average weight gain was lowest among the most active men and women and highest among the least active men and women, at every weight and age. The highest gains were among those whose activity declined. Women with no regular weekly activity had gained four pounds more at the end of the 10 years, and men an average of six pounds more, than those who were vigorously activity twice or more a week. The study controlled for smoking, health and economic factors.[35]

Many people attempt an exercise regimen, but cannot stick with it. Studies show that half of people who begin an exercise program quit within two weeks, and 70 percent quit during the first year.

Wayne Miller, PhD, an exercise physiologist at George Washington University, found 82 percent of overweight adults believe they can't maintain a healthy weight because they can't keep up a regular exercise program. So even though nearly all are convinced physical activity is needed, they are not able to make this change.[36]

For some reason, the barriers seem to outweigh the benefits. These are some of the barriers that Miller finds:

• Lifestyle change seems too overwhelming

- The benefits are not readily apparent
- It takes too much time and effort to reap the benefits
- It is confusing to know which type of activity helps most
- It is confusing how much activity should be done
- Increasing daily activity doesn't seem very helpful in weight loss
- There's no guarantee it works, especially for women

The desire to lose weight through exercise is another barrier for women. Women have been led to believe that the main reason to be active — the only reason, really — is to burn up calories and lose weight. It's what they focus on, one more unpleasant chore that needs to be done. When you put forth all this effort and don't lose weight, it's easy to get discouraged and give up. The best reasons for being active, of course, are for fun and health, but for many women these benefits get lost in the single-minded desire to be thin.

Often women associate exercise with dieting. They develop a lasting negative attitude toward it, because when they quit a diet program, they quit exercising, says Karin Kratina, PhD, RD, an eating disorder specialist and exercise physiologist in Coconut Creek, Florida.

"For many women, quitting exercise is connected with a despair over role stereotyping which encourages women to get in shape as a means of increasing personal value by becoming more sexually attractive ... (They) are often disappointed in themselves as well as with the exercise when they don't become that ideal shape," says Kratina.

Being physically active becomes a measure of self-worth, a testament to a woman's inner character, strength and value. When she fails at it, she feels worse, and is reluctant to try again.

Exercise is also used as self-punishment for not looking good enough, or for overeating.

Then there is the feeling of being conspicuous and "on display" when out running, playing a sport, or joining an aerobics class. I've heard women say that they can't go to a fitness center yet — first they need to develop a trim, fit body so they won't be embarrassed.

For larger women, embarrassment can be a major barrier. For example, some barriers to exercise reported in a Melpomene Institute study of 58 large women were the fear they wouldn't do well, that their ability to be athletic was doubted by others, and that they had experienced ridicule. A tennis player quit because she was embarrassed by her size. A woman who enjoyed swimming quit because of feeling conspicuous in a bathing suit. A biker stopped riding because she became uncomfortably aware of what others might think when viewing her from behind. Another stopped going to aerobics because she couldn't keep up, and felt self-conscious with mirrors on all sides.

Judy Lutter, president of Melpomene Institute for Women's Health Research in St. Paul, says clothes were a problem for many of the women. "Clothing, mainly bathing suits and shorts, sometimes prevented activity for 30 percent, 24 percent said clothes often prevented activity, and 14 percent said they never tried physical activity because of clothes."[37]

One woman said, "I keep trying to find a group of like-sized women and space where we're not 'the show.'"

Having been sexually abused is another reason women may dislike physical activity, Kratina points out. "Moving the body can bring up memories of the abuse, can trigger flashbacks ... Exercising is often curtailed after abuse begins, at puberty, or at some point when experiencing being sexually objectified."

Another barrier to physical activity is the safety factor. Women who once ran in public parks, may no longer feel safe, and so they curb their own activity out of fear.

"I know that concerns for my safety limit my physical activity. For instance, I'd like to be able to run after my two young children are settled in for the night. But I'd be foolish to go out alone after dark — I'd be exposing myself to unnecessary risks, and I'd be fearful and tense the whole time," said Linda Feltes, a Melpomene writer.

Feltes said there is plenty of helpful advice on precautions women can take to protect themselves. "But when you stop and think about it, you have to wonder why we have to adapt to a world that so severely limits us when, in truth, it's the world that needs to change. The world needs to stop assuming that it's acceptable to harass and harm women."[38]

Taking it to extremes

At the other extreme from being sedentary is the woman who exercises obsessively.

Kratina describes the typical scenario of a young woman with exercise dependence or activity disorder, as it is also called. "She rises each morning at 5:30, hits the pavement for a brisk three miles, rain or shine, works out 45 minutes at the fitness center on lunch break, and goes to another health club after work for an hour of aerobics, half an hour on the Stairmaster and a half hour on the Lifecycle. She appears to be a motivated, fit and happy person but her legs ache constantly as she continues to work out, despite shin splints. When she stops for a time her depression and anxiety become so overwhelming, she can't wait to get back to her workouts."[39]

Signs of this disorder, according to Kratina, are:

1. The person narrows the scope of her physical activities, and follows a stereotyped pattern of exercise with a regular schedule,

once or more daily.

2. She gives increased priority to maintaining this pattern over other activities.

3. She is able to perform more and more exercise over months and years.

4. She has withdrawal symptoms, such as depression and anxiety, when unable to follow her regular schedule.

5. She rapidly returns to the previous pattern when possible, gaining relief from withdrawal symptoms.

Weight loss by dieting may be secondary to all this, initiated to improve performance.

Or an eating disorder may be primary, the main purpose being to lose weight, and exercise dependancy secondary.

Obsessive exercising is closely linked to eating disorders, and has many of the same features. A key to when exercise becomes a problem is often when goals shift from enjoyment and becoming fit and healthy toward body reshaping. It is important for teachers and coaches to emphasize health-promoting goals, and question weight loss and muscle building.

Kratina says at least half the anorexics and bulimics she sees probably deal with some form of exercise dependency. "Stress injuries are common, and frequently the person exercises right through an injury so it can't heal properly."

Jolie Glass, MS, Director of Women's Exercise Research Center, George Washington University Medical Center, in Washington, DC, defines activity disorder as excessive, purposeless physical activity that goes beyond any usual training regimen and ends up being a detriment rather than an asset to health and well-being.

In working with patients with a history of eating disorders, Glass says it is important to closely monitor them for signs of overtraining. Exercise should not be recommended until eating behaviors are relatively stable and balanced.[40]

Female athlete triad

Amenorrhea and menstrual dysfunction are common for female athletes in many sports, often linked to weight restrictions. The *female athlete triad* links eating disorders, amenorrhea and osteoporosis and is a known risk for elite women athletes. Any component of the triad can impair health and performance, and the combination of all three compounds the risk.

The American College of Sports Medicine recently published a position stand on the female athlete triad.[41]

An obsession with a sport may be a "red flag" that an athlete is overtraining in unhealthy ways. Athletes at risk tend to talk and think about their sport constantly, often spending hours upon hours in the gym perfecting their workout at the expense of school activities, friendships and hobbies.[42]

Female athletes may have a special predisposition to eating disorders because of sports-related pressures, perfectionism, high expectations, low self-esteem, and emotional instability, experts say.

Trying to control weight while focusing on training and performance may lead to a sense of frustration, guilt, despair and failure, and to unhealthy eating.

Amenorrhea is associated with scoliosis and stress fractures in young ballet dancers. Delayed menarche, as late as age 19 or 20 for very thin female athletes and ballet dancers, usually with a restrictive diet, is linked to osteoporosis and bone fractures.[43]

Avoidance of meat is common for female athletes and is linked to menstrual abnormalities, warn Alvin Loosli, MD, and Jaime Ruud, MS, RD, writing recently in *The Physician and Sportsmedicine*. One study showed the prevalence of menstrual irregularities was less than 5 percent for 41 nonvegetarian women, compared with over 26 percent among 34 vegetarian women. Another compared regularly menstruating runners with amenorrheic runners and found 44 percent of the menstruating runners ate red meat, while none of the amenorrheic runners did. Similar results were found in a study of recreational athletes and elite female cyclists.

Another study showed that even though iron and calorie intake were the same, female runners who ate less than 100 grams of red meat per week had significantly lower iron levels than those who ate more meat. Another study showed female runners who did not eat meat, chicken or fish had lower protein levels than recommended for endurance athletes.[44]

Although it is theoretically possible to compete athletically on a meatless diet, Loosli and Ruud emphasize there is risk. They recommend that female athletes who call themselves vegetarians be screened for disordered eating and amenorrhea, and if either is found, for osteoporosis.

Red flags for athletes

Experts are calling for mandatory training for coaches to help them become more aware of exercise dependance and eating disorders, and alert them to warning signs.

Nancy Thies Marshall, chair of the USA Gymnastics's task force on eating disorders and the youngest member of the 1972 US Olympic gymnastics team, has struggled with some of these problems herself. She offers these "red flags" for athletes, coaches and parents to watch for:

- Obsession with the sport. At the expense of family, friends, hobbies and school activities, the athlete at risk tends to devote herself to her sport.
- Preoccupation with food and weight. Thinking or talking often about food, fat and calories, frequent weighing, skipping meals and binge eating. Motivation for exercise may be a belief that losing weight will improve performance or appeal to a judge's eye.
- Drinking an overabundance of fluids in the effort to feel full.
- Laxative or diet pill use.
- Bathroom visits after meals. This may suggest the binge-purge cycle of vomiting after eating.
- Wearing baggy clothing. Clothing may be used to hide weight loss.
- Dramatic weight loss.
- Physical deterioration. Malnutrition may cause chills, apathy, irritability, dry and pale skin, hair loss. Vomiting may cause callused finger, and sores on lips and tongue.
- Withdrawing from relationships. Feeling depressed, moody and lonely.
- Overexercising. Compulsive exercise beyond her regular workouts may be a sign the athlete is trying to compensate for eating.
- Menstrual dysfunction. Missing periods or delaying menarche for too long (perhaps beyond age 16 or 17) raises concerns of premature osteoporosis and bone fractures.[45]

Bodybuilding

Bodybuilding, one of the fastest growing women's sports in the U.S. today, can have aspects of extremism, and may attract women and men with body image issues. Bodybuilding itself is an integrated program of weight training and cardiovascular workout that increases strength, endurance and bone density.

But competitions in bodybuilding are not really about strength or skill. Rather, they are a form of modeling, and of reshaping the body so it is "right." Often they involve profound alterations to the natural body. There are extremely restrictive ways to eat so as to reduce fat under the skin and reveal the muscles as more "ripped" or "sliced."

The technique combines long hours of high-intensity training, extremely lowfat diet, depleting fluids in the final days before a contest, and for some, use of illegal steroids and prescription drugs. Steroid effects may be permanent and can put users at risk for heart disease and stroke. Dependency is another risk, according to Jim Wright, PhD, Health and Science editor of *Muscle & Fitness*.[46] Eating disorder specialists suggest that many young women are substituting bodybuilding for eating disorders, or combining the two.

For women contestants, familiar conflicts arise. Should they go all out for full muscular development, or emphasize their feminine traits? Some judges favor femininity, others prefer heavy muscles.

There is much potential for abuse. Some female bodybuilders seem to be just more women dissatisfied with their bodies.

Anorexia and bodybuilding have similarities, points out David Schlundt, PhD, an eating disorder specialist at Vanderbilt University, in Nashville, Tenn. "There are special diets, use of diuretics, steroid use, obsessive exercise, very lowfat diets, and so on. An obsession with changing size and shape of the body leads to extreme and sometimes dangerous changes in diet, exercise and substance abuse. This is true about anorexia, bulimia, and some bodybuilders who take it to obsessive levels."

The use of steroids and illegal prescription drugs in bodybuilding is a sensitive subject that competitors are reluctant to discuss. A writer in *Mademoiselle* says almost all the women bodybuilders she talked with acknowledged that drugs are often used to increase muscle size and strength.[47] The anabolic steroids favored can have masculinizing side effects. Women may stop menstruating, and develop masculine appearance, deep voices, facial hair, and male pattern baldness. Many women bodybuilders have breast implants, as their breasts shrink from the lack of body fat or testosterone use.[48]

CHAPTER 10

How the diet industry exerts control

■

"Diet and pharmaceutical companies influence every step along the way of the scientific process. They pay for the ads that keep obesity journals publishing. They underwrite medical conferences ... Most obesity researchers would lose a lot of money if they stopped telling Americans they had to lose weight."
— *Laura Fraser, author of Losing it*

If this industry made cars, no one would buy them, and if they did, consumer groups would force a recall. If it offered any other health service, it would be required to prove safety and effectiveness before its products could be prescribed to millions of unsuspecting consumers — as were both the disastrous very low calorie diets and fen-phen/ Redux diet pills in the last decade. It would be held accountable for the many deaths and injuries it causes. But no agency even bothers to keep track.

The problem is not that the diet industry makes large profits, pulling in $30 to $50 billion every year in the United States alone, or that it promotes itself in the most favorable light, exaggerating its successes and minimizing its failures. Many businesses do as much.

The problem is that the promotions of the diet industry are virtually *all* false promises, or at least manipulations of the truth. Its failures comprise uncounted tragedies, deaths, and injuries with no accountability and, worse, the industry exerts such control on national health policy that its agenda is literally being sold to long-suffering victims with their own tax money.

Because these victims are vulnerable and desperate, shameless exploitation is allowed. And they are vulnerable and desperate in part because of fears whipped up by the very companies and agencies who exploit them.

This industry alone among health care providers is allowed to parade pitifully weak studies without challenge at national and international conferences — meetings it often finances. I've often been disappointed at the silence of knowledgeable scientists who guard their careers by saying nothing. Others try to bring balance, speaking out when they can, publishing well-documented articles that take a broader view when and where they can. But this is a protected industry. It is allowed to publish irrelevant research, almost identical articles, over and over again in the most respected medical and scientific journals of the day. Industry-paid scientists sit on those editorial boards.

Many obesity researchers at prestigious universities have vested interests in the weight loss industry. Their research is funded by diet companies; they serve as paid consultants, advise company policy, fly the world expense-free, collect big fees to present lectures at industry-cozy multinational conferences. Sometimes they are part owners of the companies. At the same time, they may help determine federal policy.

"Diet and pharmaceutical companies influence every step along the way of the scientific process. They pay for the ads that keep obesity journals publishing. They underwrite medical conferences ... Some obesity researchers have a clear conflict of interest, promoting or investing in products or programs based on their research ... while they also sit on the boards of the medical journals that determine which studies get printed. What it comes down to is that most obesity researchers would stand to lose a lot of money if they stopped telling Americans they had to lose a lot of weight," writes Laura Fraser in her revealing book, *Losing it: America's Obsession with Weight and the Industry that Feeds on It.* (For readers who want to learn more about the players involved in all this, I recommend this book. An investigative journalist, Fraser names the names and provides their records and affiliations.)[1]

C. Wayne Callaway, a George Washington University endocrinologist and obesity expert, agrees. "The so-called clinical research in this field has been largely paid for by the formula and drug companies."

What was true a decade ago has mushroomed 10-fold today, now that the Food and Drug Administration (FDA) has opened the door for diet drugs. Large multinational drug companies stand wedged in the door, determined to make huge profits by rushing their diet pills to market before the next shoe falls. Today, many obesity experts are no longer beholden to just one or two companies, but sometimes six or eight. And these same experts advise U.S. health policy by sitting on federal advisory boards paid for and trusted by the American public.

They represent a powerful segment of this field. These are respected scientists making health decisions in the national interest according to their highest ethics, and they may argue that other academics make accommodations to the issues of research funding, financial affiliations, consultancies, and the politics of power. Yet there is a special vulnerability in this field.

Members of the federally-funded National Task Force on the Prevention and Treatment of Obesity, which sets U.S. national policy, for instance, are well funded by the diet industry. This Task Force is organized by the National Institute of Diabetes and Digestive and Kidney Diseases (NIDDK).

In 1996, the nine members of the Task Force disclosed for the first time their financial affiliations. This landmark disclosure was required for an article on diet drugs they published in the *Journal of the American Medical Association*. One can only guess at the power struggle that went on at that literary institution. I had three times requested this disclosure information under the Freedom of Information Act, and three times Van Hubbard, MD, PhD, Director of Nutrition Services at NIDDK, had explained the impossibility of this.

No wonder. The list reads like a Who's Who of the diet industry. Of the nine members, eight are university-affiliated professors and researchers who have financial ties with from two to eight commercial weight loss firms each. They are consultants, serve on advisory boards, conduct industry research, and receive honorariums and grants from weight loss companies and drug manufacturers of diet pills, most of this support being current at that time or within the year.

The eight were William H. Deitz, MD, PhD, Tufts University School of Medicine; F. Xavier Pi-Sunyer, MD, Columbia University; James O. Hill, PhD, University of Colorado; Rena R. Wing, PhD, University of Pittsburgh; Judith Stern, DSc, University of California, Davis; Roland L. Weinsier, MD, DrPH, University of Alabama; Barbara Rolls, PhD, Pennsylvania State University; G. Terence Wilson, PhD, New Jersey State University. The diet and diet pill companies providing funds for these eight members included Knoll Pharmaceuticals, Hoffman-LaRoche, Roche Laboratories, Wyeth-Ayerst, Lilly Pharmaceuticals, Genentech, Neurogen, Procter & Gamble, International Life Sciences, Amgen, Parke-Davis, Ross Laboratories, Sandoz Nutrition, Weight Watchers, and Duke Diet and Fitness Center. Most of these funded several Task Force members. Five, a clear majority on any vote, listed financial affiliation with Knoll.[2]

The question is, what officials are responsible for appointing these kinds of advisory boards? Why do they not obtain financial affiliations from all candidates at the beginning?

Did the same people select the 24 NHLBI panel members who put together the influential 1998 *NHLBI Clinical Guidelines on the Identification, Evaluation, and Treatment of Overweight and Obesity?* Probably. Disclosure of financial affiliations was not required from members of the NHLBI Guidelines panel, chaired by F. Xavier Pi-Sunyer, director of the federally-funded Obesity Research Center, St. Luke's/Roosevelt Hospital Center in New York City. However, the make-up is similar to that of the Task Force.[3] Pi-Sunyer's financial affiliations listed in the *Journal of the American Medical Association* included being on the advisory boards of Wyeth-Ayerst and Knoll pharmaceuticals, and being a consultant to Lilly Pharmaceuticals, Genentech, Hoffman-LaRoche, Knoll, Weight Watchers, and Neurogen. Others on both the NHLBI panel and the Task Force are William H. Dietz, James O. Hill, and G. Terence Wilson, each listed as having at least two financial affiliations with these same companies.

This is an industry that does not hesitate to give liberally and to forge partnership links, as universities and their scientists seek ever more private funding. Especially now when diet drugs loom so tantalizingly on the horizon.

The latest revelations come with fen-phen/Redux lawsuits out of Dallas. According to evidence given at a May 1999 injury trial, the makers of Redux (dexfen) paid ghostwriters for 10 articles promoting obesity treatment and creating market demand for Redux and then arranged for prominent researchers to publish the work under their own names. Two of the articles were published in medical journals before the drugs were pulled off the market; the other eight were scrubbed. Evidence at the trial showed that Wyeth-Ayerst paid Excerpta Medica Inc. $20,000 each for the ten articles and to retain the obesity experts, offering them $1,000 to $1,500 each. Exerpta arranged to submit most of the papers to medical journals owned by its parent, Reed Elsevier Plc, according to documents.[4]

Prominent obesity experts listed in the documents as authoring the ghostwritten articles are: F. Xavier Pi-Sunyer, Thomas A. Wadden, Richard L. Atkinson and Albert Stunkard.

Jerome Kassirer, editor in chief of the *New England Journal of Medicine* said this conduct appalls him. "The fact that Wyeth commissioned someone to write pieces that are favorable to them, the fact that they paid people to put their names on these things, the fact that people were willing to put their names on it, the fact that the journals published them without asking questions."

"This is a common practice in the industry," responded a Wyeth spokesman.

Unfortunately, his words ring all too true, from my vantage point of 16 years observing the industry.

As timely as ever is the 1990 protest of Thaddeus Prout, MD, former chair of the FDA Committee on Anorectic Drugs, and of the Committee on Drugs for the American Board of Internal Medicine, when he gave this testimony before the Congressional hearings investigating drugs in the weight loss industry:

"The same faces, the same people who have been doing industry-paid research for two decades are before us ... In July of 1983 we discussed this same question ... We listened to their data, looked at their paltry studies. We are hearing all the exaggerated claims of success again ... The medical profession has learned that they need not waste the time or postage [with] an entrenched and persuasive pharmaceutical industry. What can we do? Shall we wait another decade and have a new generation of concerned physicians wringing their hands and bumping their heads against the stone wall of industry?"[5]

Government parrots industry needs

The heavy hand of the $30 to $50 billion diet industry is evident in most federal reports on obesity. In these, the diet industry needs government to keep repeating these points:

1. Huge numbers of Americans are overweight.
2. This is a severe health risk.
3. Losing weight will improve their health.
4. Current weight loss methods are safe and effective.

And so it does, especially, it seems, when the reports link back to NIDDK, the agency in charge of diabetes. (One might think that NIDDK would champion the health of large people and people with diabetes, instead of offering them up as sacrificial lambs.)

The diet industry also needs government to ignore dysfunctional eating and eating disorders, or discount them as unimportant. And it does.

Following are current examples of government reports and their pretense that all is well with obesity treatment.

● *The Clinical Guidelines on the Identification, Evaluation, and Treatment of Overweight and Obesity* — often called the NHLBI

Guidelines — seem to have the not-very-hidden agenda of getting more people on weight loss programs regardless of health consequences, and persuading insurance to pay for it. The 1998 Guidelines define 55 percent of American adults at risk for weight-related diseases, and urge physicians to motivate their patients to lose weight by telling them about the risks of overweight and explaining how this new plan will be different. No effective plan is offered, however, so this seems to encourage doctors to manipulate their patients with scare tactics and false promises. The Guidelines fail to warn of the risks of weight loss treatment, or to advise screening for eating disorders. They were developed by the National Institutes of Health, National Heart, Lung, and Blood Institute and NIDDK.[6]

- "Almost any of the commercial weight loss programs can work," declares a consumer brochure on *Choosing a safe and successful weight-loss program* by WIN, the Weight-Control Information Network. Yet it provides no credible evidence for this statement. WIN is an educational program of NIDDK that provides information to the public and the media. It has often seemed inappropriately aimed at keeping up consumers' and clinicians' flagging interest in weight loss treatment.[7]

- Weight cycling, or yo-yo dieting, was deemed relatively harmless in a special report by the National Task Force on Prevention and Treatment of Obesity of NIDDK. It reached this questionable conclusion by a selective review of research, extensively discussing and discounting concerns about a drop in metabolism rate, but ignoring what many consider the major problems, increased cardiovascular disease risk and increased mortality with weight cycling. The report urges people *not* to let their concerns over weight cycling deter them from efforts to lose weight. It is promoted and referenced heavily by the diet industry, the Task Force and WIN.[8]

- *Weighing the Options: Criteria for Evaluating Weight-Management Programs.* This book reviews available weight loss programs, and finds nearly all safe and effective. It also seems to suggest that many more people should undergo stomach reduction surgery than currently. The book defines long-term weight loss as a period of only one year, which might begin on sign-up day and include months of weight loss. (The American Heart Association says weight loss is not long term unless maintained for at least five years.) *Weighing the Options* is published by the National Academy of Sciences, a nonprofit group chartered by Congress to advise the federal government on health policy.[9]

- The healthy weight table in the 1995 *Dietary Guidelines for Americans* sets a narrow standard for thinness. All adults with a body mass index of 25 or over, or who have gained 10 pounds after reaching adult height, are told bluntly, "You need to lose weight." It removed the 10- to 15-pound age allowance after age 35, set in 1990, despite strong evidence that a wider weight range is healthy as people grow older. The dietary guidelines are published by the Department of Agriculture and the Department of Health and Human Services on order of Congress.[10]

Obesity is a concern, but balance needed

Certainly many scientists and health leaders have a genuine concern about obesity and the rising diabetes rates and other problems that accompany its increase. Many well-intentioned individuals who work on these reports may honestly believe that emphasizing the risks of obesity is the best way to deal with it. Perhaps they fear if they don't — if they discuss the problems of undernourished kids, of eating disorders, or of the risks of weight loss — then our health services will be overwhelmed by a rising tide of excess weight.

Perhaps this is the fear of William Dietz, now director of the Nutrition and Physical Activity Program at the Centers for Disease Control and Prevention (CDC), who will be influential in what happens to kids. His comments are sobering.

I asked why the Third Nutrition Monitoring report, which documents the severe undernutrition of teenage girls and which he helped write, does not mention a concern for this in its own summary.

"Because obesity is more important. We need to focus on obesity," he said.

"Yes, obesity is a concern," I agreed, "What about teen girls' undernutrition?"

"Later, perhaps, after we get obesity under control."

"Are you having success on that front?"

"No, it's increasing."

So, when do we get around to the undernourishment of teenage girls?

This kind of thinking and pressure from the diet industry kept eating disorders off the nation's Healthy People 2000 agenda, and shunts them off to a mental health area for Healthy People 2010. There they'll be as far from the obesity objectives in nutrition as possible, a shocking and inexcusable ploy, in my opinion. Healthy People is the document that sets the nation's health goals for each decade. That eating disorders have become even a tiny part of Healthy People 2010, is only due to the dedicated efforts of many women professionals.

Thus, the health community jeopardizes the health of America by overemphasizing the dangers of obesity, at one extreme, without warning of dangers at the other extreme.

A balance is needed. These kinds of problems need to be discussed openly by leaders without vested interests, by laying all the cards on the table, without industry controlling the play.

But at the many national and international obesity conferences I have attended, never has the tone been: We have a problem with rising obesity rates — what can we do about it?

No. Instead the theme is invariably: This works, and this works, and it's almost certain, if *they* would just cooperate, this would work, too. The issues are approached from the view that problems are already solved. The answers are at hand, so where's the problem?

Yes, I'm concerned about rising obesity rates, but I'm even more concerned about what health agencies will do about it, especially as it affects children.

How reports manipulate the truth

Government obesity reports often say one thing in the body and another in the conclusion. It's as if they are written by two opposing factions — one documenting the facts, the other masking them.

Wayne Miller, PhD, professor at George Washington University School of Medicine, points out these contradictions from the report of the 1992 NIH Conference on Methods for Voluntary Weight Loss and Control, which investigated the weight loss industry. One statement truthfully sums up the conference: "Long term weight loss following any type of intervention was limited to only a small minority." Then comes the non sequitur, the inference that does not follow: "Regardless of products used, successful weight loss and control is limited to and requires individualized programs consisting of restricted caloric intake, behavior modification and exercise."[11]

How's that again?

Miller says, "It is puzzling how the NIH could come to any effectiveness conclusion based on the paucity of data they received which they themselves judged to be inadequate, questionable, and inconclusive."

From the evidence given, he points out that only two conclusions were possible. Either there could be no conclusion, because there was no data on which to base it; or no commercial program is effective at producing long-term weight loss, because no company could provide data to show otherwise.[12]

Reports cautioning about the risks of diets or diet pills often end with a paragraph warning that it can be dangerous — except when used on severely obese people. This is hardly logical. If it is risky for healthy people, why is it not even more so for high-risk individuals? If it doesn't work for moderately overweight people, why would it work for larger people?

This last paragraph, the non sequitur that doesn't follow, has been called by size activists the *P.S. phenomenon* that says: P.S. Keep dieting. We hate you.

The 119-pound bombshell

In September 1995 one of those well-staged media events hit virtually all American women in one day like a bombshell. JoAnn Manson, PhD, of Harvard University and her colleagues announced that the Nurses' Health Study showed a five-foot-five woman risked higher death rates if she weighed more than 119 pounds. A woman's healthiest weight, they said, is between a very thin body mass index (BMI) of about 19 and 22. After that risk of death increased.

Women were appalled and frightened. The health community was rocked.

"Even mild to moderate overweight is associated with a substantial increase in risk of premature death," Manson reported. Carrying an extra 10 or 20 pounds was a risk, she said, based on data from the 16-year Nurses' Health Study of 115,195 women.

Women who read the study soon found reports of their impending deaths were greatly exaggerated. First of all, these were fairly young women, initially age 30 to 55, and not many had died. Further, of non-smoking women, only a few died of heart disease, the only disease clearly associated with weight. And their increased risk was slight, almost none up to a BMI of 30.

Fraser says that Manson later told her she was actually talking about a "statistical trend" when she said there was increased risk under a BMI of 27 — the point where risk is barely noticeable. When Fraser pointed out that the Nurse's Study showed being 20 to 40 pounds overweight makes little difference, Manson admitted, "It's insignificant."[13]

In fact, the study findings were quite different from what she reported to the press. They showed that a stable weight after age 18 is beneficial, but gains up to 22 pounds do not increase risk. The women who gained this much had the lowest mortality from cardiovascular disease, and no higher mortality from all causes than those with a stable weight or who had lost weight. Women who had lost 9 to 22 pounds had higher risks, even though the message most women got from the story was that they should lose weight. A low death rate at the lower weight was true only for a small subgroup. Furthermore, some categories had been collapsed to attain significance in a way that seemed misleading.[14]

Fraser suggests that Manson's financial interests may have influenced how the study was fed to the press. At the time FDA was considering approval of Redux by Interneuron, for which Manson was consulting, and subsequently FDA granted approval.

Similarly, Harvard researchers Anne Wolf and Graham Colditz have used figures like these from the Nurses' Study as they calculated obesity costs, figures that are being extrapolated worldwide.[15]

The Nurses' Study is based on self-reported, mailed-in questionnaires from mostly-white nurses in 11 states. While it provides useful information on many topics, it is not based on a representative sample and thus may not be appropriate for figuring prevalence and risk ratios. Experts are questioning why Nurses' Health Study data is being inserted so widely into government reports for these purposes.

David Allison, PhD, a Columbia University obesity researcher, suggests this makes unwarranted assumptions and gives imprecise estimates. "Why not use data from good national health studies, the NHANES follow-up, or the American Cancer studies?" he asks.

Allison observes that Nurses' Study findings often differ markedly from what is found in those other studies. Perhaps this is precisely why it is being used so much.

The fen-phen and dexfen tragedy

Dexfenfluramine should never have been approved in the United States. By the time it was, in April 1996, two of its terrible effects were well known, and a third was soon to come.

The drug, sold here under the brand name Redux, had been used liberally in Europe for over ten years — a strong argument for its approval. But bad things were happening there. France had already cut back to one-year prescriptions, and an international study was investigating deaths in several countries.

Still, the pressure was on. Michael Weintraub, a University of Rochester pharmacologist who had done the study that launched fen-phen pills was installed at FDA, so it was only a matter of time. FDA had held out for 20 years without approving any new diet drugs, and its own advisory board voted "no." But Redux was approved over this negative vote during a questionable meeting about the drug's safety from which doctors and scientists from health-advocacy groups were excluded. *U.S. News & World Report* says pressure and political donations to California Rep. Tom Lantos helped close that FDA meeting.[16]

By this time the fen-phen era was in full cry. While the fen-phen combination never was approved by FDA, it was prescribed widely "off label." This means both drugs were approved for other purposes, and doctors can use their own best judgment in prescribing.

Fen-phen's popularity was based on publicity given the four-year Weintraub study, which combined two drugs. In this study the majority of subjects dropped out, many because they could not tolerate the side effects, and only 26 of 121 kept off as much as 10 percent of their weight.[17] The study seemed so unimpressive that I laid it aside and decided not to review it for *Healthy Weight Journal.*

My mistake. The Weintraub studies were soon being pumped up and quoted everywhere in academia and the scientific press. It was obvious a new drug era was about to begin.

Fenfluramine and dexfenfluramine are isomer cousins, two forms of the same drug. Fenfluramine was sold under the brand name Pondimin by R. H. Robbins. Dexfen or Redux was sold by Interneuron Pharmaceuticals and Wyeth-Ayerst Laboratories. They act on serotonin in the brain to suppress appetite. Phentermine (the phen in fen-phen) seemed to make them both work better, although the makers of Redux warned against the combination.

Once approved, Redux pills flew off the shelves. Many people lost a lot of weight, but it was the same old story: most of the weight was lost through dieting, and that part returned whether or not the pills were continued. The drug itself kept off an average of only about five and a half pounds over placebo.[18] And it was a Catch 22 scenario. FDA listed the drugs as safe for only one year, but if you stopped taking them the five pounds returned, so to be effective they had to be taken long-term, like for the rest of your life.

Reading the Redux package insert was sobering. It listed many risks, adverse reactions and complications, and warned, "The safety and effectiveness of Redux beyond one year have not been determined at this time."

In the past this has often meant that long-term results are not good. After all, if there were no long-term studies, why not? The drug had been used over a decade in European medical clinics and was tested before approval there. Known risks were primary pulmonary hypertension, a lung disease fatal within four years for nearly half of its victims, and brain damage, found in more than 80 animal studies.

In a sizzling diet pill market, sales of fen-phen and Redux to U.S. pharmacies totalled over $214 million in wholesale dollars during the first half of 1996, filling 87 million prescriptions, according to IMS America, a firm that tracks drug sales.[19] Diet pills were prescribed in medical clinics, in weight loss centers, and even at California flea markets.[20]

Meanwhile, the prestigious *New England Journal of Medicine* was caught in an ethics crunch. It published the European study showing that patients who took a form of the fen drug were 23 times as likely to suffer pulmonary hypertension as matched controls who did not, and the longer they took the drugs, the greater the risk.[21] However, in the same issue an editorial by JoAnn Manson and Gerald Faich criticized the European study and basically told physicians not to worry because the risks of being obese were far greater than any risks from the pills.[22] The editorial was probably why Interneuron's stock rose 13 percent in the next few days, said one critic.[23]

Then the *New York Times* reported that Manson was a paid consultant to Interneuron, and Faich was paid by two companies marketing the fen and dexfen drugs.[24] The editors of the journal, Angell and Kassirer, apologized and said this was the first violation in six years of their policy of requiring the authors of editorials to be free of associations with companies that stood to gain from a product mentioned. They faulted the writers for not disclosing their financial sources, but confessed that only the year before they had printed an article by Manson in which she disclosed her connection with both Interneuron and Servier (the French company marketing dexfen).

Reasonable health leaders watching the diet pill scene felt most discouraged at this time. Common sense seemed swept away.

Yet, in early 1997 during the heat of the fen-phen/Redux craze, California dietitian Joanne Ikeda predicted that it would not last, that industry-paid obesity specialists who pretend to be neutral, would be exposed. "Their day will come," she said. "Associating with the pharmaceutical industry will become a liability rather than an asset one of these days. In fact, I think the tide is turning as the public suffers the consequences of the new drug treatments for obesity. These scientists are losing their professional reputations for scientific objectivity. They will soon be considered 'bought and paid for' ... I am just sitting by the sidelines enjoying watching it happen!"

Ikeda could not have been more prophetic. What happened next was a shock.

Abruptly, on Sept 15, 1997, FDA issued a news release asking the makers of fen and dexfen to take the pills off the market. Within hours both drugs were gone, and it is unlikely they will ever be back.[25]

I am proud to be associated, if only by geography, with the drama behind this action.

Without a doubt, sonographer Pam Ruff, of Fargo, N.D., is the unsung hero of America's sordid flirtation with fen-phen and Redux diet pills. Ruff noticed it first in December 1994: an abnormal heart valve coated with a glistening white substance that prevented it from closing fully, unlike anything she had seen in more than 10 years as an ultrasound technician. Curious, she asked the patient if she took diet pills, and was told, yes. The same day she saw another nearly identical abnormality, and again was told the patient was on fen-phen. For nearly two years Ruff and her fellow sonographers at the MeritCare echo lab kept records on the strange heart valves, now numbering nearly two dozen, all patients using fen-phen.[26]

At length, they were able to interest Jack Crary, MD, a MeritCare heart surgeon. He called a friend at Mayo Clinic in Rochester, Minnesota, who found a few more cases. The article they wrote for the *New England Journal of Medicine* so startled the editors that they contacted FDA.[27]

The FDA was so alarmed that it notified the companies and released the news report even before the article was published. Later FDA said 25 to 30 percent of patients who took the drugs may have abnormal echocardiograms. The damage sometimes worsened after the pills were stopped.

A senior official at FDA says, "Clearly, had the drugs stayed on the market longer, we would be seeing many more and more-serious cases of heart valve damage and pulmonary hypertension."

How many hundreds or thousands of users can thank the modest Pam Ruff that they are still alive? Without doubt, but for her, the tragedy would have extended much longer, perhaps years. I think it's an amazing story, and it confirms my belief that one person can make a difference — and two or three can make a miracle. But what an unnecessary tragedy it was, the many deaths, bereaved families, young children with a mother now gone.

Even before Redux was approved, the companies and FDA knew about heart valve damage, says a 1999 expose' in the *U.S. News & World Report.*[28] The article says Wyeth-Ayerst also knew of 101 more cases of pulmonary hypertension than the 132 cases they reported for FDA approval. Over 1,000 lawsuits are pending.

The story is not over. Just two months later, in November 1997 the FDA approved sibutramine, sold under the brand name Meridia by Knoll Pharmaceutical, again over a "no" vote of the FDA scientific advisory council.[29] An agent at FDA told me that even though this drug does not work very well either, and may be unsafe (it, too, has only one year safety and effectiveness data), it is needed by desperate patients and their doctors. "We need to give them some kind of a drug ... The decision for its use will be between patient and doctor."

His explanation had a false ring to it that made me long for the old tough FDA. Is it too much to expect that those desperate patients and their doctors might move ahead to health-centered treatment and a measure of size acceptance instead of one more round of likely failure?

NHLBI Guidelines fail purpose

The 1998 NHLBI Guidelines for physicians on how to treat obesity are an example of the unfortunate advice that evolves from the intimate three-way relationship of government, industry and obesity specialists.[30]

Purpose of these guidelines, developed by the National Heart, Lung, Blood Institute, is to give the best information on who is at risk and how they can best be treated. But I believe they fail in both these objectives. In the end, they seem to serve the diet industry better than they serve consumers or health professionals.

The Guidelines lower the so-called "healthy weight range" to a BMI of between 18.5 and 24.9, and label everyone over this weight as at risk. This puts 55 percent of American adults in this category. This is foolish, as any number of researchers are quick to point out.

"It's an absurd goal. Many people are at natural and healthy weights over a much wider range than this," warned Cliff Johnson of the National Center for Health Statistics earlier when obesity specialists began toying with these definitions. His agency set the definition of overweight for national health studies at 27.3 for women and 27.8, and assured Americans that health risks did not necessarily start at this point.

So what is the evidence all these people at a BMI of 25 are at risk? Not much. The Guidelines themselves hardly defend this decision. Instead, they almost exclusively discuss risks beginning at about a BMI of 30.[31] The only exception they find is that the Nurses' Health Study appears to show that higher risks begin at a BMI of 22. The Guidelines repeatedly boast of being based on research from 236 solid, randomized controlled trials, so why bring in this self-reported, non-randomized, non-controlled study at all? The truth appears to be because this is the only study that lets them claim risks at a weight this low.

Far from finding any real risks at a BMI of 25, the Guidelines actually show this is the level of least risk. And for African-Americans, Native Americans, and older adults the point of lowest risk is shown to be even higher. This is especially true for women.

Two other reasons for selecting a BMI of 25, rather weakly offered by long-time proponent George Bray, MD, of the Pennington Biomedical Research Center are that, first, cutoff points of 25 and 30 are easy, and second, because others do it.[32] He fails to mention that some other countries do it because obesity experts worldwide are a small tight

network, all strongly influencing each other and fed by the same industry.[33]

False claims of effectiveness

The Guidelines define success as keeping off lost weight for only
one year.

This is meaningless, as the experts who set this criteria well know.
One of them complained to me it was because it's so hard to find longer
studies. Of course. Longer studies are embarrassing, so most researchers don't publish them.

We do have better definitions, so why not use them? Long-term
weight loss means keeping off lost weight for two years after the end
of any maintenance program, according to the Federal Trade Commission. The American Heart Association guidelines call for five years, and
say bluntly, "If there are no data to demonstrate that program participants maintain their weight losses for five years or more, there is no
scientific evidence of long-term results of the program."[34]

The NHLBI Guidelines recommend losing about one to two pounds
a week for six months, and then beginning a weight maintenance program. There is almost no chance this can work.

"No plan has demonstrated significant success in weight maintenance beyond 6 to 12 months," writes Ann Coulston, MS, RD, senior
research dietitian with the General Clinical Research Center at Stanford
University Medical Center.[35]

Putting a spin on prevention

The Guidelines also give us a new twist on obesity prevention. In
the real world, prevention involves three levels, primary, secondary and
tertiary. Goals are: at the primary level, to prevent excess weight in the
general population; at the secondary level, to prevent additional weight
gain and related risk factors for overweight persons; and at the tertiary
level, to treat obesity and its related problems.

The new spin brings failed obesity treatment in at the secondary
level. The Guidelines claim that secondary prevention includes "avoidance of weight regain following weight loss." This is not prevention, but
treatment. We should not confuse the two. Weight loss treatment is
responsible for its long-term results.

Combining maintenance with prevention serves the weight loss industry well, as it can continue to claim short-term success, while avoiding responsibility for maintenance. It puts honest prevention on hold,
once again. A sounder public health policy than we have in place today
would require weight loss therapy to prove long-term maintenance be-

fore any weight is lost, thus avoiding more weight cycling.

Guidelines promise harm

Unfortunately, the NHLBI Guidelines recommendations can do a great deal of harm, and there is no evidence they will benefit people in any lasting way.

If these new federal guidelines are followed and physicians instruct millions of already weight-obsessed Americans to lose weight, these are likely outcomes:

1. Many more people will be injured or die from hazardous attempts to lose weight.
2. Weight cycling and its risks will increase.
3. Eating disorders, binge eating, and dysfunctional and disturbed eating will increase.
4. Teenage girls and children will be most severely affected, with more disturbed eating patterns, undernourishment and malnourishment, stunted growth, arrested development, and fragile bones.
5. More women will limit their mental and physical potential by living in "starvation mode," with its attendant body shutdown and physical, intellectual, emotional, social, and spiritual costs.
6. More large patients will avoid or delay health care.
7. More people will begin smoking, and fewer smokers quit.
8. Health professionals, the media, and the public will continue to focus on weight, rather than health.
9. Media and advertising will increase the pressure on women to be extremely thin, and continue to promote female role models who are weak, passive, self-absorbed and vulnerable, with emphasis on appearance, rather than character, talent or achievement.
10. Prejudice will increase against people who do not conform to size standards.
11. Costs will rise (and industry will profit greatly), as FDA approves more diet drugs with only short-term safety and effectiveness data, and doctors prescribe more of these drugs.
12. Health insurance will be forced to pay for ineffective and potentially harmful treatments, as well as the resulting injuries, increasing health costs for everyone.
13. Preventive efforts will remain stalled.

It seems unlikely that many experienced physicians will follow the NHLBI Guidelines' advice. The six weight loss methods described have been in use for many decades and have often failed both patient and doctor. For those who do, the most likely result will be one more round of weight cycling — or as often happens, a ratcheting-up of the patients' weight even higher than before.

The Guidelines bring together valuable background information, but can hardly be helpful because they serve the failed goal of weight loss rather than improved health.

Entrepreneurs in quackery

The questionable and fraudulent segment is as much an integral part of the diet industry as are the big legitimate companies. Business is booming for these players — diet gurus, con artists, miracle pill entrepreneurs. Some make enormous profit in a short time with full-page ads sporting big bold headlines, extravagant promises, before-and-after photos and testimonials.

Why does the legitimate diet industry never speak out against this quackery and fraud? I've wondered that this industry with its disparate parts sticks so closely together, never criticizing, never plumbing each other's shadier aspects.

I suppose the scientific branches know that public faith is fragile, and fear to shake it. They may even like having the con artists out there — forever whipping up excitement, fantasy and hope. No doubt they gain fallout from this, and it makes a nice contrast to the crisp scientific stance.

Attempts at control

In 1990 Congress began the hearings Deception and Fraud in the Diet Industry. Chaired by Democratic Rep. Ron Wyden of Oregon, these hearings exposed many deceptive promotions, unfair business practices, lack of accountability, high failure rates, and injuries.[36]

Wyden charged that the industry provides "A new mix of questionable products, untrained providers and deceptive advertising, exposing our citizens to unexpected health risks."

Up until then, advertising was wide open, with diet companies large and small making extravagant promises. The three regulatory agencies — the FDA, in charge of content and false labeling; the Federal Trade Commission (FTC), in charge of regulating advertising and marketing; and the Postal Service, with authority to prevent using the mail for fraudulent purposes — investigated and eliminated, on a tedious case-by-case basis (as they still do), only the most fraudulent and dangerous of these products. Promoters found guilty often bounced back quickly with a new company name, a new twist on the product, sometimes an ownership transfer to a family member.

Before the hearings, the very low calorie diet companies made these kinds of claims: "The one that's clinically proven safe and effective" (Optifast/Sandoz); "You will not experience a rebound phenomenon after you attain your goal" (Medifast/Jason Pharmaceutical); "With the support of the *Ultrafast* Program (National Center), you get a new attitude. The weight stays off."

Now FTC took on these big guns. In 1992 and 1993 the agency charged 17 companies, including all the major commercial diet companies and weight loss centers, with making false and deceptive claims about safety and effectiveness. In addition to the above three, they charged Diet Center, Diet Workshop, Weight Watchers, Nutri/System, Physicians Weight Loss Centers, Jenny Craig, Beverly Hills Clinics, Doctors Medical Weight Loss Centers, Quick Weight Loss Centers, Formu-3 International, Abbott Laboratories, United Weight Control, Health Management Resources, and Pacific Medical Clinics.[37]

FTC obtained consent agreements that these companies would no longer make claims they could not back up with reliable studies. This has helped. Advertising claims are improved for all the big companies and many small supplement companies. However, numerous weasel words and creative spins are being used to fool the unwary.

In 1992, the FDA banned 111 diet pill ingredients, mostly herbals, after a review the agency had stalled for nearly 20 years.

FDA also agreed to review the safety and efficacy of PPA (phenylpropanolamine), approved for over-the-counter sales in 1979. Not so easy, as this took on powerful drug companies and products like Dexatrim, Accutrim, and Dex-A-Diet. Wyden repeatedly asked FDA to speed up this investigation, but in May 1993 he received a letter from Donna Shalala, Secretary of Health and Human Services, that he could expect more delays. They were still looking at the risk of stroke, she said. In the meantime, "The agency does not believe ... there is a basis for removing PPA from the marketplace while this additional information is being collected."[38] So the PPA review is stalled indefinitely.

In 1992, the NHLBI held an assessment conference to investigate Methods for Voluntary Weight Loss and Control. Conclusions were that there are few credible studies evaluating safety and effectiveness, that available studies indicate people tend to regain the weight they lose, and that weight loss strategies have caused medical harm.[39]

In 1997, another NHLBI conference report stated bluntly that, "Little information is available showing that intentional weight loss improves long-term health outcomes ... In fact, a growing number of critics in both the scientific community and the lay press are questioning whether obesity should be treated at all."[40]

In 1999 FTC announced its Partnership for Healthy Weight Management, bringing together a consumer, science and industry group, aimed at developing industry standards and educational messages for the public. It remains to be seen how compromises can be worked out with the industry in policing itself. I'm not optimistic from what I have seen of their compromises so far, yet I have some faith in FTC as an agency that took on the powerful and their high-priced lawyers before, and did not back down.

Women can refuse to be victims

The questions I keep asking are: Why does the government keep promoting failed diets? Why are undernourished and malnourished women and girls being so steadfastly ignored at federal levels? Why are eating disorders ignored?

And the answer that keeps surfacing is: because it serves the industry. Because women and girls who are dieting and dissatisfied with their bodies are important to the weight loss industry, and to those obesity specialists and federal officials who feed off them.

In 16 years of reviewing weight loss treatment programs worldwide, I've continually searched for the truth and often found it being manipulated and obscured. All of this pretense, deception, half-truths, misinformation, and manipulation of data gets in the way of solving urgent problems. As long as obesity experts and federal health officials insist that failed treatments are safe and effective, we are prevented from moving ahead. This keeps health providers confused and hoping, just as it does the public and the media.

As long as we have people in power in our institutions and federal agencies who are keeping up the fiction that obesity treatment is safe and effective, we can't move ahead in solving our critical weight and eating problems. We only move from one miracle cure that fails to the next, and progress is blocked.

It's time to confess we don't know the answers. Time to get serious about solving weight problems instead of letting weak or unethical leaders, a relentless diet industry, doctors who dispense "rainbow pills," exploitive advertisers and the media lead us into ever deeper trouble.

Do these people ever say, *I'm sorry,* to bereaved families? Children growing up without mothers? Disconsolate husbands? Bewildered parents?

I don't think so. They leave disaster in their wake and it rolls off them like a duck's back.

This is why women need to stop participating in all this, to refuse any longer to be the willing victims of this industry. We can say no.

PART II

CHAPTER 11

Health at any size

■

Health at any size is about wellness and wholeness,
eating in normal, healthy ways, and living actively. It's
about self-acceptance, self-respect, and appreciation
of diversity in others. Everyone qualifies!

It's time to move ahead with vision and direction, to focus in positive ways of living a healthy, happy lifestyle. This is an urgent challenge for America and countries around the world.

The old dieting mentality and its traditional ways of dealing with weight and eating have not worked. They need to be replaced by a new paradigm, a new and different world view, that helps people and does not harm them.

In the obsession with thinness that grips our culture today, many women are making their bodies their life's work. As they and others eat in increasingly disturbed ways, problems like overweight, eating disorders, and dysfunctional eating are increasing at alarming rates, and they are severely affecting children at younger and younger ages.

We can do better than this. As women we can live up to our rich potential as strong, capable, loving, generous individuals, and inspire others to do the same.

A new movement is emerging to deal with the weight and eating crisis in better ways. Leaders in this movement say it is time to throw out the old, failed weight-centered model, and move on to a new health-centered paradigm that helps people and does not harm them. This movement — health at any size — is coming into its own.

It's a movement that meets people where they are in their health journey. The World Health Organization describes health as a state of well-being, of feeling good about oneself, of optimum functioning, of the absence of disease, and of the control and reduction of both internal and external risk factors for both disease and negative health conditions. It's health at any size.

Nutrition and health leaders are saying that women everywhere are ready for a "health at any size revolution." The '60s gave us the civil rights movement; the '70s, feminist breakthroughs. And while the '80s and '90s brought a setback with weight obsession and woman as waif, contrasted with this came a remarkable cracking of the glass ceiling by stronger women. Entering the 21st century, women have broken through barriers and are ready for the health at any size revolution.

The goal of the new approach is to promote health and well-being, wellness and wholeness, for everyone of every size. It encourages people to eat well, live actively, and feel good about themselves and others.

A focus on health at any size sets women free. It frees women who have kept themselves thin, but limited, by living in starvation mode — and now understand they can move on to a more enriching life. It frees large women who have known society's scorn, have waited to be thin, and are ready to get on with their lives.

By contrast, the current control paradigm says: All bodies should be at an "ideal" weight and large people must lose weight to be healthy, even though they cannot do this in a healthy and lasting way.

The new approach recognizes the body cannot be shaped at will. It does not demand that women waste their lives trying to reshape their bodies into what someone else thinks would be ideal for them.

Women hold the key to moving ahead in refreshing ways. Women understand the problems of the old control paradigm well. They suffer its worst effects. And women see clearly its devastating effects on children, teenage girls, boys and men.

What we need to do is this: Consider the four eating and weight problems together as interrelated issues. We need to understand how they affect each other, and we need to be wary of the harm so easily done to vulnerable women and girls. Overweight, eating disorders, dysfunctional eating and size prejudice are not separate issues, they're all part of the same problem and they're all influenced by our unnatural obsession with thinness.

Understanding this helps us to realize we can't rush in to "fix" one problem without affecting, and perhaps intensifying, others. We can't diet without disturbing normal eating patterns — and once disturbed, normal eating patterns are not easily restored, even after the diet ends.

This new approach asks: How can we be healthier at the weight we are now? How can we gradually shift to healthier habits that will last a lifetime? How can we prevent eating and weight problems?

It rejects the false notion that all thin people are healthy and large people unhealthy. It reminds health professionals of the Hippocratic oath to "do no harm," recognizing that much harm has been done in trying to help large people lose weight.

Shifting from a weight-centered to a health-centered approach is a good way to begin.

Following these four guiding principles will help us make this shift:

1. **Eat well.** Eating well encompasses both healthy nutrition and normal eating patterns. Choosing foods from all five groups — fruits and vegetables, whole grains, meats and alternates, and milk products — ensures us of a balance of the many nutrients needed for health, energy, and our protective immune system. Eating in variety means enjoying many different foods and a variety of fruits and vegetables. When we eat moderately we avoid the disruption of extremes, neither overeating nor undereating, neither overindulging in high-fat, high-sugar foods nor fearing to eat these foods, which may be favorites and can certainly fit into a healthy diet.

   Normal eating means eating at regular times and responding to internal signals. If Americans would do this, we could prevent many of the eating and weight problems that plague our culture today. Normal eating enhances our feelings of well-being, promotes clear thinking and mood stability, and promotes stable weights, which appears to be the healthiest course for people of all sizes.

2. **Live actively.** Being active is the natural way for people to live, so enjoy physical activity, without being obsessive about it. Take pleasure in being active in your own way, every day, as a normal part of your life. Make fitness a family activity. Reject the notion that losing weight is a major reason for women to be active. It's not: engaging in regular activity is important for many reasons, only one of which is its beneficial effect on weight. Live actively because it's a great and wonderful way to live.

3. **Feel good about yourself.** You're okay just as you are, so respect, accept and trust yourself. You are unique, with your own special talents and traits, and this is a marvelous thing. If you've been waiting for thinness to get on with life, don't wait any longer but do it now. Free yourself to move on with health-centered changes that improve your life. Feel good about yourself, avoid negatives,

and keep up the positive self-talk.

4. **Feel good about others.** Respect and accept the people around you, and appreciate their size diversity. Be tolerant and nonjudgmental of appearances. Rise above prejudice. Insist on zero tolerance for size bias in school and the workplace. Each person needs acceptance, and deserves a sense of well-being, peace and tranquility. In the family, support those you love by making it unconditional, "I love you no matter what."

When you follow these guidelines you'll begin the shift from a focus on thinness to being healthy at the weight you are, physically and mentally. You'll put these issues into healthy perspective, and prevent eating and weight problems for yourself and your family.

Some people will lose weight when they make this shift. Others will stay the same weight, but they feel lighter once they lift the load of guilt and find self-acceptance. Still others who have kept themselves at an unnaturally low weight may gain a few pounds. Note that if you — or someone you know — are staying below your natural weight by keeping undernourished, in a starvation syndrome defensive mode, this is paying too high a price. You are sacrificing your unique self, your personality and your human potential.

Instead of struggling against our natural setpoint, we can recognize and work with it. A change in attitude toward acceptance can be very freeing. It liberates women from "waiting to be thin" or thinner, and helps them move on with health-centered changes that make life infinitely better. We need to throw out our reliance on the scale and the

---

Health at any size, the new health-centered paradigm

The health at any size approach helps prevent weight and eating problems through encouraging:

- Normal eating balanced by active living
- Normal growth for children, stable weight for adults
- Self-acceptance, self-respect and empowerment
- Respect, acceptance, and an appreciation of size diversity in others.

The new paradigm embraces the Canadian *Vitality* message:
Enjoy eating well, being active and feeling good about yourself.

WOMEN AFRAID TO EAT 2000

numbers on that scale.

In this way women can get on with their lives. Weight will tend to be stable as we keep regular eating and activity patterns, feel empowered, and stop weight cycling or waiting to be thin. The new paradigm recognizes that everyone, at every size, deserves a high quality of life, a sense of well-being, self-acceptance and self-respect. It includes an appreciation of size diversity, tolerance and respect for others, whatever their size or shape.

If you're a traditional thinker, making this mental shift may take time, so don't expect to do it overnight.

Defining healthy weight

Today many specialists are calling for a new, broader definition of healthy weight than set by the NHLBI Guidelines (body mass index of 18.5 to 24.5). It is clear factors other than BMI need to be considered.

Obesity is properly defined as excess body fat, according to most texts. The problem with arbitrarily designating a weight is that it does not allow for frame size or muscle. For example, a man with a BMI of 27 might have as little as 10 percent or as much as 31.7 percent body fat, according to researchers at Southern Illinois University.[1]

Defining a BMI of 25 and above as at risk includes huge numbers of individuals with low body fat, who are healthy and strong, who would not normally be called overweight and are in no way at risk. Athletes are a prime example.

Some experts say that obesity should be defined as the level at which health risks begin. This would differ for individuals, depending on their genetics, family history, culture, fat distribution, dieting history, lifestyle, and physical activity.

Others say healthy weight should be defined as the natural weight the body adopts, given a healthy diet and meaningful levels of physical activity.

Or should we define healthy weight at all? This may be a moot point — if, as current research suggests, and several studies confirm, weight is less relevant, after all, and it's fitness that counts most. Perhaps *healthy weight* has little more relevance than terms like *healthy age, healthy gender,* or *healthy nationality.* These denote very different concepts than healthy lipids, blood glucose levels, blood pressure, or even healthy nutrition or physical activity, factors which are critical to health.

Metabolic fitness is a term being proposed to take the place of a weight focus. Defined as the absence of any metabolic or biochemical risk factor for chronic diseases, its goals are reachable independent of weight loss.[2] It recognizes the good general health of many obese persons.

The relevant question, after all, is, "How can we be healthy at the weight we are?"

Shifting to health at any size

How can we make this shift? Health Canada has shown leadership with its Vitality public awareness campaign that gives this simple and eloquent advice: Eat well, live actively, and feel good about yourself. To this I like to add two words: and others.

Vitality is an integrated approach to healthy living that shifts the focus away from rigid goals, dieting and prescriptive exercise toward the acceptance of a range of body sizes and shapes and an emphasis on healthy eating, active living and positive self and body image. Vitality encourages us to be healthy at the weight we are, get on with life, and stop obsessing about weight. It's a message of preventing problems before they happen. It is also the basis for new treatment programs with its three-pronged approach of eating well, living actively and self-esteem.

The Vitality chart on the next page demonstrates this shift from a weight-centered to health-centered approach in eating, activity and self-image. Instead of dieting and counting points, women can move on to eating to satisfy hunger. They can enjoy a variety of foods, and trust their bodies. Instead of exercise prescriptions focused on burning calories, they will move ahead to living actively for the pleasure and health of it. From being obsessed with weight and dissatisfied with their bodies, women can move on appreciating themselves and others. This is the new paradigm of health at any size.

Some women embrace this new approach almost immediately with a refreshing enthusiasm. They've been immersed far too long in the weight-centered mode, and are more than ready to move on. For other women, the shift comes gradually. They may read about it, think it over, and slowly begin the process of change. It's like planting seeds that take time to sprout and flourish.

Others refuse to think about it: "I have to keep control of my eating. If I didn't diet, count calories, keep track of fat grams, I'd be totally out of control. I'd gain weight."

Yet the seeds are planted.

I've seen this process unfold many times in professional groups. The seeds lie dormant, then unexpectedly burst into life, grow, and bear the fruit of leadership.

The goal of the health at any size approach is the well-being of all people of all sizes and helping them to embrace their intellectual, physi-

The shift to *Vitality* from a weight centered approach

Weight centered approach	VITALITY
DIETING	**HEALTHY EATING**
• Restrictive eating	• Take pleasure in eating a variety of foods
• Counting calories, prescriptive diets	• Enjoy lower-fat, complex-carbohydrate foods more often
• Weight cycling (yo-yo diets)	• Meet the body's energy and nutrient needs through a lifetime of healthy, enjoyable eating
• Eating disorders	• Take control of how you eat by listening to your hunger cues
EXERCISE	**ACTIVE LIVING**
• No pain, no gain	• Value and practice activities that are moderate and fun
• Prescriptions such as three times a week in your target heart-rate zone	• Be active your way, every day
• Burn calories	• Participate for the joy of feeling your body move
• High attrition rates for exercise programs	• Enjoy physical activities as part of your daily lifestyle
DISSATISFACTION WITH SELF	**POSITIVE SELF/BODY IMAGE**
• Unrealistic goals for body size and shape	• Accept and recognize that healthy bodies come in a range of weights, shapes/sizes
• Obsession and preoccupation with weight	• Appreciate your strengths and abilities
• Fat phobia and discrimination against overweight people	• Be tolerant of a wide range of body sizes and shapes
• Striving to be a perfect "10" and to maintain an impossible "ideal" (thin or muscular) body size	• Relax and enjoy the unique characteristics you have to offer
• Accepting the fashion, diet and tobacco industries' emphasis on slimness	• Be critical of messages that focus on unrealistic thinness (in women) and muscularity (in men) as symbols of success and happiness

The VITALITY approach calls for a shift from negative to positive thinking about how to achieve and maintain healthy weight.[1]

VITALITY 1994/WOMEN AFRAID TO EAT 2000

cal, emotional, social and spiritual health. We can visualize this as in the Healthy People diagram on the facing page and the first chapter of this book.

To achieve the goal of healthy people of all sizes, we need consistent messages that encourage normal eating, active living, self respect and an appreciation of size diversity. If women and girls (as well as men and boys) receive these messages consistently from national health policy, health care providers, teachers, their family and the media, then I believe the four weight and eating problems will be diminished or prevented.

This is an approach that does no harm. Rather, the consistent effort acts on and responds to negative aspects of culture in positive and effective ways. It keeps a healthy perspective while challenging the detrimental effects of traditional thinking and health politics aimed at size alone.

We can help women shift out of the diet mentality, develop self respect, assertiveness, healthy coping skills, and learn to trust themselves. We can help them find their unique potential as lovable, capable, valuable individuals, so they take pride in themselves and their bodies at whatever size they are.

This approach shifts the focus away from thinness to being healthy, active, and well-nourished at our natural or normal weight. This is within everyone's reach.

Canada's *Vitality* program puts it this way: "To overcome the influence of a media-dominated culture that judges women on how they look, we must encourage women to accept a wide range of healthy body weights and shapes, to love their bodies as they are, to value slimness only as it relates to overall health, to refrain from dieting and to reject societal pressures to conform to an unrealistic body size. In doing so, women will improve their self-images and be more realistic in their assessment of body image.

"One of the results of living in a thinness culture is the belief that health is improved with weight loss and achieving a low body weight. This basic assumption has been challenged and the negative effects of dieting and weight cycling are now being examined closely.

"While a reduction in weight will improve the health of some overweight people, a fixation on weight reduction and ideal body shape can lead to yo-yo dieting, weight cycling, restrictive eating, obsessive exercising and negative perceptions of body image. Furthermore, pursuit of a rigid standard for size and shape inevitably fails for most people over the long term."[3]

The health-centered approach grows out of the nondiet movement,

Healthy people

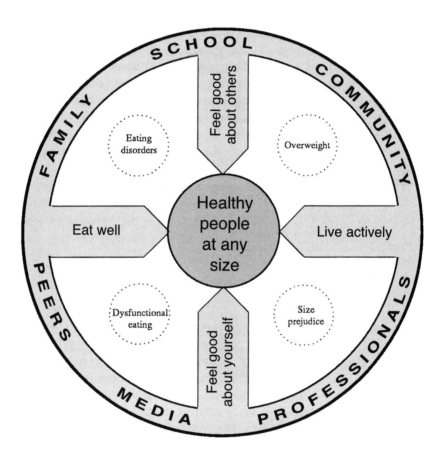

To achieve the goal of healthy people at any size, a comprehensive health approach is needed, whereby all receive consistent messages that encourage eating well, living actively, and feeling good about yourself and others. If family, teachers, health professionals, peers and the media consistently give these messages, then the four major weight and eating problems (dysfunctional eating, eating disorders, overweight and size prejudice) will be diminished.

led by nutrition specialists who reject the traditional thinking that everyone should be thin and large people should always be trying to lose weight, and instead advocate normal eating, active lifestyles, and stable weight.

The new health paradigm unites the work of visionary leaders from many fields: nutrition, eating disorders, medicine, exercise science, obesity, psychology, size acceptance and others. It is research based and practical.

Most nutritionists and dietitians now seem to accept the new paradigm, to at least some extent. They are among the first professionals to revise their traditional role in weight loss treatment. The new thinking is now reflected in policy decisions of the Society for Nutrition Education, which has a special Weight Realities division that explores these issues. It is widely accepted in Canadian nutrition and dietetics groups, and is reflected in American Dietetic Association position papers.

This is no new radical approach to living. The concept of health at any size is natural, nurturing, and wholesome. It recalls a time before this debilitating thinness obsession began, perhaps the 1950s when war-weary citizens were happy to nourish themselves and their children, and only yearned to do it better, and the early 1960s, when wellness and healthy lifestyle meant well-being, being your best self, not thinness for its own sake.

Yet, there is an important difference from that earlier time: Women now have a freedom to be themselves that they never had before. Women are empowered to be at their personal best if they choose, without constraints on how they "should" look, or act, or what "their place" should be. Women need no longer be treated as objects, someone's playthings, if they are willing to shake loose from these constraints. Women do have the power to accept the truth and lead others to health at any size.

Research supports the health-centered approach

Research confirms the wisdom of this new approach. Good health is associated with a positive attitude, optimism, healthy lifestyle and fitness, rather than weight loss, "ideal" weight, and worry.

There's a great deal of scientific evidence that shows health is improved when people feel good about themselves and have a positive outlook. In fact, people who expect to be well generally are. Having an optimistic attitude predicts better health and survival 20 or 30 years later.

We are far more resilient and capable of managing our health than medicine has given us credit for, say Robert Ornstein, PhD, and David

Sobel, MD, in *Healthy Pleasures*. They cite much research that shows keeping a positive mood and feeling good about life helps us live longer, healthier lives. "The human organism is not a helpless, defenseless victim attacked at every turn by agents of disease, whether germs or stressors. We resist breakdown and disease through a remarkable internal health maintenance system regulated by the brain. The essential link is a pleasure-presuming frame of mind and a healthy capacity for sensual enjoyment."

Optimism and feeling good about ourselves seems to guard our immune system. In one study cited by Ornstein and Sobel, the attitudes of patients about to undergo a coronary bypass were measured before the operation. Those with more hopeful, positive attitudes showed fewer complications during surgery, and less evidence of heart muscle damage. They also recovered more quickly, sat up in bed sooner, and were able to walk around the room earlier. The patients who expected an improved quality of life tended to get just what they expected.[4]

Another study of patients with advanced breast and skin cancer found that a joyful attitude and optimistic attitude were the strongest psychological predictors of how long they would remain cancer-free.[5]

A Canadian study asked 3,500 older men and women about the state of their health. Those who rated their health as excellent were almost three times less likely to die during the next seven years as those who rated their health as poor. Yet many who viewed themselves as healthy had doctors who turned in negative reports on their health, and many whose doctors found them healthy said their health was only fair or poor. The patients' perception proved more accurate in predicting death than did the medical testing of their doctors.[6]

Optimists expect good things to happen, and they usually do.

What does this mean for perfectly healthy large people who are continually being told by our health authorities that they are at risk? Do they start to believe it and make it a self-fulfilling prophecy? There is no justification whatever for this treatment. It's barbaric, false, and needs to end.

There's much evidence that keeping a stable weight through adult life is healthy for women and men of all sizes, and that large people can be very healthy, of course. The risks of overweight have been greatly exaggerated, and the risks of underweight and losing weight minimized.

Recent research shows fitness to be more important than weight in good health and longevity. Steven Blair and his colleagues at the Cooper Institute for Aerobics Research in Dallas studied 22,000 men for 18 years, and found it was lack of fitness, not weight, that was linked to mortality, illness, and functional limitations. Fit men outlived those with lower levels of fitness, regardless of weight. And fit obese men lived just as long as fit lean men. Their studies show similar results for women.[7]

People come in a range of sizes. Some are naturally short, others tall, and most somewhere between. If you graph it, it makes a nice bell curve. Similarly, some people are naturally thin, some naturally large, and most in between.

And that's okay. It's not true that thinner people are healthier, even though some of our health leaders seem to think so. This is a false belief. Fit people are healthier at any size.

The opposing debate

Arguments against health at any size focus on the concern that if the public is allowed to lose its fear of fat and accept size diversity, we'll see a tremendous increase in overweight, which is already on the rise. Another argument is that the public needs to keep believing in current ineffective obesity treatments because someday there will be drugs that work and people must be kept in a mood to take them. Then, there's fear the weight loss industry may be damaged by a more open approach. Finally, some obesity specialists say publicly that eating disorders can be discounted because they affect so few people.

These are weak arguments based on fallacies, not research or reality. First, the fear of fat has not prevented obesity. On the contrary, it may have made weight problems worse during the last three decades by causing increasingly dysfunctional eating and even more weight cycling. Second, people will recognize and respond to honesty in an area where they have so often been deceived. It is untrue that the health-centered approach opposes reliable obesity treatment. Rather, when such treatments become available and are proven long-term safe, effective and health-promoting, they will fit into this sound, healthy approach, and size-accepting people will certainly use them when appropriate. Third, yes, there may indeed be loss of profits for weight loss companies, but those willing to develop sound lifestyle programs based on health at any size can benefit. Fourth, eating disorders are not insignificant. They affect an estimated 10 percent of young people with death rates as high as 18 to 20 percent for anorexia and bulimia. This is much higher incidence and higher risk than many diseases that get far more attention.

A better vision for women

Working together and supported by a health-centered policy that deals with size, weight and eating issues, we can bring about the healthy change needed for our future.

As we search individually for answers, it is helpful to keep a balanced perspective. We need to remember that weight, eating and health are only part of what makes life worthwhile. Wellness and wholeness are not about attaining perfect health or longevity as ends in themselves, but about improving the quality of life, so we can each accomplish what we want, and live well emotionally, intellectually, physically, socially and spiritually.

In the family, caring parents and significant individuals who understand the issues set the stage with unconditional love and acceptance, no matter what, from infancy on. They give reassurance that every child and every adult is okay, just as she is, and they model and teach normal eating, active living and a positive outlook on life.

Schools and colleges provide the intellectually stimulating environment needed for learning when they are accepting and safe — safe from emotional violence, harassment and bullying, as well as from physical violence or sexual abuse. And students, in turn, gain most from the academic process when they are well nourished, with minds ready to learn, not focused on food, hunger, weight or appearance.

As women embrace this new approach, they make changes in five major areas: attitude, lifestyle, prevention, health care and knowledge. Shifting toward a health-centered approach in these areas furthers the goal of healthy people of all sizes. It sets people free and helps them live happy, productive, fulfilling lives.

All women can join in, and provide leadership in this health at any size revolution. This is a cause that allows us and those we love to enjoy life as it was meant to be.

I like the poster in my dentist's office that says, "One person can make a difference — two or three can make a miracle!" I really believe this, that you and I can make a difference, all alone, wherever we are — and that working together, we can make a miracle!

"Never doubt that a handful of committed citizens can truly change the world," said anthropologist Margaret Mead.

Together we can change the world.

CHAPTER 12

It's about you

■

Our healer within continually guides us in self-acceptance, self-love, intuition and wisdom, if we let it do its healing.

You're okay just as you are.

You're a unique person, capable and loveable, with special talents and traits, and this is a marvelous thing. No need to work on perfecting yourself. In fact, it can be self-defeating. It keeps a person locked in the anticipation trap, waiting and hoping to be "better."

Many women who struggle with eating, weight, and body image spend inordinate amounts of time and energy trying to improve themselves. They believe they must be perfect, or at least much closer to it in how they look, what they say, how they feel, and what they do. They hate what they consider their flaws, and invest great amounts of time in trying to fix those flaws. But fixing one thing is never good enough. It only leads to more striving.

Having flaws is not a reflection on who we are. A flaw is not a secret shame — it's just part of being human.

It's been said that "women need to stop renovating their bodies and move in."

Your body is okay. Your size is okay.

In their book *When Women Stop Hating Their Bodies*, Jane Hirschmann and Carol Munter urge women to stop trying to measure up to society's standards of female beauty, which are "ridiculous and impossible." Instead, they insist, women need to look in the mirror and like what they see. We need to accept our bodies, our feelings, and ourselves unconditionally.[1]

Some women really feel "they are supposed to hate their bodies because they don't fit the ideal," says Memphis dietitian Millicent Lasslo-Meeks. "When you introduce them to this new paradigm (nondiet, self-acceptance, health at any size) a light bulb comes on, and they feel a new freedom that someone said it was okay to be the way they are."

The good news is that you can change how you feel about your body without changing your body or looks. Just change your opinion.

Accept that your body has a setpoint that affects your size and weight. Get comfortable with the real you, inside and out. Your weight is not a measure of your self-worth. What you are is much greater than this. Recognize how destructive is the obsession with being thin, and how it affects others around you, especially children.

Choose self-care

Ask yourself: "Can I accept myself as a well-nourished person at what seems to be my natural weight? Am I willing to stop focusing on weight, stay out of the starvation mode, keep a stable weight, and get on with my life?"

If the answer to both questions is "Yes," you're well on your way to healthy self-care. If not, you may want to work on some body distortions. Keep your body well-nourished and it will work for you, helping you achieve what you want and deserve in life.

It's time for self-acceptance. Time for healing. So take time for self-care. We need to respond to our healer within, while reining in our inner critic.

Self-care involves wellness, wholeness, and well-being, a balance of physical, intellectual, emotional, social, and spiritual health. It means investing in small things that increase your well-being, reduce stress, and enrich life: a nourishing meal, a phone call to a friend, reading to a child, a nap after lunch, a stretch break at your desk, laughter with your spouse or best friend, taking time to enjoy a sunset, the pleasures of smells, tastes and sounds.[2]

The airline attendant giving emergency instructions on every flight tells passengers to first secure their own oxygen masks before trying to help others. It's a simple truth: we need to take care of our own needs first, before we can be fully helpful to others.

The steps to self-care are:

1. Listen to yourself and learn what fills you.
2. Take action to care for yourself. Do something that fills your

needs; don't wait for someone else to do it for you.

"You may need excitement, freedom, laughter, tenderness, or seren-ity ... But you can't fill yourself until you know what you need," say Donald Tubesing, PhD, and Nancy Loving Tubesing, EdD, in *Seeking Your Healthy Balance*[3].

To attend to self-care we need to stop trying to be perfect.

The fact is you won't ever be perfect, no matter how hard you try. No one will. We could probably engage a retinue of plastic surgeons to make us look more perfect on the outside, but it still wouldn't be enough. Do you really care?

The problem is, the "fixing what's wrong" approach is misguided. It emphasizes what is not good enough, rather than celebrating what's great.

We're not in a contest, but life. Since this is the only life we'll have on this earth, it makes sense to live it with joy and relish. Not as a perfect object for others to admire, but as human beings of value, worthy of respect and acceptance from ourselves and others.

Set aside time each day for yourself. This is a self-care time; give yourself permission to take it.

Many women set standards for themselves that are unrealistically high and impossible to attain. They even may insist that others meet these expectations, imposing impossible standards, and causing anger and stress, especially for family members.

Perfection is a myth. It doesn't exist in the real world where we live.

Instead of focusing on your flaws, honor and respect yourself by accepting your emotional and mental self. You'll find it's a relief to finally give up a judgmental attitude and accept yourself just as you are.

Tools for creative change

We each carry around two powerful instruments that can bring about positive, creative change in our lives:

- Images, the pictures we carry in our heads.
- Self-talk, the inner dialogue that goes on in our heads all day long.

Together these pictures and words send a powerful message to the subconscious of who we are and what we can or can't do. They determine the course of our lives. With these instruments we can change our beliefs and lifestyle habits.

Positive images and self-talk can be fine-tuned and improved upon; they can replace negative thoughts.

They're like seeds planted in a garden. When we plant good seeds and tend them well, they produce abundant harvest. But if we plant infertile seeds, or allow weeds to flourish, the harvest will be a mixed bag.

We can also think of the subconscious mind as a computer. If we program in good information, we get good results. If not, it's "garbage in, garbage out."

Make sure you plant good seeds in your subconscious; program in positive, helpful information.

Get over any sense you may have of not being good enough.

Where did these messages come from?

Many parents give their children strong, confident, helpful self-images and self-talk messages that translate as, "I am loveable and capable. I can get along fine just as I am."

But some parents give children negative labels that stick with them all their lives, reminding them what they lack, what they are not able to do. It can be a self-fulfilling prophecy as they live out these predictions.

Fortunately, we're not stuck with childhood scripts going through our heads. We can program in new messages that tell us what we want to hear.

Eric Berne, author of *Games People Play*, has called the way we view things and respond to them as our script or story. It's as if we are each acting out a play and dutifully following the script as written. But Berne says we can change our script if we choose. We just need to rewrite the story ending the way we want it.[4]

When you change your mental image and rewrite the self-talk, the entire story of your life is changed. You are free to do this, to take a new course.

Here's how you can put your subconscious to work with both imaging and self-talk.

First, visualize yourself acting confidently and successfully in the many ways you live actively, eat well, feel good about yourself and others.

Second, write and program in the self-talk sentences that affirm your success and pleasure in living positively.

Set yourself up for success. When you want to change a habit, break it down into smaller parts and work on one segment at a time. Begin with one small step that you're sure you can achieve.

Visualizing

What we picture in our mind's eye has a big effect on our feelings.

You can transform your body image by learning to visualize it more accurately and more attractively. Thoughts can change the images you see in your mind.

Begin with a mental picture or vision of one thing you want to happen.

One way is to relax and visualize. Relax completely. Close your eyes, and picture exactly what it is that you want to do. You might see yourself walking down a country lane, enjoying the fresh spring air. You may watch yourself walking into a room, meeting friends and strangers assertively, feeling easy and confident about yourself.

Visualize yourself doing this one thing successfully and joyfully. If the end result is not clear, keep working on the mental pictures until you get a clear, precise image. Keep that vision in mind, and repeat the process over several days or weeks until the scene comes easily to mind.

The mental pictures you keep in mind have a profound effect on what really happens.

The power of mental imagery is being used to improve athletic skills. A skater may first imagine herself doing a perfect spin, and then follow through with a flawless performance.

In one study, a group of students practiced shooting basketball free throws for 20 minutes every day for 20 days. A second group of students did not practice or even touch a basketball, but spent 20 minutes every day imagining shooting free throws; when they missed their mental shots, they imagined correcting their aim so the ball shot straight into the basket. Testing at the end showed the second group, which practiced only in their imaginations, had almost identical scores with the first group; both improved their free throw scores by about 24 percent. A control group did not improve.[5]

A noted Dutch piano teacher advises his students to practice the piano in their heads. Any new piece, he maintains, should first be studied, memorized, and played in the mind, before the pianist ever touches the keyboard.

Instead of trying so hard to act just right, and worrying about all the things that can go wrong, Maxwell Maltz, MD, in his book *Psycho-Cybernetics* urges people to rely on winning mental pictures.[6]

He says when we mentally picture the desired end, we are forced to use positive thinking. Our creative success mechanism takes over, and our subconscious mind works at making it happen. The brain and body make up a highly complex machine that is constantly trying to reach the target we have set for it. This machine only needs us to define that goal clearly, program in appropriate self-talk, and it will take us to that goal.

Sweet-talking

How do you talk to you *about you*? Is it respectful, considerate of your feelings?

Self-talk consists of the thoughts and conversations that go on in your head. It's like a cassette tape that runs all day long.

These internal dialogues, or conversations of our minds, require no conscious thought at all. This has both advantages and disadvantages. It helps us effortlessly do several things at once without really thinking about them, such as driving a car or brushing our teeth. It keeps what we do consistent with our belief system, and if our beliefs are positive, our self-talk will be, too. But it can also keep us in a negative groove.

Research confirms that how we talk to ourselves in our internal dialogues can have a powerful effect on how we feel and act.

If you want to check your self-talk right now, look in the mirror. Listen to what you are saying. Is it, "I look pretty nice today," or "Oh, I look terrible, I can't go out!"?

Get rid of *too* thinking: *My hips are too big;* and *wishful* thinking, *I wish I had a beautiful complexion.*

While you are in a relaxed state, program in some positive self-talk messages. Clinical psychologist Stephen Timm, PhD, of Fargo, N.D., calls this sweet-talking. Add the sweet-talking words to visual pictures, he says.

If your self-talk tends to be filled with *shoulds, musts, oughts,* take them all out. Instead of telling yourself: *I should start exercising; I should write a letter to Aunt Sue,* change the self-talk to, *I can start exercising if I choose to; I can write a letter to Aunt Sue if I choose to."*

This gives us a feeling of empowerment and personal freedom. We know we can do these things, and we are asserting our freedom to do them or not, as we choose.

Keep on sweet talking — and don't allow scolding, or guilt trips to creep into your private internal conversation.

Dale Carnegie, author of *How to Win Friends and Influence People*, was a great believer in promoting positive self-talk and banishing negative thoughts.

He wrote, "If we think happy thoughts, we will be happy. If we think miserable thoughts, we will be miserable. If we think fear thoughts, we will be fearful. If we think sickly thoughts, we will probably be ill. If we think failure, we will certainly fail. If we wallow in self-pity, everyone will want to shun us and avoid us."[7]

Your belief system can be changed by self-talk, as well as the other way around. The positive beliefs you create from positive self-talk create higher self-esteem and self-worth.

Some call these statements affirmations.

Affirmations

Affirmations are positive self-statements that can effectively change your beliefs.

Write down the self-talk you'd like your subconscious to process: positive self-statements that affirm you are strong, capable, loveable, and free to make your own choices.

These may focus on self-acceptance, feelings, body-image, making mistakes:

"I accept how I'm feeling right now"

"I accept and enjoy my body the way it is today."

"I made a mistake and I'm still okay."

"I'm the same person no matter who I'm standing next to."

"My body is healthy and comfortable."

"My body deserves appreciation for all the things it does. These are great legs. Look where they've taken me — they get me wherever I want to go. Great hips. Great stomach that takes what I give it or don't, with almost no complaint. These hands — what they can do! My eyes — how wonderfully they work for me. My smile — it's nice how this smile can warm those I love."

Create affirmations that allow you to accept your flaws, without belittling or rejecting yourself.

Write your affirmations on sticky notes in various locations, and repeat them several times every day. Memorize these messages and keep repeating them to yourself. Give them time to work. Some people record their statements, repeated five or six times, in their own or another's voice, and listen at least once a day for three or four months, until they come naturally and easily to mind.

When the old tape begins to run in your head, just punch the eject button. Say *stop* and insert your new tape. This takes practice and persistence — because the old tape is on automatic start, and doesn't shut off, but just keeps on running unless you eject it.

Your new self-talk messages will get stronger and more persuasive the more you use them.

Carnegie said that he had many times seen people transform themselves in this way, by changing their thoughts. "I know men and women can banish worry, fear and various kinds of illnesses, and can transform their lives by changing their thoughts. I know! I have seen such incredible transformations performed hundreds of times. I have seen them so often that I no longer wonder at them."

Be your own best friend. Keep your mind working for you with positive images and positive self-talk.

Changing distorted thinking

If you feel a strong sense of body-hatred or dissatisfaction with yourself, you may want to work on changing these distortions.

Visualizing and self-talk are powerful tools that can help change aspects of life that are not working for you. They can heal the past, help you view the world through more positive and realistic beliefs. It's a winning cycle — these tools can change beliefs, and new beliefs can change them.

To overcome perfectionism, self-criticism, and body dissatisfaction, we need to alter our beliefs and thoughts. Many upsetting thoughts and beliefs are simply bad habits. They can be examined, disputed, and replaced by positive habits.

The first step in changing negative and self-destructive beliefs, as recommended by psychologists, is to listen to the internal dialogue, and become aware of those critical self-statements. Write them down and think about their meaning and exaggerations. Identify the thoughts and feelings you'd like to change. Begin with an easy problem, or one that interferes most in your life.

Next, develop those positive statements and other ways of viewing the situation which are nonjudgmental, forceful, and more compassionate of the self. Practice substituting these for the negative thoughts. Repeat over and over. The subconscious will take all this to heart and adjust your beliefs to fit. They will be believed, and the habit can be changed.[8]

Allow yourself to experience and acknowledge your full range of feelings: anger, resentment, excitement, anxiety, worry, despair, disappointment, sadness, joy, affection, arousal, love. This takes the fear and anxiety out of negative feelings, makes them less threatening, and opens the door to compassion for the self.

Don and Nancy Tubesing say it's tempting to want to screen out "bad" feelings and recognize only the "good" feelings. But when we do this, they often go underground only to burst out at some other time and place.

Emotional health requires an awareness of these feelings, but they remind us we needn't be at the mercy of our bodily sensations and emotional impulses. "Angry feelings can be experienced without being expressed directly or destructively. Sexual attraction can be enjoyed without being indulged ... Feelings are controlled by our mind, not by external events."

The Tubesings suggest that people stretch their feeling capacity — find the vocabulary to express just what you are feeling and acknowledge it. Then look for the silver linings. Choose to be positive and laugh rather than complain. "Love and thankfulness will open your life and fill it with vitality and healing. A positive, hopeful, open attitude will fill us with warmth... Obsession with hate and revenge erodes our bodies, our minds, and our spirits — not to mention our relationships with others."

Instead of giving in to body-hatred, consider the good things about each body part: These are good, strong legs and hips that take me wherever I want to go.

Psychologist Thomas Cash suggests using mental imagery to desensitize negative feelings about your body.

He advises that, while in a state of pleasant relaxation, you first picture an area of your body you find satisfactory. Imagine this part clearly for about 15 seconds, being aware of how you feel. Return to total relaxation for 30 seconds, and again clearly imagine this body area. After a third time focusing on the area, move on to another body part and repeat the process. Continue your mental examination, from body parts you like to those less liked, while keeping relaxed, and just being aware of how you feel, and accepting these feelings. This may take several days. Repeat several times. This process weakens the connection between your negative feelings and your mental images of your body.

"You actively use your relaxation skills to maintain feelings of calm and contentment and to melt away any feelings of tension, distress, or discontent," says Cash.[9]

Many women are making their bodies their life's work. Is this a worthy project for you? Do you want to spend your life's energy this way?

Bodylove

The healing antidote for body dissatisfaction is body love, an aura of positive emotions, attitudes and actions.

"Bodylove has little to do with how you actually look," says Rita Freedman. "It's not beauty, but self-esteem that builds bodylove. That's because body image is quite independent of physical appearance."[10]

Hirschmann and Munter suggest carrying on a gentle and sympathetic conversation with each body part that concerns you, until you can resolve your feelings about it. Writing both sides of the discussion might go like this:

Mary: My stomach is disgusting. I hate it. I think it's grotesque.

Mary's stomach: I am a baby place. I gave you children. I deserve

Loving your body

Loving your body is hard in our fat-phobic, diet-obsessed world, but it is worth every ounce of effort that you put into it. It means accepting the diversity of human bodies. It means recognizing that no one should be discriminated against because of the shape her or his skin. Appreciating your body means learning to celebrate your unique abilities, and finally making friends with the mirror on the wall.

💜 Throw away the scale. Focus on fitness and weigh yourself only when medically necessary. Even then, you can choose to ignore the number if you want.

💜 Reject fat prejudice in yourself and in others. Recognize that healthy, beautiful bodies come in all shapes, sizes, and weights.

💜 Invest time and money in yourself rather than the diet industry. Spend your money on beautiful clothes, jewelry, haircuts, manicures and massages — not on diets.

💜 Surround yourself with size-friendly people. Choose friends, therapists and doctors who accept you the way you are and support the lifestyle changes you want to make.

💜 Stand tall and proud. Straighten your shoulders and your stance. Feel energy, strength and confidence flow from your head to your toes.

💜 Put your mind in touch with your body. To heighten your confidence and body awareness, check out yoga, walking meditation, t'ai chi, or movement therapy.

💜 Clothe your body in beautiful, comfortable clothes that fit now. Search out stores and catalogs that cater to people of your size, shape and fashion style.

💜 Join groups that promote size esteem. Look for local and national organizations that provide resources and support the natural diversity of sizes and shapes.

💜 Read magazines that feature women of all sizes and shapes doing a variety of activities.

💜 Be patient with yourself. Old habits die hard and changes may take a while to become permanent fixtures in your thoughts and in your life.

By Dayle Hayes, MS, RD, Billings, Mont. Reprinted with permission. Copyright 1999.[1]

respect.

Mary: I've never thought of that before. I've always hated you so much.

Mary's stomach: But not when the babies were in me. Then we were friends.

Mary: You're right. I'm truly sorry. I'll try to remember.

Their cure for body bashing is to legalize one's body, give up false hopes, give up the disguise that hides real concerns and anxieties, give up misdirected anger, give up mother bashing, give up the sisterhood of fat talk, give up self-punishment for secret crimes, and move beyond these losses to self-care. They urge women to have the courage to feel deeply, think independently, solve problems and let go of them, face up to disappointment, speak up, and move on. It's all part of befriending one's own body.

Journaling can be another technique to improve your relations with yourself. Keep a journal of all the joys and gratitude in your life, along with exploring your thoughts and feelings.

Cash suggests writing a letter to "Dear Body of Mine," that begins this way: "I want to begin by saying I'm sorry. I've owed you an apology for a long time. I've been unfairly critical of you over the years"; and ends by saying, "I'm working on being less critical of you and on our doing more fun things together. I'm feeling better about me by being nicer to you. Thanks!"

In today's popular culture the female perfection that many strive for is to be thin, young and beautiful. Thin means long, bony legs and long, bony arms. Fashion photographers may call this look "great bones," but osteoporosis specialists see a future of weak and brittle bones, stress fractures, and collapsed spines. An obsession with youth may keep us from gaining the rich benefits of maturity. Thus, what some women strive for is a false goal, which needs to be examined and discarded.

If you can't quite give up that goal of weight loss and there's a new method that has your friends and local physicians dizzy with excitement — my best advice is to wait two years. Wait two years after your friends are dropping weight, and doctors are delighted their treatment is working so well, and newspapers are featuring photos of husbands and wives gleefully standing inside one trouser leg and holding out the excess before them.

Wait another two years after all this. Watch what happens to these people in 12, 18, and 24 months. By then you'll know the truth, and so will they, likely to their chagrin. Yes, of course, you're in a hurry, but you do have time to wait.

This has proved to be good advice for all of the last 15 years I've offered it. It has saved emotional turmoil, time and energy, money, the risks of weight cycling, and I believe it has saved lives. People who waited to take the fen-phen/Redux pills are tremendously glad they waited. So are those who awaited long-term success for the very low calorie liquid diets. Remember that any method works short-term, and none works long-term. And that's the truth.

Remember that keeping a stable weight is a reasonable and healthy goal (allowing for some gain at midlife).

If you can't bear to wait two years, can hardly wait till Monday to start that new diet you saw in a magazine, may I suggest a six-month break? If you've been a chronic dieter, take a few months off to live more normally, enjoy your world, welcome your family back into your circle, find a more worthwhile purpose in life, recover your sense of humor, laugh, live well, accept yourself wholeheartedly, and accept others. You may never go back.

The healer within

Psychologist Deirdra Price, PhD, says that our self is made up of the healer, the critic, the child, and the adolescent.

Our healer within believes we're okay just as we are. This healer continually guides us in self-acceptance, a sense of self-love, intuition and wisdom, if we let it do its healing.

Listen to this voice, says Price in her book *Healing the Hungry Self*. "The healer gives many suggestions and words of encouragement ... is compassionate and patient. Sometimes it takes listening closely, especially when working through negative beliefs and critical thinking ... Listen beyond the critical messages. A subtle thought will bubble up. This is the healer offering helpful guidance."[11]

But it's hard to hear the healer if you've let the critic take over too often, loudly enforcing negative beliefs. Dieting promotes these negative beliefs that we're not okay. If we let it, the critic is ever ready with a barrage of negative messages: "My thighs are too big," "I'm unloveable," "I can't make a mistake," "I must please everyone."

These are beliefs, and beliefs can be changed. We need to deal assertively with the critic, discount those negative beliefs, and strengthen beliefs that support the healer.

Our belief system comes from childhood and adolescence when we had both pleasure and pain, according to Price. Wounding experiences told the child she was inadequate in some way, and this brought pain and shame. Shame is easier to bear than pain, so the pain gets buried, while shame continues to be felt through life.

"The way to release shame is to go back to the shaming situation, visualize it, then give it back to the people who gave it to you in the first place (your parents or other significant persons). You process and release the feelings ... in your imagination, feeling whatever comes up and seeing yourself express your feelings," says Price.

You can imagine a different outcome for painful experiences. Create a different ending in your mind.

Want what you have

Contentment is seldom taught today, yet being content has long been advised in world religions and philosophy. Learning contentment can help women overcome the drive to perfect their bodies.

The secret to happiness is not to get what you want, but to want what you have, insists Timothy Miller, PhD. In his book *Wanting What You Have*, he says that a lifetime craving things you don't have, and may never have, harms your quality of life as well as quality of life for the people around you. Realizing how much you already have brings true happiness. Don't put happiness on hold.

We can learn contentment by being more compassionate, attentive, and grateful, Miller advises. These are traits that can help us feel good and add to life's joy. Compassionate habits of thought recognize how unique and important is each person, and they also include compassion for ourselves, giving up harsh judgments about ourselves, our feelings, and mistakes we've made. Being grateful celebrates the many good things we already possess, and helps us enjoy the small pleasures of life, while working through any anger or resentment.[12]

Attentive habits keep us in the present moment, the here and now. They prevent us from playing the useless anticipation game — in which women keep hoping and believing that *someday* they'll get what they are after, and be free of problems, failure and pain. They stop us from brooding about the past and worrying over the future. We can bloom where we're planted.

Miller assures us that "Life's magic and grandeur are not located in the future or in an alternate reality — they're right here, right now."

Price notes that the diet mentality keeps women stuck in the anticipation trap.

"Practice living in the moment by consciously redirecting your attention back to what is happening right now," she advises.

Learn relaxation techniques

It's easier to tune in to body sensations and signals when we are relaxed. Relaxation is also a way of self-care.

Learning to relax gives a woman a sense of balance and enhances her life. It's like re-booting a stressed-out computer. Everything works better afterward.

Stress is a real physical reaction that sends adrenalin and other stress hormones into the blood stream, causing the heart to beat faster and blood pressure to rise as arteries constrict and direct blood to the brain and vital organs. The body gears up for "flight or fight." But if there's no release, no physical exertion, the pressure continues to build inside. Chronically high levels of stress chemicals can keep blood pressure and heart rates dangerously high. This stress overload is linked to such problems as exhaustion, insomnia, headache, diarrhea, anxiety, restlessness, depression, abuse of alcohol, increased risk of heart attack, and weakened immune system.

Relaxation has a positive effect on this stress overload.

One popular method to relax and relieve tension is progressive relaxation. The technique is to first take several deep breaths. Deep, slow breathing enhances your sense of control and deepens relaxation. Then tense and relax each body part slowly and progressively, from your toes up to your shoulders, out to your fingertips, and up to your forehead.

Another method is to simply let your body go limp for one minute several times a day.

You might make or purchase your own relaxation tape.

One of the best ways to relieve stress is to exercise, work it off; run, walk, play tennis or shoot baskets. This is the "fight or flight" reaction your body has geared up for and wants.

Other tension-relieving tactics are to sing, laugh, cry, take a nap, listen to music, talk it out with someone you can confide in, hug a friend, play with children, pet your dog, and just let go of those worries and anxieties.

Live assertively

An assertive state of mind will give you a sense of freedom. Your efforts to live assertively are very worthwhile and rewarding.

Assertiveness allows a woman to express her honest feelings, thoughts, beliefs, and opinions comfortably, to be direct and straightforward, and to obtain her personal rights without denying the rights of others and without experiencing undue anxiety or guilt.

The assertive woman respects herself, speaks calmly and clearly, maintains eye contact, projects her voice, and smiles sincerely when she means it. She avoids disclaiming or minimizing her feelings or statements. In conflict situations she finds it better to use "I" statements, such as "I feel angry," rather than "you" as in "You made me angry."

When offered a compliment, she says, "Thank you," without minimizing, justifying, or disputing.

"There is so much more to be gained from life by being free and able to stand up for oneself, and from honoring the same right for others," say Alberti and Emmons in *Your Perfect Right*.[13]

If you normally respond to others in passive or aggressive ways, you may want to learn how to be more assertive, perhaps through taking a class or self-study.

Women who act passively fear rejection, try to avoid conflict and being criticized, and strive to be liked by everyone. They let others push them around, yet may be manipulative in trying to solve problems and deny responsibility for their actions. Often they over-apologize, smile too much, and express effusive thanks when inappropriate. This is in a sense a self-betrayal.

Women who act aggressively, at the other extreme, are pushy, forcing their own opinions and desires, and showing little respect for the feelings of others. They may even be violent, getting their way through blame, threats, screaming or hitting. Aggressive women may act directly to resolve conflicts and achieve goals, but in the process violate the rights of others. They lose out because they foster fear, resentment and avoidance in those closest to them.

Many people slip back and forth between these behaviors, perhaps being assertive with a salesperson, passive with a co-worker, and taking out aggression at home on spouse or children.

Learning to be assertive takes practice. Your body language, posture, facial expressions, voice, and gestures, are as important as what you say. It may take time to coordinate these with your newly assertive feelings, beliefs, and words, just as it does to drive a car or learn to rollerblade. Note that a person may overcompensate in trying to move from being passive to assertive, and act aggressively at times.

Living assertively also helps women get out of the Compassion Trap. This is defined as a trap that keeps women believing they exist to serve others and must provide tenderness and compassion to everyone at all times. Getting out of this trap means valuing your own feelings and being responsive to them, as well as being considerate of others, say Stanlee Phelps, MSW, and Nancy Austin, MBA, in *The Assertive Woman*.[14]

Understanding this means viewing the suggestions offered in this book as friendly guidelines. You don't need to accept them at face value. Listen, think, and take what seems best for you at this time in your life, and leave the rest. After all, that's being assertive!

Dress for success

Living assertively means dressing in ways that make you feel good.
"Clothe your body in beautiful, comfortable clothes that fit now,"
says dietitian Dayle Hayes, of Billings, Mont.[15]

Clothes should help us stand out, make our own statement, be
unique, be noticed, be who we are as individuals, says Carol Johnson.

She deplores TV home shopping hosts who often repeat the dismal
message that the clothes they sell will cover up "figure flaws" and help
women "look slimmer" so they can "recede, hide, cover up, be unobtru-
sive, be monochrome."

A more powerful message that she'd like to hear: *This outfit will
accentuate every curve on your body, make your presence even
more commanding and call attention to your body in all its magnifi-
cence!*[16]

Don't buy or design clothes to hide who you are, but as a personal
statement of who you are as a unique individual.

You may want to clean out your closet of clothes that don't fit, or
that you can wear only when you've been dieting. If you can't bear to
give them away, store them elsewhere. This makes more room for
clothing you will enjoy wearing.

Strengthen your social support

We all feel better if we can include pleasant and stimulating interaction with others in our day. Maintain nourishing intimate relationships
with family and friends; experience and express your emotions to them,
and respond to their feelings in appropriate ways. We each need one or
more special friends or family members we can trust and share almost
anything with.

If you seem to be missing out on relationships you'd like to have,
getting involved in volunteer work can help. Working with others on a
project is one way we bond. Lend a helping hand and a helping heart.

Friendship is richer if you avoid comparing yourself to other women.
This has a bad outcome: others seem either better or worse, superior or
inferior, by comparison. It's a no-win judgment. In the same vein, avoid
poring over photos of thin models. If you're vulnerable those images can
haunt your thoughts.

You might want to form an awareness or support group in which
you examine traditional values, dissect stereotypes about weight and
eating, and share personal experiences in a supportive atmosphere which
is conducive to helping women grow and change.

Don't forget to have some fun in your day. Laugh out loud. Enjoy
others, yet keep a bit of solitude to renew your soul. Listen to your kind

of music. Hug and be hugged — if you don't have a person handy, how about a pet?

Nourish your spiritual health

Finally, let's look at other aspects of what is really important in our lives.

In this book we focus on eating, weight, body image, and related issues. Learning to love your body, rejecting perfectionism, and growing more assertive are all part of a process toward personal freedom and growth.

Yet we need to keep our perspective, keep in mind the big picture. Our culture seems to teach that attaining perfection and material wealth will solve all of life's problems. But the drive for perfection and wealth never brings the happiness we hope for. There's a lot more to life than this.

Spiritual abundance is another dimension that gives us a profound sense of who we are, where we came from, where we're going and how to get there. It recognizes a power beyond the natural and rational, and accepts on faith what is unknown and unfathomable.

Thinking about your spiritual abundance can put body dissatisfaction into perspective. In the bigger picture, considering the meaning of life and what is going on in the world, why would a person waste time on body hatred?

Price points out the need for spirituality. "Tending to your soul means developing your spirituality and having a sense that there's something bigger than you in the universe, and you're a part of it. You'll discover a feeling that you're not alone in your existence, but are connected to a larger whole ... When you ask for help or guidance, it's there for you. You access it through meditation, prayer, quiet contemplation, and by asking directly ... Listen, and you'll hear your soul telling you that you need to pay attention and look inward."

Shape a healthy balance

Putting all this together brings us to a sense of wellness, wholeness and well-being.

Many women try to do it all — excel at a career, be a supermom, care for home and family, socialize with friends, work out, and take care of personal needs. The problem is finding time and energy for everything.

The answer is not to do it all, but to find a reasonable and satisfying balance that works for you.

Self-care, caring for others, and work are each an important part of life, say the Tubesings. This is a triple agenda that can seem overwhelming at times. Yet it challenges us to seek personal wellness and wholeness, recapture the values of family and friendship, and strive to find stimulating work where we can make a contribution to the wider society in which we live.

"The challenge is, in light of your values and beliefs, to invest yourself where it counts — to invest yourself in a balance between self-care, other-care, and meaningful work that you believe in, that you can live with and be proud of, and that ultimately you will be willing to die with as your legacy. Invest yourself so that you can look back on your life and say that in your own way you did what you could to make the world a better place," they advise.

We all need a reason to get up in the morning, a purpose outside of ourselves.

Women who are truly whole, well-nourished, and healthy have a broader agenda than taking care of themselves. They focus on people and purposes beyond themselves. They have work and community commitments, they reach out to family and friends, and they invest whole-heartedly in some causes for which they have passion.

The benefits they gain are immeasurable.

We can make the connection between health and pleasure for ourselves and others. So how do we create an atmosphere that makes healthy choices easy and fun, and the natural way to live?

The Canadian Vitality program gives us an excellent road map: "Feeling good about yourself starts by accepting who you are and how you look. Healthy, good-looking bodies come in a variety of shapes and sizes. A good weight is a healthy weight, not necessarily a low weight, so don't let your self-worth be determined by the bathroom scales.

"Think positive thoughts. Laugh a lot. Spend some time with people who have a positive attitude — the type who look at the cup as being half full, not half empty. Positive vibes are contagious. Enjoy eating well and being active. Feel good about yourself. Have fun with family and friends, and you'll feel on top of the world!"[17]

CHAPTER 13

The joy of active living

■

"Imagine being able to enjoy physical activity just for
the sheer joy of it, without worrying about doing
enough, being competent, or losing weight."
— *Gail Johnston*

Life is more fun when we live actively.

It's the natural way for people to live. Being active is a pleasurable experience in a balanced life. It's something you do for yourself, for the sheer joy of it, to increase your enjoyment of life, your mental well-being and self-esteem as well as to improve your health, your strength and your endurance. Even problems come into better perspective when we're active.

The new approach to physical activity is more light-hearted than in the past. In living to be healthy at any size, activity should be a pleasure in itself, not pursued just for good health, and not for weight loss. It does not become an obsession, but a regular part of a balanced and pleasurable life.

The goal is to live actively in a way that makes you feel good and fits in with the way you want to live your life. Some people enjoy and are challenged by strenuous workouts, aerobic classes, weight-lifting or marathons. Others find the benefits by incorporating activity into their everyday life. All are worthwhile, just different choices.

"Fitness should be a healthy pleasure. Gentle exercise can make you feel terrific. You need to decide for yourself what kind of action can give you pleasure, and set aside some time for it. Above all, pick activities that you enjoy. And remember, this is supposed to be fun!" say Robert Ornstein, PhD, and David Sobel, MD, in their book *Healthy Pleasures.*

It's ironic that of all healthful behaviors women could choose to practice, the one that is actually fun to do and that leads to improved mental health is the one women are least likely to do. We can change that, starting now.

The Vitality program explains, "Being active means enjoying physical activity and finding fun ways to be active every day of the year — at home, at work, within your community. Whether it's bowling, mowing the lawn or playing hopscotch with the kids, an active lifestyle pays off. Make fitness a family activity: go ice-skating at the local rink, take an after-dinner walk together. Plan an active living vacation — a weekend hike, cross-country ski holiday, a canoeing getaway."

Young children are the most active of all. Kids spend, on average, one or two hours a day in moderate and vigorous physical activity. They are active in other ways, as well, because they want to be, not because it's good for them.

We need to strengthen and extend this active joy of living, and carry it into adulthood. After all, it's just for fun that friends play softball all afternoon. It's for fun and exhilaration that skiers and hikers challenge a mountain. It's for the social enjoyment, and rhythmic, musical pleasure that young people dance nonstop for hours on a Saturday night.

In this approach, everyone can succeed. You don't need to measure target heart rate, calories burned, study activity like a science, develop a fitness plan, or lose weight to achieve the benefits of exercise.

Focusing on weight loss can backfire and take all the fun out of it.

Ornstein and Sobel point out that much popular health advice ignores the less intense, more enjoyable forms of activity, in favor of urging vigorous exercise. Many people feel discouraged and end up doing nothing.

Gail Johnston, a health and fitness consultant in Walnut Creek, Calif., holds a new vision: "Imagine being able to enjoy physical activity just for the sheer joy of it, without worrying about doing enough, being competent, or losing weight. Imagine a world where men and women of all sizes walk into a health club and see healthy active role models of all sizes."

Johnston in her book, *If I Know I Should Be Exercising, Why Aren't I?* says we can take this new path of making physical activity accessible to all people if we move away from charts and graphs and incorporate activity into the total human experience. "In some undefinable way, exercise helps us be the best we can be. But only when we are given the best opportunity to succeed."[1]

"The good news is that recent studies show that even mild physical activity is helpful," points out Linda Omichinski, a registered dietitian and author of *You Count, Calories Don't.* "So if you have been laughing at your neighbors as they garden or rake leaves while you are riding your stationary bike, take a second look at who is getting hooked on an active lifestyle. Changing your attitude and your lifestyle by adopting a more light-hearted approach can make you happier and healthier. Make that special time for yourself."

So if you've let this area of your life slide, make the decision to recapture that feeling of exhilaration. Don't let barriers — like being too busy, having to take care of others, or no place to exercise — stand in the way of this healthful, pleasurable habit that women are least likely to develop. You can work around those barriers, whatever they might be.

Find the natural rhythms of your body, and let them invigorate you. Reconnect with the wonderful things your body can do for you.

Just do it

So how can you change behavior?

Like the Nike slogan says, just do it.

That's right. You don't need to study the health benefits first. You don't need to make a complex plan. You don't even need to change a skeptical attitude. Learning theory tells us the first step is just to begin in a small way, and succeed at that. After people have tasted success, they start to believe, and they change attitudes without effort. Once attitudes are changed, behavior is changed for good.

If you're ready to begin, right now, I suggest you turn to the walking plan on these pages, and walk for five minutes, either indoors or outdoors.

Keep it simple. Just do it. Stick to your first step for one week, then continue for three more. Give yourself plenty of room to succeed.

Trust yourself

The new approach to health at any size focuses on developing inner control and self-trust. You can further your self-empowerment and inner control in these ways:

- Take a self-trusting approach to exercise. Trust that you have the ability to know what's best for you, what is enjoyable, what feels right. You are the expert on your own health and well-being.
- Listen to your body's internal signals. Your body will tell you when you need to be more active or less. When you need more

challenges, more intensity, when to ease back. We need to respond to these signals, find the rhythms of our own bodies.

- Focus on the enjoyment of the activity and the social benefits you get from being active with others.
- Reinforce and reward your activity. Tell yourself how much you are enjoying the activity. Praise your progress. Reward yourself by thinking about active pleasures you've enjoyed during the day.

Find the activities that are right for you.

If you are physically challenged in some way, you can definitely be active. In fact it can be doubly rewarding, because you will see your life change dramatically. You may need to experiment, and think about how you can work through a problem. You can find a way to move your body — and do it three to five minutes every day for four weeks.

If you have mobility problems, try walking around a table or counter, holding onto it as you move around. Walking too difficult? Then choose a sitting activity. Make up your own routine: swing your arms and legs, march directing a band, or row a boat to music. There's a wonderful video we've used called *Chair Dancing*.[2] You can even do exercises while lying down.

Keep up your activity, resist the urge to let it slide. If it seems too much, then it's better to drop back a few levels, and begin again at a level that is more comfortable.

How much is enough?

As you become more active, you decide how much is enough, and what's right for the woman you are.

If you're a social person, it might be an active life in sports. Or an hour at the fitness center. You may most enjoy quiet solitary walks. Indoor activity at home may be most appealing, walking room to room, dancing or marching in place before the television, setting up and following your own parcourse, using exercise equipment.

Becoming more active is even more important for the usually inactive woman than for others, because it gives her a greater leap in health benefits.

The President's Council on Physical Fitness & Sports urges inactive people to take on the challenge: "By making the relatively small change from an inactive lifestyle to one that includes moderate but regular physical activity, even the most sedentary Americans can prevent disease and premature death and improve their quality of life."

Whatever you choose, I encourage you to resist the urge to set those goals too high or too far out ahead. Many people set ambitious goals that lead to failure and discouragement. You need to taste success and gain rewards each time.

One week goals are enough, I think, perhaps beginning with a five-minute commitment. Start the action. Establish the habit.

We need to avoid attaching moral values to physical activity and other health habits. People are not "better" if they exercise, and less worthy if they don't. It is false and foolish to feel either morally superior or inferior because one runs six miles a day and another lives a sedentary life. It's not a question of morality, but of well-being.

Break up day-long inactivity

Can you get more activity into your day?

Research finds the major cause of weight increase in this generation may well be the almost total inactivity of many children and young adults. Studies in several countries show people don't eat more calories (they may eat less), and certainly eat less fat — but they are far less active than 30 years ago.

Experts have taught that to reverse this weight gain, it is necessary

---

How to set up a parcourse in your home

The parcourse, developed in Switzerland for outdoor exercise, can be easily adapted to indoors. Here's how to design your own parcourse:

1. Find a set of 10 or more exercises you like, preferably with pictures. These can be found in various pamphlets or health bulletins.
2. Number, beginning with stretches, and cut them apart.
3. Tape them up around the house. The sequence may follow a course from one end of the house to the other, including basement and upper floors. Or group odd numbers at one side of the house or apartment, and even numbers at the other, as far apart as possible.
4. Turn up your favorite lively music and enjoy your own personal Swiss parcourse by doing each exercise five to 10 times in sequence, then walking or jogging for the distance between them. Or march in place.To increase, add more exercises, or the activity between them, or go twice around the course.
5. Take the parcourse three or more days a week, alternating with other activities.

WOMEN AFRAID TO EAT 2000

to add a period of time during the day when people actively exercise — hence the recommendation that everyone accumulate at least 30 minutes of moderate or vigorous activity on most days. But some health leaders now say this will not be enough if there's relatively little movement the rest of the day.

We probably need to look at those other 23½ hours in the day. It may be inactivity during all those hours that takes the biggest toll on health. A half hour burst of sudden activity may not reverse this.

How can you keep your day relatively active?

You may need to create your own opportunities for movement, especially if you sit at a desk or in front of a computer all day, as many of us do. This is not the normal activity of humans. Even 100 years ago, everyday work meant keeping a fire going, chopping wood, carrying water, gardening, preserving food, scrubbing clothes, or holding a lurching plow in the ground, walking behind a horse all day.

Working in a home office, staying home all day, cuts down even more drastically on the natural activity that goes with getting to and from work, walking from subway stop or parking, moving through offices, and up and down stairs.

You'll need to be creative. Try some of these ideas:

- Stand up, stretch and walk around at least every hour.
- Stroll while talking on the telephone if the phone is cordless, walk in place if it's not.
- While seated, march in place, "direct" an unseen orchestra, and stretch at odd moments, while pondering that computer screen (if privacy and consideration of co-workers allows it).
- Volunteer for carrying jobs and running errands.
- Instead of a coffee break, take an activity break. Walk up to the top floor, or down to the lowest, down a long hallway, twice around the block. Or find a quiet spot to run in place. Ask co-workers to join you.
- Walk wherever you can, or bike to work.
- Park the car farther away, or get off the bus at an earlier stop, and get in the habit of walking the extra blocks. In shopping, park the car at the outer edge of the lot.
- When shopping at a mall, walk through the entire building.
- Houseclean with extra vigor and speed. Use large movements. Jog, dance or march in place while folding clothes or vacuuming the living room. It can add zest and humor to the work.
- If cleaning work is quickly done, go on to sweep the sidewalk.
- Watching TV or a movie, find time to stand up, move around, dance, jog, jump rope, or walk around the edges of the room.

(This can be distracting or annoying to others, so be considerate, or persuade them to join you.) During commercials, run up and down the stairs.

- Don't sit too long without moving.
- Walk your dog.
- Dance around the house, play active games with children.
- Enlist the family and get everyone involved in a big cleaning or yard project. Turn on lively music and move to the rhythm.
- Use fewer labor saving devices.
- Spend more time in outdoor work you enjoy.
- Gardening is a great activity. So is lawn work. How about using an old-fashioned push mower?
- Prefer active sports to spectator sports.
- Go dancing.
- On trips, stop periodically to walk or go on a short hike.

You may find that increasing your activity throughout the day is all that's needed to move you from being a sedentary woman to an active one. Be flexible, and make activity enjoyable and relaxing, not frenetic. You'll have more energy, feel better, and be empowered to make other changes in your life.

After a few months of learning curve, try to get in the habit of accumulating about 30 minutes of activity into your day, perhaps during two or three periods, and also being more active throughout the day.

We can fool ourselves

The 30 minutes of moderate activity that people should accumulate most days need not be all at once, according to the Centers for Disease Control and the American College of Sports Medicine. The good news is that big chunks of time are not needed. Three 10-minute periods of moderate activity can be as beneficial as one 30-minute period, when done five days a week.

But be honest. Don't cheat yourself by imagining that increasing activity is so easy it doesn't matter. Busy women are not necessarily as physically active as they think.

I know this from my own experience. I remember well when I decided to begin walking. We were planning a trip to Europe to visit friends and relatives in Norway, England and Switzerland. We'd been there before and knew we'd do plenty of walking — people there walk a lot more than we do. So I started one Sunday afternoon in spring by trying a half-mile run with my daughter, who was in junior high track.

We live at the edge of town, with a small pasture and on the other side of that is a half-mile road. We set off across the pasture and hit the road about in the middle. We started to run and I was soon winded — I couldn't believe it. My heart was beating wildly, I gasped for breath, had a stitch in my side, my legs ached. I had to stop, catch my breath, and walk awhile. Kathy waited patiently till I could run again, but soon I told her to go on and I sat down on a rock till she came back.

I was in good shape, I thought, strong and healthy, in my 30s. With four children I was busy and on the go all the time, often carrying the youngest. As a child on a Montana ranch I had run a lot. I liked to run. Yet I couldn't run one-fourth of a mile to the end of the road! I couldn't even run one-eighth of a mile. I walked back to the starting point, and waited till Kathy ran to the other end of the road and back.

It was a rude awakening, and it prodded me into walking a mile a day. Before long I was running that mile and adding another to it. I like to run, and kept it up for three months until our trip, which as I had anticipated included many long and wonderful old-world walks. Then I quit running. I had accomplished my purpose. Again I was busy, no time for indulging myself.

But something was missing. It was that wonderful break in the day when I'd run out the door, our yellow Lab, Sham, loping along beside me, sniffing out the ditches, laughing up at me, a meadowlark singing, wild flowers waving, a watching deer trembling in the trees, breathing in that fresh, cool air. So I started again and have been running or walking a couple of miles a day ever since. The rewards are so great I can't even begin to express them.

If this sounds like you, I'd like to inspire you to give walking a fair trial. You won't know those rewards till after they become a part of your life. Then tell me you don't have time for this!

Benefits of being active

Only 40 percent of American adults are regularly active and only 15 percent engage regularly in vigorous physical activity three times a week for at least 20 minutes during leisure time, according to the Surgeon General's report.

Author John Steinbeck had a term for sedentary living: the "sweet trap." He said people who fall into the "sweet trap" are living the life of semi-invalids.

Can it be true that today nearly two-thirds of our population chooses to live like semi-invalids? Steinbeck would likely say so.

"Most of us don't wear out, we rust out," observes a U.S. Public Health booklet for seniors.

There are enormous health benefits in being active. But women agree that other benefits are even more important to them. A boost to self-esteem and mental outlook is usually number one on their list. Active women feel empowered to take charge of their lives, and more confident about making other changes.

In a Melpomene Institute study of 58 larger women, nearly all said their self-image improved with increased physical activity. They were enthusiastic about these kinds of results:

"Feeling strong, graceful and having fun."

"A sense of accomplishment and self-pride."

"Knowing you can do something. I always think what a failure my body is, but if you exercise, that's not true."

"Feeling better, not getting short of breath after a slight amount of exercise."[3]

The good news is we don't have to reach competitive heights to achieve major health benefits from physical activity. We can improve the quality of our lives — put more years in our lives and more life in our years — by living actively in moderate ways.

Being physically active improves health in all sorts of ways. It lowers blood pressure. It improves cholesterol levels, increases "good" HDL cholesterol, reduces heart rate and lowers the risk of cardiovascular disease. It improves blood glucose levels and reduces risk of diabetes. It increases longevity. The effect on bone density is particularly important for young women, because this is the time in life when bone mass peaks. Think of your bones as muscles; if you actively use or stress them, the bones will grow stronger. Tennis players, for instance, have much thicker and stronger bones in the "tennis" arm, the arm used most often, than in the non-tennis arm.

Being active may even make young people smarter. Brain research suggests that exercising the large muscles during adolescence helps increase nerve connections for higher brain development. This supports studies that suggest students involved in sports do better in academics. Regular exercise lifts the mood, and is especially helpful for women who are depressed or anxious. It relieves tension and anxiety, lowers stress, and helps put your problems in perspective. Best of all, it enhances the quality of life.

And as people reach midlife and beyond, it's even more clear that living actively adds more years to life and more life to those years. Here are just some of the benefits you can enjoy from regular, moderate activity:

- Improves your self-image
- Boosts your self-confidence
- Gives you more energy and zest for life
- Helps you look your best

- Reduces stress and tension
- Helps counter anxiety and depression
- Refreshes, relaxes
- Increases resistance to fatigue
- Improves sleep
- Increases lean body mass and reduces body fat
- Keeps weight stable, helps prevent overweight, may improve weight loss
- Increases strength and endurance
- Helps you be more productive at work
- Keeps heart and lungs working more efficiently
- Lowers blood pressure and hypertension risk
- Lowers risk of cardiovascular disease
- Improves cholesterol levels, increases "good" HDL cholesterol
- Reduces heart rate
- Improves blood glucose levels and reduces risk of diabetes
- Reduces risk or symptoms related to some types of cancers
- Improves muscle function and joint problems
- Increases longevity.
- Helps prevent heart disease, and diabetes
- Builds bone, slows bone loss, helps prevent osteoporosis
- Improves strength and function of elderly
- Provides social benefits: brings family and friends closer through shared activity, an easy way to meet and enjoy new friends

Surprisingly, it's never to late to begin. In a nursing home in Boston, 100 women and men dramatically increased their strength in 10 weeks through a high-intensity resistance training program of the hip and knee extensors, working out 45 minutes three days a week. Their average age was 87! Initially these men and women, ranging up to age 98, were quite frail — 83 percent required a cane, walker or wheelchair, and 66 percent had fallen during the year. Half had arthritis, and nearly as many had pulmonary disease and osteoporotic bone fracture; one third had hypertension; one fourth had cancer; half had mental impairment, and over one third had depression.

In just over two months of resistance training, these elderly women and men walked faster, climbed stairs with more power, and increased muscle strength by 113 percent. Risk factors improved, and many with arthritis increased their range without pain. Some who could hardly get out of bed, now did so easily. Some left their walkers for a cane. It was the weakest who gained the most strength. Most importantly, these elderly people enjoyed an improved quality of life.[4]

Don't focus on weight loss

Regular physical activity can prevent obesity and keep your weight stable. Fitness is a key factor in long-term weight regulation. Being more active also is the most promising way that some people can lose weight and apparently lower their setpoint. In doing so, they lose more fat relative to muscle, which is a healthier way to lose weight.

In two studies of weight-loss maintainers, being more active was cited as critical in keeping off lost weight. Women in a 1990 California study who had lost 20 or more pounds and maintained it for at least two years, said they were more active and had changed some eating habits. They were more likely than controls and regainers to be eating regular meals.[5]

People in the National Weight Control Registry who have maintained an average weight loss of 30 pounds for an average of five years say their success is due to high levels of exercise and eating a lower-fat, lower-calorie diet.[6]

However, people differ in the effect exercise has on their weight. Some lose, others don't. Men are more likely to lose than women, probably because they have more lean mass.

Often what women lose first through being more active is not weight but size. After a few months of increased activity, women commonly remark, "I haven't lost any weight, but I can buy clothes two sizes smaller."

Size is reduced because muscle mass is smaller but heavier than fat, in the same way a textbook is smaller but heavier than a pillow.

Isn't reducing size what women really want? Of course it is, yet it's appalling what power those numbers, those pounds, can have. Far too many women drop an activity program they enjoy and are gaining enormous benefits from, simply because they can't count the pounds lost. Weight benefits don't show up as quickly from increased activity as through dieting, but they are lasting.

Women need to lighten up on weight loss. The main reason for being active is not to burn calories. A goal of determined calorie-burning often leads to dropping out — or to obsessive exercise. Keeping track of the calorie dials and numbers on fitness equipment, supposedly adding up how many pounds will be lost, does not work, and is self-defeating. It's only theoretical, so don't expect to lose weight based on those numbers. If it were true, some people would disappear altogether. Doesn't happen. We humans regulate our bodies far better than this.

The role of exercise in weight loss has often been exaggerated, bringing much disappointment and discouragement, warns Chester Zelasko, PhD, director of the Human Performance Laboratory at Buffalo State

College in Buffalo, N.Y.[7]

In 1993, the National Institutes of Health Technology Assessment Conference Panel concluded that no diet or exercise program yet available could produce sustained weight loss for most people.[8]

Instead of to lose weight, Zelasko says we should exercise for the right reasons: "For the health of it! To improve the cardiovascular system; to improve the strength, endurance and flexibility of the muscular system; to effect positive changes in other body systems such as skeletal, digestive and immune systems; for other manifestations of improved health such as lower serum lipids and lower blood pressure."

Weight loss only works when increased fitness is part of it, so it makes more sense for us to bypass the weight loss attempt altogether and go straight to increased fitness. Let weight come off as a side effect. If it happens, it happens. This is far better than the course most women take: lose 30 pounds, struggle to keep it off through frantic exercise and diet, watch it all return and more. If they continue exercise, they may keep off five or 10 pounds, which they could have done in the first place without the diet and the weight-cycling stress.

Let's be realistic in our advice, warns Roger L. Hammer, PhD, professor of Exercise Science at Central Michigan University. People should not expect dramatic changes in weight loss, fat loss, fat free mass, or resting metabolic rate when they increase activity. What they can expect is increased aerobic exercise capacity and cardiovascular endurance, a small change in weight and fat loss, prevention of major weight gain, improved maintenance of weight loss, an improved blood profile, and decreased risk of disease.

"As professionals we need to de-emphasize the preoccupation some of our obese patients may have with achieving an ideal weight. We need to teach those we work with to learn to live a healthy lifestyle and to be satisfied with whatever end weight is subsequently achieved," says Hammer.[9]

What really matters: fitness not fatness

The good news is that exercise is a far more effective and safe way for us to improve health than is weight loss.

Exercise improves the fat to lean ratio and increases cardiovascular fitness. New studies are challenging some of the risks traditionally blamed on obesity. These risks may have more to do with lack of exercise than with weight. Large people who are fit seem to have no greater risks than thin people who are fit.[10]

The long-term Cooper Institute studies in Dallas demonstrate that it is fitness that makes the difference. In this research, Steven Blair and colleagues tested and followed-up 22,000 men for over eight years and found higher death rates and risk factors were related to lower physical activity and fitness, not weight or body fat levels.[11]

Blair finds the same for women. Of 3,120 healthy women, at every weight, those with moderate and high fitness had much lower death rates than women with low fitness.[12] In another long-term study of women who remained obese, exercise normalized their abnormal plasma glucose, insulin and lipid levels.[13]

Furthermore, new research suggests that unless people can maintain lean body mass while losing fat, they increase their overall risk in losing weight. Failure to do this is thought to be why most large long-term studies show increased risk of death with weight loss.[14]

The research is so strong and so unequivocal that it's amazing the public and the media haven't noticed: Being active and fit means we gain better health and longer life, while weight loss alone fails to improve health in most cases, and is linked to higher death rates.[15]

The conclusion is inescapable: The health community needs to encourage large people to live actively, and shelve the weight loss talk —

Tips to encourage lasting activity habits

Jolie Glass, MS, director of Women's Exercise Research Center at George Washington University Medical Center gives these tips for staying involved in an exercise training program:

• Choose an emotionally safe environment. The atmosphere should be comfortable and encouraging and not intimidating or competitive.

• Find an exercise specialist who is sensitive to women's weight and body issues. Specialists should show true concern for the whole woman, not just the physical woman.

• Plan for exercise. Schedule sessions and pack apparel in advance.

• Minimize the effort required to prepare for exercise. Choose a place that is easily accessible and exercise during a convenient time.

• Make exercise fun. Choose a mode of exercise that is enjoyable and find an exercise partner or group.[1]

WOMEN AFRAID TO EAT 2000

Walking for a lifetime

A WALKING PROGRAM

Make walking a lifetime habit by starting today with a five-minute walk. That's right — just five minutes. It's enough. Too many people begin with a brisk two-mile walk — and never come back!

Walking is an excellent, pleasurable aerobic activity. It can be a friendly social event, or a quiet interval of solitude in your busy day. By walking regularly you can improve your health, your endurance, your self-esteem, your enjoyment of life, your appearance, and your mental well-being. Walking is almost injury-free. And no matter your age, it's never too late to start walking.

It's easy to begin. You can walk anywhere, down the street, in a park, at the mall, in a gym or health club, or in your own home by walking down the hallway and around the rooms, or marching in place before the television. You need no special clothing, just shoes you can walk in and whatever else you're wearing. It's something you do for yourself, so enjoy the time. You deserve it.

These suggestions can help you begin and continue a walking program for a lifetime:

1. Start slowly. Begin walking 5 minutes a day at a moderately slow and easy pace. Use positive self-talk: tell yourself how much you like walking; reject any negative thoughts.

2. Benefit from the four-week routine. It takes four weeks to develop a habit. Remember this is your objective, to establish the habit, not to get fit as quickly as possible. Enjoy walking this way for four weeks, five minutes a day, shifting it to different times in your daily schedule to find what works best for you. Don't be tempted to increase the time, unless this is truly too brief for you. Be content to progress slowly. Half of those who begin an activity program quit the first week. They set goals too high, and soon get tired, discouraged, gain sore muscles, and can't imagine keeping this up longterm. Instead, you can succeed in these four weeks.

3. Try one-week contracts. Goals, contracts, and records are part of making it happen for many people, but others don't

work well with these kinds of pressures. If you do, set short-term goals and write them into a contract. Add a reward, then sign your name. For example: "I will walk five minutes a day, at least five days this week. My reward will be a new cassette tape." Find what works for you.

4. Proceed at your own pace. After four weeks you may be ready to increase time or intensity. Or maybe not. Increase to eight minutes, then 10, and later, to 15 minutes. Keep in mind that you're not in a race. You're making a lifestyle change of critical importance in your life. By six months you may be walking 20 or 30 minutes a day, or a couple of miles. This may be a good level to continue long term. Or it can be increased if it suits you and your lifestyle.

5. Walk five to seven days a week. Walk daily, or almost daily, and it is most likely to become a lifetime habit.

6. Consult your doctor. Walking is safe for nearly everyone, but consulting a doctor is advised if you are very sedentary or at medical risk.

7. Keep a simple record. Mark each day on a chart and watch the miles add up. Some people chart their miles on a state map. Or try another country, learning about the towns you "walk" through. It's a great feeling when you've walked 300 miles. Who would have thought it possible? Again, records are not for everyone, but they can be fun.

8. Reward yourself. Promise a reward and at the end of the week pay up. It's another way to make your walking program fun. Make rewards special: something you buy for yourself, places to go, or things to do. (Not food rewards, though; avoid using food for emotional purposes.)

9. Find activities that are right for you. Walking is great, but you may prefer swimming, biking, running, dancing, playing softball, or gardening. Try a variety. If you have physical disabilities, there are many enjoyable activity programs just right for you. Investigate, and try out the possibilities.

10. Keep up contracts, records, and rewards about four months, if this works for you. The secret is: It takes four weeks to change a habit; four months to make it a lifestyle change; four years — and it's a vital part of your life.

Live actively

35 EASY WAYS TO INTEGRATE
MORE ACTIVITY INTO YOUR DAILY LIFE

At home

- When you're on the telephone, walk around, pace back and forth. Do the same at least part of the time when you're watching TV.
- While television watching is a good time to get in 20 to 30 minutes of exercise by jogging, marching or dancing in place. Or walk around the edges of the room, back and forth, during your favorite program. During commercials run or walk up and down the stairs. Don't sit too long without moving.
- Clean house a little every day.
- Houseclean with extra vigor, use large strong movements.
- Wash your car with the hose instead of at the car wash.
- Dance or march in place while folding clothes; you'll find it adds zest to the job.
- Enlist the family and get everyone involved in a big cleaning or yard project. For children, turn on lively music and tell them to move their bodies as much as possible.
- Sweep the garage.
- Sweep the sidewalk in front of your house (even if it doesn't need it).
- Gardening is a great way to stay active.
- Dance around the house, play active games with your children.
- Spend more time doing outdoor work you enjoy.
- Use fewer labor saving devices; a hand mower instead of a gas powered mower.

At work

- Walk or ride a bicycle to work and elsewhere.
- Get off the bus two or three stops before your corner.
- If you drive, park two or three blocks away. If you enjoy this short walk, you may want to park farther away.
- Walk up and down the stairs instead of taking the elevator.

- Leave the elevator two or three floors early, and take the stairs.

- Instead of a coffee break, walk inside or outside the building with co-workers. Find a quiet corner or back room and run, march or dance in place to lively music for 10 minutes.

- Walk through your building two or three times during the day, especially if your work is mostly sitting. Walk upstairs and downstairs.

- Stand instead of sitting while talking on the telephone.

- Stand up and move around every hour or so, if your work is mostly sitting down. Or spend five minutes cleaning a storage closet.

- Brown bag your lunch and take it to a nearby park to eat. Or take your lunch to eat at a friend's house, then go for a walk together.

- Take a walk at your coffee break or before lunch.

Recreation and community

- When sight-seeing, take a hike in the area.

- Take a walk when picnicking.

- When shopping in a mall, walk through the entire mall at least once.

- Walk any distance that is four blocks or less (or better yet, a mile).

- Park farther away from where you are shopping, instead of driving around looking for the closest parking spot. Park once for all your needs when possible.

- Increase your interest in active sports. Find what's available. Play group sports, or with friends and family at an enjoyable level of competition.

- When you go to the beach, instead of just sunbathing, go swimming or walk along the beach.

- Go dancing.

- Golf without a cart.

- Use stairs instead of elevators or escalators.

- Walk your dog.

until they have something far better to offer than in the past, and can show proof that it improves health and longevity. If health is really the desired outcome, then a physical activity program makes much more sense than one more failed weight loss program.[16]

What kind is best?

Much misinformation is being circulated as to what kind of activity is most effective for weight loss and fat loss.

Will you lose more with high intensity exercise for a shorter period of time better, or low to moderate intensity for a longer time? Is weight training exercise more effective than aerobic exercise?[17]

Wayne C. Miller, PhD, of the Exercise Science Programs, George Washington University Medical Center, Washington, DC, reviewed the research in a recent issue of *Healthy Weight Journal*, and reported that as yet this cannot be determined. It is not yet clear how much or what kind of exercise works best for either weight loss or fat loss. However, for the larger person, low intensity aerobic exercise over a longer period is probably most appropriate.[18]

The American College of Sports Medicine makes a general recommendation that it is the overall energy cost that counts, and any intensity that promotes a high caloric deficit is useful.[19]

A few studies show heavy resistance training promotes short-term weight loss in obese persons. Miller said this type of exercise can help maintain lean body mass and metabolic rate throughout the weight reduction period, and is valuable in building strength. However, it needs to be performed safely. This type of exercise presents the highest safety risk, has not been shown to lower obesity risks, and has only been shown to be effective in short-term studies on obese persons.

Safety in exercise

A moderate activity program that progresses gradually is generally safe for everyone. But we need to be aware of possible risks. Exercise may cause muscle soreness, injury, light-headedness, or cardiovascular problems.

To avoid soreness and injury, begin each exercise session with a brief low-intensity aerobic warm-up, and stretching. Cool down slowly by decreasing intensity and staying in motion for a few minutes to avoid light-headedness. When exercising outdoors, dress appropriately for the weather, and wear layers of clothing that can be removed as body temperature rises. Drink plenty of fluids to prevent dehydration and overheating.

If you feel chest pain, dizziness, confusion, cold sweating or abnormal heart activity, stop. If symptoms persist, seek emergency care.

On whether to check with your doctor before beginning an exercise program, Miller suggests two "rules of thumb" on this:

1. If you are apparently healthy and 65 years old or younger, you can probably start an exercise program without a visit to the doctor. Some type of medical clearance is advisable, however.

2. If you have any abnormal discomfort, pain, or dizziness during exercise, do not continue until you consult your physician.

CHAPTER 14

Eating well

■

Food is not our enemy, but our friend. Enjoy it for
taste, texture, good health and the pleasure of eating
with family and friends.

Eating well means having a normal eating style. Eating well means
tuning in to inner signals of hunger and fullness, taking pleasure in eating
meals with family and friends, and enjoying balance, variety and moderation in food choices. Eating well means integrating all this with active
living, which ensures that appetite mechanisms and other body functions
are activated in a natural body rhythm.

Normal eating means usually eating at regular times, typically three
meals a day and one or two snacks to satisfy hunger. It means choosing
foods you like, ones that satisfy and taste good to you. It means enjoying
food and eating in moderate, relaxed ways. It means you can eat your
favorite foods now — or later. In normalized eating, no foods are
"good" or "bad."

Normal eating enhances our feelings of well-being. We eat for
nourishment, energy and health, sometimes for pleasure and social reasons. After eating, we feel good. Normal eating is regulated by internal
signals of hunger, appetite and satiety — we eat when hungry and stop
when satisfied. Normal eating means that food choices more likely meet
the sound nutrition principles of balance, variety and moderation.

Normal eating nurtures clear thinking, the ability to concentrate,
mood stability, energy and good health. It fosters healthy relationships in
family, friends, work, school and community. Thoughts of food, hunger,

weight, and body image are relegated to the "back burner," and take up only a small part of the day. Normal eating promotes stable weight, within a wide range, expressing both genetic and environmental factors. If modern women could eat this way, and balance eating well with active living, we would prevent many eating and weight problems that plague our culture today.

"Normal eating is three meals a day, most of the time, but it can also be choosing to munch along. Normal eating is flexible ... giving yourself permission to eat sometimes because you are happy, sad or bored, or just because it feels good. ... Normal eating is trusting your body to make up for your mistakes in eating," writes Ellyn Satter in *How to Get Your Kid to Eat . . . But Not Too Much.*[1] While written to help parents nurture their children, her book can also help women to nurture themselves.

Normal eating is natural and simple. It is trusting yourself. People who eat normally will not all be thin, as weight is influenced by a variety of inherited and environmental factors. But they will usually have stable weights, a valuable goal in itself. They'll be fully nourished, with the strength and energy to do the important things in their lives. They will be healthy at any size.

There are two aspects to eating well: how and what.

First, let's look at how to eat in normal, healthy ways.

Normalizing eating

Normal eating gives structure and good habits that become natural. Habits are enormously useful — consider brushing your teeth or fastening your seat belt. Making normal eating a habit will mean you don't waste time or mental energy thinking about it; you just do it.

Eating should be a perfectly natural part of our lives, contributing to our sense of wellness and wholeness. Nevertheless, it is only one small part, and should not dominate.

Learning how to eat well again begins by stopping all diets. Normalizing one's eating habits happens through eating at regular times, reconnecting with inner signals of hunger and fullness, and enjoying balance, variety, and moderation in food choices. While this can take time, it is a pleasurable journey, if you relax and allow yourself flexibility.

Restoring normal eating is a priority for those who have restricted their eating and for those who habitually overeat. Women need to do this not only for themselves but for others who are affected by their attitudes and behaviors.

Learn to view food as a friend, as health promoting and energizing, as enjoyable and to be savored without guilt. Reject perfectionism and come to regard food in a flexible way. Tell yourself, "I can eat it if I want it, now or later."

Many dieters fear that without limits they will overeat. They panic at the thought of relying on internal signals. It may take time to overcome this fear and learn to trust yourself, but you will. Dieting can be hard to give up. For some people it involves a kind of grief, a giving up of the lifelong dream or fantasy that "when I'm thin, my real life will begin." It also means relinquishing the excitement and drama of the diet that begins next Monday morning.

What will replace this? Maybe your real life can begin.

If you're a dieter, you may be making rules for yourself right now on how much to eat today, how much tomorrow. Maybe you'll weigh yourself first, then decide if this should be a semistarvation day or not.

Normal eating

Normal eating means eating at regular times, typically three meals a day and one or two snacks to satisfy hunger. It means choosing foods you like, ones that satisfy and taste good to you. Normal eating enhances our feelings of well-being. We eat for nourishment, energy and health, sometimes for pleasure and social reasons. After eating, we feel good.

Normal eating is regulated by internal signals of hunger, appetite and satiety — we eat when hungry and stop when satisfied. It means that food choices more likely provide the sound nutrition principles of balance, variety and moderation. It promotes clear thinking and mood stability, and fosters healthy relationships with family and friends. Thoughts of food, hunger, weight and body image take up only a small part of the day.

Normal eating nurtures good health, vibrant energy, and the healthy growth and development of children. It promotes stable weights, within a wide range, expressing both genetic and environmental factors.

WOMEN AFRAID TO EAT 2000

If you make these kinds of eating plans, it's time to stop. It's time to get on with your life, starting today. It's time to learn to trust your body.

Eating at regular mealtimes is a healthy and satisfying habit that does much to normalize eating. People will tend to feel hungry at these times if it's a habit, responding more easily to their natural hunger and satiety cues. Meals are also more likely to include the food variety and balance needed, to give us the five food groups that provide high quality nutrients — protein, carbohydrates, vitamins, minerals and fiber.

"Grazing" can work in the same way. But too often women who graze instead fill up on crackers, chips, cookies, candy and bakery goods that are low in vitamins, minerals and fiber, and high in sugar, fat and salt. Women who let snacks like these take the place of well-balanced meals end up with diets lacking nutrition and loaded with calories.

Eating attentively

Learn to pay attention to what you eat.

Linda Omichinski, author of *You Count, Calories Don't*, says any bite of food that goes into your mouth deserves attention. When you eat, do nothing but eat, even it it's a handful of raisins. "Sit down, take a deep breath, relax, and focus on the raisins. ... Experience the different taste sensations, textures, and aromas."[2]

Nutritionists call this attentive, intuitive, or purposeful eating. It is a way to eat deliberately, with full intent, being conscious the whole time of taste, texture, and body responses. This minimizes haphazard, casual, and indiscriminate eating, and helps you feel satisfied, that you enjoyed what you ate, and that the meal will last a few hours.

"Having enough food available helps you feel comforted, well taken care of and secure. Not having enough of what you want to eat may make you feel deprived. Enjoying your food means enjoying the taste and flavor. Eating foods you don't enjoy leaves you feeling unsatisfied after the meal," says dietitian Karen Siegel.[3]

Ronna Kabatznick, PhD, author of *The Zen of Eating*, extends this farther. She suggests we pause and pay homage to each food on the table and its ingredients, that we marvel at the abundance and variety, recognize where these foods came from, honor the hard-working people who produced them, then take time to savor each bite.[4]

Eating with this kind of leisure, appreciation and respect, helps us keep in touch with our internal signals of hunger, appetite and satiety.

How do you learn to eat when hungry and stop when satisfied? How do you get in touch with your natural body signals?

Once it came naturally. As babies, when our stomachs were hungry, we cried. We ate. It felt good, and as we grew full, we stopped eating. Simple as that.

Unfortunately, in our society today many people of all ages have lost that natural regulation and eat in dysfunctional, disturbed ways. They respond to inappropriate internal and external signals instead. Children learn to ignore and override their internal signals when told by overanxious parents that they must eat more — or less — than their bodies tell them they want. Dieting teaches women to ignore and override these cues, to distrust their own bodies.

To get back in touch with their hunger and satiety cues, women need to accept their setpoint weight range, say nutritionists Karin Kratina, MA, RD, and Nancy King, MS, RD. "If a client is keeping her weight unnaturally low through restriction of calories or excessive exercise, her body is in a state of depletion, resulting in distorted hunger and satiety signals."

Using a hunger scale in which 0 represents empty, 5 is neutral, and 10 is stuffed, they ask women to record their level of hunger throughout the day, before, during, and after eating. This helps them understand through subtle shifts when it is time to eat, how much food is needed to feel satisfied or full, and how long before they feel hungry again. In doing this, women should slow down, relax, and be flexible. There is no specific number at which they should begin or stop eating. Quitting at a 6 may mean being hungry again sooner than if eating to an 8.

Exploring the desire to eat without real hunger can be a journey of self-discovery and self-acceptance that should be undertaken in a relaxed and uncritical way.[5]

Many people who try a new, more relaxed style of eating begin feeling stomach sensations they've never felt before.

Women tell me that they are afraid to stop dieting — if they don't diet, they'll eat out of control. But it doesn't happen. If you learn to trust your body, you'll feel when it is time to stop eating. You'll want to stop at that point. There's no reason to overeat, because you can eat again whenever you want to.

If you've been living in the starvation mode, don't expect to recover instantly even when you begin eating normally. Remember that it took about nine months for the men in the Minnesota Starvation Study to stabilize their eating and return to normal weight.

Don't worry if your appetite seems to increase somewhat as you begin normalizing your eating. Overeating for a time is a perfectly natural response to food deprivation. But the urge to binge will soon stop when plenty of food is available and you give yourself permission to eat it. Be assured that it is worthwhile and ultimately satisfying to go through this process.

Eating well brings freedom to women who have limited themselves by living in a food deprived state, within a protective shell, and in an emotional, physical, mental, social and spiritual shutdown. They recover their personalities and become whole again, moving beyond those feelings so closely linked with hunger — moodiness, anxiety, irritation, guilt, shame, apathy, depression, intolerance, rigidity, and self-centeredness — and instead choose to be strong, capable, energetic, friendly, optimistic, generous and compassionate.

Physicians who unthinkingly have prescribed medications to depressed, hungry women will find drugs are not needed. Food was the medicine needed all along.

Messages from many lands

Taking pleasure in eating, and enjoying taste, flavors, and home cooking are part of the recommendations for good nutrition in many countries. For example, the first point in the British dietary guidelines is "Enjoy your food." In Japan, national guidelines urge people to "make all activities pertaining to food and eating pleasurable ones." Vietnam recommends its citizens partake of "A healthy family meal that is delicious, wholesome, clean and economical, and served with affection." In Thailand, people are advised, "A happy family is when family members eat together, enjoy treasured family tastes and good home cooking."

Of Norway's *Ten Good Eating Rules*, two of the foremost are:
• Enjoy your food
• Eat until your stomach is "just right"

The National Nutrition Council gives Norwegians this equation: FOOD + JOY = HEALTH.[6]

Family meals, with the television off, are an important time for sharing. Eating mindfully allows your family to feel relaxed, comfortable, and in touch with their internal cues of hunger, appetite and satiety. Women need to be aware that the way they relate to food, eating, weight and body issues affects everyone around them. This has been ignored in the past 20 years of focusing on dieting, as if each woman stood alone and affected no one with her chaotic eating. Now we find there were always little eyes and ears paying close attention. My earlier book in this series, *Afraid to Eat: Helping Children and Teens in Today's Weight Crisis,* documents problems that often result from chaotic eating in the home, and offers positive guidelines for parents, teachers, counselors and health providers.

What to eat

Healthy food choices keep us feeling at our best. This means enjoying a variety of foods — and emphasizing fruits and vegetables, whole grains, lean meats and low fat dairy products.

Balance, variety, and moderation are the guiding principles of good nutrition. A balanced diet (which may be balanced over several days) provides adequate nutrition from each of the five groups.

The Food Guide Pyramid helps us visualize these five groups: bread and grains, vegetables, fruits, meat and alternates, and milk. Eating a variety of foods from each of these groups ensures that we will get the many nutrients essential for health and energy.

Eating moderately, until the stomach is "just right," avoids the extremes of either eating too much or too little. It also reminds us to be moderate in eating high-fat and high-sugar foods, not overeating nor rejecting them entirely if we want them — which can lead to feelings of deprivation and bingeing.

Nutrient-dense foods, rather than calorie-dense foods, should be selected most often from each of the five groups. These are foods high in nutrients and low in calories, fat, and added sugars. Many are bulky, high in fiber, and filling, such as apples, corn and beans. Others pack a lot of nutrition into small size and are very satisfying, such as eggs, fish and lowfat meats.

Calorie-dense choices and foods from the tip of the pyramid, fats, sweets, alcohol, are better consumed less often and in smaller quantity. Unfortunately, trends today are to eat more and more processed high-fat, high-sugar snack foods, crackers, desserts, candy and soft drinks, and less fruits and vegetables, less milk, less meat and eggs than even 15 or 20 years ago.

The Dietary Guidelines for Americans offer this sound advice for healthful eating:

- Eat a variety of foods
- Choose a diet with plenty of grain products, vegetables and fruits
- Choose a diet low in fat, saturated fat, and cholesterol
- Choose a diet moderate in sugars
- Choose a diet moderate in salt and sodium
- If you drink alcoholic beverages, do so in moderation[7]

In addition, it makes sense to use local foods whenever you can. They are fresher, and often taste better, are more nutritious and cost less. Buying local foods saves on wasteful packaging. It saves transportation resources, compared with foods which are shipped back and forth across the country. In addition, buying locally supports your own producers and your local economy.

Bread and cereals

Bread has long been known as the staff of life, and that's why grains — breads, cereals, rice, pasta — make up the broad base of the Food Pyramid, our foundation for healthful eating.

The guidelines tell us to eat at least 6 to 11 servings from this group.

Foods in the bread and cereals, or grains, group provide complex carbohydrates and are an important source of the energy and vitamins and minerals, and fiber we need every day. They are also high in fiber when we include some whole-grain foods — and most of us need much more fiber than we're getting.

Vegetables and fruit

In looking at improving how we eat, a good place to start is with those five-a-day fruits and vegetables — and no need to stop with five (five to 11 are recommended). Most Americans eat less. Include all kinds, the cancer-protective vegetables from the cabbage/broccoli family, deep-yellow and dark-green leafy, starchy potatoes, corn and beans. Add two or more servings of fruit, including citrus.

Remember, variety is important, so learn to enjoy something new.

Five a day isn't so much. It only means a glass of orange juice with breakfast; an apple at lunch; a salad, green beans and mashed potatoes for dinner. That's easy.

Fruits and vegetables are excellent sources of so many nutrients — vitamins, minerals, carotenoids, antioxidants, phytochemicals, protein, starch and fiber — that we need to be including them at every meal (and snacks). People whose diets are high in fruits and vegetables seem to have lower risk for heart disease, diabetes, and certain types of cancers.

Not only do many people not eat enough, but they may eat only two or three kinds of vegetables and fruits. Yet it is from variety — all kinds of dark-green leafy, deep-yellow, cabbage-family, starchy, and citrus vegetables and fruits — that we get the many different nutrients we need.

It should be so easy, but if people eat a great many highly-processed foods, they may not be eating much variety. Even though it seems like foods come from lots of different packages and brand names, they may be basically combinations of the same ingredients.

Most of us also need more fiber, both soluble and insoluble, which comes from fruits and vegetables and whole grains. Fiber not only provides the "roughage" we need for good digestion, but also seems protective in lowering cholesterol levels and preventing certain cancers.

Current research shows that people who eat plenty of fruits and vegetables have lower rates of heart disease, diabetes, and certain types of cancers. A reason may be that our bodies produce free radicals, which can cause damage, and these appear to be blocked by the defenses of antioxidants like vitamin C, vitamin E, beta carotene and other carotenoids, and certain minerals found in fruits and vegetables.

Milk

Milk and milk products like cheese, yogurt, puddings, ice milk and ice cream provide us with our best source of calcium, as well as eight other essential nutrients. Other compounds found in milk such as conjugated linoleic acid (CLA) in milk fat, sphingomyelin and vitamin D may have anti-cancer effects as well.[8] Fat free or low-fat milk products are both low in calories and satisfying.

We never outgrow our need for milk. But unfortunately, there's a sad and recent decline in drinking milk. Women up to age 50 need 1,000 milligrams of calcium a day, and after that 1,200, under the new recommendations.[9]

How can we possibly get all this calcium? Since one cup of milk contains about 300 mg of calcium, it's a good idea to drink two or three glasses a day, in addition to eating other milk products, such as yogurt and cheese, and to add calcium from plant sources.

Some people are allergic to milk, or feel uncomfortable when they drink it. Experiment with drinking small quantities, with milk for lactose-intolerance, and with yogurt and buttermilk, which are often more acceptable. If you don't drink milk, you'll want to plan your calcium intake with even more care than others.

One set of nutrition guidelines does not necessarily fit everyone. We are all different, and need to listen to our bodies as well as to sound nutrition information.

Women often lack the calcium they need to protect themselves from osteoporosis, which is a loss of bone mass and weakening of the bones. More than 25 million Americans suffer from osteoporosis, most of them women, causing 1.5 million bone fractures, costing $10 billion annually, and severely reducing quality and length of life.

Of course, it helps to inherit good bones. Genetics is the most critical factor in bone mass, and helps determine whether bones are large and dense or thin and fragile. But good nutrition, lifelong exercise, and maintaining a sturdy frame play key roles.

Estrogen drops during menopause, causing accelerated bone loss. Smoking and drinking excessive alcohol also increase the risks. Many doctors recommend estrogen replacement therapy after menopause to help prevent bone loss.

Food Guide Pyramid
A GUIDE TO DAILY FOOD CHOICES

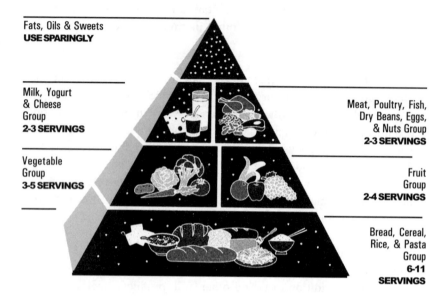

Fats, Oils & Sweets
USE SPARINGLY

Milk, Yogurt
& Cheese
Group
2-3 SERVINGS

Meat, Poultry, Fish,
Dry Beans, Eggs,
& Nuts Group
2-3 SERVINGS

Vegetable
Group
3-5 SERVINGS

Fruit
Group
2-4 SERVINGS

Bread, Cereal,
Rice, & Pasta
Group
**6-11
SERVINGS**

Use the Food Guide Pyramid to help you eat better every day. Start at the pyramid base with plenty of grains, breads, cereals, rice and pasta, six to 11 servings, depending on your appetite, hunger, satiety. At the second level add vegetables and fruits — five to 11 or more, together. Moving up, add two or three servings of milk (three to five for older children and teens) and two or three servings from the meat and alternates group. Go easy on or avoid the extra fats, oils, sweets and alcohol at the tip of the Pyramid, foods that provide calories but few other nutrients.

Eating well focuses on balance, moderation and variety. Balanced food choices come from all five food groups. Eating in variety from each food group ensures you'll get the many nutrients you need for health, energy and growth. Eating moderately means eating enough for good nourishment, not past the point of satiety, and choosing foods moderately low in fat and sugars.

In using the pyramid, remember that the suggested serving size and number gives a general guide for minimum amounts to get the nutrients most people need. However, people will differ in the amount of food they choose and that satisfies their needs, depending on their size, activity and temperament. Eating well means using sound nutrition recommendations, and at the same time, trusting our bodies to respond to their natural signals of hunger, appetite and satiety.[1]

What counts as one serving?

THE FOOD GUIDE PYRAMID

Bread, cereals, pasta group (6-11 servings)
- 1 slice of bread
- 1 ounce of ready-to-eat cereal
- 1/2 cup of cooked cereal, rice, or pasta

Vegetable group (3-5 servings)
- 1 cup of raw leafy vegetables
- 1/2 cup of cooked or chopped raw vegetables
- 3/4 cup vegetable juice

Fruit group (2-4 servings)
- 1 medium apple, banana, orange
- 1/2 cup of chopped, cooked or canned fruit
- 3/4 cup of fruit juice

Milk group (2-3 servings)
- 1 cup of milk or yogurt
- 1 1/2 ounces of natural cheese
- 2 ounces of processed cheese

Meat and alternates group (2-3 servings)
- 2 to 3 ounces of cooked lean meat, poultry or fish

Equals 1 ounce of meat:
(double or triple this amount to make one serving)
- ½ cup cooked dry beans
- 1 egg
- 4 ounces tofu
- 2 tablespoons peanut butter
- 1/3 cup nuts

You may choose to add a calcium supplement, taking care that this supplements an already adequate diet, and is not relied on as the major source of calcium. The American Dietetic Association points out that "when milk is the calcium choice, rather than a supplement, the overall nutrient quality of the diet is enhanced."

Meat and alternates group

Foods in the meat and alternates group pack a great deal of nutrition into a small package — protein, B vitamins, iron, zinc, and other vitamins and minerals. Heme iron from animal sources in this group helps your body better absorb non-heme iron from plant sources.

The Food Guide Pyramid suggests you eat two or three servings each day of foods from this group, or about 5 to 7 ounces of cooked lean meat, poultry or fish. Count 2 to 3 ounces of cooked lean meat, poultry or fish as one serving — about half a chicken breast, an average hamburger, or two eggs. If you don't eat meat or animal foods, take care to eat equivalent amounts of the alternates: legumes, soy, eggs and nuts. Remember that it takes one-third cup of peanut butter, or one and a half cups baked beans to equal a 3-ounce serving of meat.

Long valued in weight management programs, lean meat, poultry and fish are low in calories and highly satisfying. A Swedish study found that women who ate a lunch time casserole that included meat were satisfied longer, rated their meal higher in taste and satisfaction, and ate 12 percent fewer calories at the evening meal, than did women who ate a similar all-vegetable casserole.

Women who avoid meat, poultry, fish and eggs, in efforts to be thin, are often severely restricting other foods, as well, and this can be a serious health issue. Many women fast and binge, alternately eating almost nothing and then bingeing on cookies, desserts and candy. If instead, you will snack on a boiled egg or roast beef sandwich you'll more likely feel satisfied and filled with energy.

Men can probably adapt better than women to a diet without meat or animal products. Because women's bodies are continually preparing for childbirth and experiencing monthly blood losses, they require more of certain nutrients than do men, yet they usually eat less. Thus, women are more likely to suffer deficiencies.

It's a good idea to eat fish several times a week. Fish and fish oils seem to have a beneficial effect in several disease states, including heart disease, vascular disease, cancer, and immune function. People who eat large amounts of fish lower risk of heart attacks.

Soy also has many health benefits. Research suggests soybean foods may be helpful in lowering the "bad" LDL cholesterol levels, in heart disease and cancer prevention, in delaying bone loss, and may even improve memory in older people. Soy can be incorporated into a variety of foods, as tofu, soy flour and other forms.

The challenge here is to get enough foods from this group to keep us at our best, while at the same time reducing fat intake. We can do this by choosing lean cuts of meat, trimming visible fat, removing skin from chicken, and avoiding high-fat cooking methods, especially deep-fat frying.

The vegetarian choice

There are many ways to eat vegetarian style. Some vegetarians eat no meat, poultry or fish, but eat dairy foods and perhaps eggs. Some eat no animal products at all, including foods made with ingredients such as milk or eggs. Semi-vegetarians base their usual eating on plant source foods, and occasionally eat meat, poultry or fish.

For vegetarians who consume dairy foods and eggs, planning a healthy diet can be much like that for non-vegetarians. As with any kind of eating, choose a balance of foods in variety, and eat them in moderation — and remember that moderation means eating sufficient fat and calories, as well as not overeating. To improve iron absorption eat plenty of plants containing iron, such as legumes and dark-green leafy vegetables, and include a food rich in vitamin C, such citrus fruit, at each meal.

If you are a vegetarian who eats no animal products, take time to learn the best way to put together a sound eating plan that will provide the nourishment and protective factors you need. You'll want to consider a reliable source of vitamin B_{12}, an essential vitamin missing in plant foods. Other nutrients that will need special attention are vitamin D, calcium, iron and zinc.

Vegetariansim can be beneficial when meals are well balanced and contain a wide variety of foods. A vegetarian diet is usually lower in saturated fats and higher in fiber. Vegetarians often have lower blood pressure than non-vegetarians.

The challenge is to get enough good-quality protein, iron and zinc to build, maintain, and repair the body tissues, and to keep the immune system functioning well. A common error for new vegetarians is to incorrectly replace meat, chicken and fish with foods from other food groups, such as primarily substituting cheese from the milk group. Legumes, tofu, soy milk, eggs and nuts are in the meat and alternates group, and should be eaten every day in equivalent amounts.

Vegetarian eating can supply you with the nutrients you need. A vegetarian cookbook that includes nutrition information, and is written by a licensed nutritionist or dietitian, can be helpful.

The more varied the diet, the less likely the vegetarian woman is to suffer from vitamin or mineral deficiencies. If you have concerns, consult a dietitian. Supplementing may be an option.

The important thing is to keep well-nourished and to fit normal eating into your lifestyle for your own good health and well-being. Common sense is always the best guide.

What about fat?

Excess fat in the diet should be avoided. Guidelines emphasize the continued importance of choosing a diet with less total fat, saturated fat, and cholesterol. When fewer calories come from fat, it also means there's more room for healthy food choices.

However, America has sadly overreacted to the lowfat message. How can we lower our fat intake without going to extremes?

Vitality tells us, "Your overall pattern of eating can include foods high, moderate and low in fat. If you want to enjoy a higher-fat food, balance it with staying active and enjoying a wide variety of foods the rest of the day."

Some dietary fat is needed for good health. Fat is not a four-letter word. It's an important nutrient that helps cells use vitamins and minerals more effectively. Fat may also be protective, as with CLA in animal fats.

The Dietary Guidelines advise reducing fat intake to 30 percent of total calories (but not lower). American women are close to this level now, at an average of 32 percent, according to NHANES III. For those who are above recommended levels, total fat can be easily lowered if we bring less fat into the house, add less fat in cooking, and use less fat at the table. In eating out, it helps to indulge less in deep fat fried foods and other high fat choices.

The problem is one of extremes. On average we're doing just fine. But many women (especially college women) have dropped their fat intake to dangerously low levels; and many others still have diets extremely high in fat. Can you look at your food choices and consider whether your fat intake is at the too-much or too-little extreme, or comfortably in the middle?

Improving deficiencies

American women and teenage girls consume far less calcium and iron than they need. Most get less than two-thirds of the RDA. At the lower end, the hungry one-fourth are sadly deficient in these and many other nutrients to an extent that can cause long-term physical and mental problems. How can these women be encouraged to eat what they need to improve their lives?

Calcium is essential for healthy bones. It is important to have plenty of this mineral during the critical bone-building years, and throughout life to avoid degeneration of the skeleton. Calcium does more than build bones and teeth. It also contributes to bone mineralization, blood clotting, heart muscles contracting, nerve cell transmission and enzyme activity. Low calcium intakes are related to osteoporosis, kidney stones, colon cancer, hypertension during pregnancy, and other health problems. Calcium may play a role in preventing high blood pressure and some forms of cancer.

Easily available in milk and milk products, our best source, calcium is also found in sardines, canned salmon with bones, dark green plants like broccoli, kale and spinach, and calcium-fortified foods. However, calcium may be poorly absorbed from vegetables that are rich in oxalic acid or phytic acid (spinach, beans, grains, nuts, soy isolates).

Recommendations for calcium intake have recently been raised. Women after menopause may want to consider a combination of calcium-rich foods, calcium-fortified foods, and a calcium supplement. If you don't drink milk, supplementation may be even more important.

Lack of iron is one of the most common nutrient deficiencies for women worldwide, due to inadequate diet and monthly menstrual blood losses. Iron deficiency and anemia cause fatigue, apathy, nausea, a chilled condition, and a compromised immune system that means a person may be more easily infected and sick more often. Half of American women get less than three-fourths of the iron they need. Again, the hungry one-fourth at the bottom are sadly deficient.

Iron comes from plant and animal foods and fortified foods in the bread and grains group. The problem is that iron is not easily absorbed, and 90 percent or more may be lost. Absorption is aided by vitamin C consumed in the same meal, but is inhibited by substances that bind to iron and calcium in whole grain cereals and legumes (phytate). Foods from the meat and alternates group (particularly red meat) are a major source of bioavailable iron in the diet. If red meat is eaten and two to three servings from the meat group included daily, iron intake and absorption is probably sufficient. If you don't eat red meat, be especially attentive to iron availability in your diet and consider supplementation. (A risk in iron supplementation is overdosing, so follow directions carefully.) It is believed that our bodies may compensate to some extent by absorbing more iron when stores are low.

Fiber is another nutrient in short supply in many American diets. Found only in plant foods like whole-grain breads and cereals, beans and peas, and other vegetables and fruits, fiber helps our bodies work better and may lower the risk for heart disease and some cancers. Most of us need to be eating more of these foods.

Supplements

Should I take supplements or not? This is a question each woman needs to answer for herself.

Most women who regularly eat a healthy, balanced diet will not need to supplement that diet. You'll have the many nutrients you need in balance and variety. If you are not fully nourished, improving food choices is the place to start. We need to be clear that a poor diet with supplements is still a poor diet.

However, if you have concerns, an all-purpose multivitamin which provides no more than 100 percent of the recommended daily allowance (RDA) is a good choice. You may also decide to choose a calcium supplement. It's a good idea to ask a pharmacist for the kind of supplement best absorbed in the body. If you have special needs, check them out with a dietitian.

Real foods are better than supplements for at least three reasons: first, the nutrients from food are usually absorbed better in the body; second, each food contains many needed nutrients, some we may not even be aware of; and third, the nutrients from food are in natural balance, so we are not in danger of overdosing.

"Nutrients depend on one another for effectiveness. Many tend to occur together in foods, a naturally beneficial coincidence. People who try to outguess nature by taking single vitamins in pill form seldom hit on such winning combinations," writes Eleanor Whitney, PhD, RD, in *Nutrition Concepts and Controversies.*

Many people, knowing their diets are deficient, rely on often-expensive food supplement pills. The truth is food is much better. Numerous studies confirm this. The idea that it's okay to create deficiencies by avoiding important protective foods — and then substitute with pills is sheer folly. Healthy diet needs to come first.

We don't know all the benefits of foods. Take phytochemicals, one of the hottest new areas in cancer research. It's estimated that in just one serving of vegetables there may be over 100 different phytochemicals, compounds that plants produce to protect themselves against viruses, bacteria and fungi. We haven't identified them all, much less which ones are most effective against cancer, and possibly heart disease. If you take a pill instead of eating a balanced diet, you lose out.

There's a great deal of confusion right now in the supplement, nutraceuticals, and natural foods businesses, with some movement toward standardization. At this time these products are largely unregulated and non-standardized. (Check for labels giving measured amount of each ingredient.) They may vary in potency, and there is risk of getting a substance that is harmful or in a dosage so high it may be toxic.

Even fiber, which is hardly toxic, can cause digestive and nutrient deficiency problems when a person takes too much in supplement form. The nutrition committee that set the RDAs recommends that fiber come from fruits, vegetables, legumes, and whole-grain cereals and breads, rather than by adding fiber concentrates to the diet.[10]

Functional foods are the latest growth area in food sales, and are expected to be marketed heavily in the next few years. These are foods that offer improved health, enhanced performance or increased general wellness. We saw some of this during the oat bran craze, when some breakfast foods containing oat bran were suggested as being preventive against heart disease.

Concerns are being raised about the extent of and support for health claims being made for these foods and, even more disturbing, the effect that their usually single-food-focused messages might have on sensible, balanced eating. On the other hand, there is no reason such foods cannot be beneficial if used well and honestly promoted.

Good foods, bad foods

When making food choices, let's remember there are no good foods or bad foods. We can eat whatever we want. All foods can fit in a healthy eating plan. The idea that some foods are healthy and others unhealthy is false and promotes the unscientific notion that some foods can be used like medicine and others produce disease. Trust reliable nutrition information and your own good sense.

In making a shift toward health enhancing lifestyles it's helpful to move gradually into new patterns. A national group that advocates the approach of enjoying food, taste and physical activity is the Dietary Guidelines Alliance, a coalition of health organizations, government agencies and food producer groups.

The key messages of the Alliance campaign are:

- **Be realistic:** Make small changes over time in what you eat and the level of activity you do. After all, small steps work better than giant leaps.

- **Be adventurous:** Expand your tastes to enjoy a variety of foods.

- **Be flexible:** Go ahead and balance what you eat and the physical activity you do over several days. No need to worry about just one day or one meal.

- **Be sensible:** Enjoy all food, just don't overdo it.
- **Be active:** Walk the dog, don't just watch the dog walk.[11]

It's sound advice for today's woman.

Americans have never been healthier than today. We live longer than ever before. Our food supply has never been safer, more nutritious, or better tasting.

Food is not our enemy, but our friend. Enjoy it for taste, texture, good health and the pleasure of eating with family and friends.

CHAPTER 15

Celebrating size diversity

■

"Whatever size you are, have a wonderful life."
— *Barbara Bruno*

We are coming to a cultural turning point on body and size issues – finally.

We are coming to a point where we as individuals can celebrate the bodies we have now. We can honor them as part of our inheritances from our ancestors. We can declare peace and accept ourselves now, at whatever size we are.

There are also some positive signs that suggest that society is ready to accept more sizes, more bodies, more diversity.

People are unquestionably fed up with dieting, and they are recognizing the harmful link with anorexia and bulimia. That change is showing up in some segments of the media that are embracing a wider variety of sizes, and as well as rare, but notable, size-positive advertisements.

Beauty, health and strength come in all sizes.

Real beauty is being strong and healthy, being generous, loving and compassionate, and accepting yourself just as you are — goals that every woman can achieve.[1]

"I often had daydreams of what my thin life would be like — I'd be successful, admired, sought after, and confident. Now I am all those things — I'm just not thin," writes Carol Johnson, author of *Self-Esteem Comes in All Sizes,* recalling a time when she believed that her "real" life would begin when she lost weight and became thin.[2]

Self-acceptance can be a powerful force, say Steven Jonas and Linda Konner in their book *Just the Weigh You Are.*

"You'll be discovering a new serenity, an unexpected peacefulness within you that you never knew existed. You'll finally be able to get on with your life, focus on the Big Picture, and figure out what really matters to you. ... Congratulate yourself for giving yourself a well-deserved break, and for having the wisdom and courage to follow your head instead of the herd."[3]

For too long, popular culture has taught us to emphasize and admire the package, rather than the contents. It's certainly time to reject that narrow view and give more appreciation to what's inside. We can't allow our size and weight to measure our self-worth, or keep us from the things we want in life.

"You can think for yourself," Carol Johnson reminds us. "You can create your own ideal based on your own knowledge and self-discovery. Reject the foolish notion of one culturally imposed ideal and realize that there can be just as many ideals as there are women. ... Allow your beauty to spring from your individuality. Beauty encompasses more than physical characteristics. Let it include your zest for life, your fun-loving spirit, a smile that lights up your face, your compassion for others."

We can set a positive example, and be that needed role model for others. We can radiate confidence and self-respect. Through self-acceptance, we will experience a sense of wholeness, of being complete, the aggregate of all those qualities that are uniquely gifted in each of us.

Granted, self-acceptance may not come easily — or quickly. Often it's a process: seeds are planted, we contemplate these issues and the seeds take root, we read and talk with others and sprouts begin to show, we change a few behaviors and the plants flourish. As seasons pass, we grow as hardy plants and trees and smile to remember how tentatively we began.

Support valuing women of size

We can move society further down the path of size acceptance if women and men join together to confirm these truths and work to help the public shift toward an appreciation of people for themselves, not how they look.

We need to move on from size prejudice to a society that is more respectful, more accepting of the many ways women differ, into a society that refuses to suppress liberty, or withhold the promise of happiness from anyone on the basis of size or other criteria.

"If we accept that even one woman should be oppressed for her body size and shape we are all oppressed by body size and shape —

because that is the gauge by which we are all measured," writes Mary Evans Young, a British size activist.

Think of the women you know. Aren't they all sizes, shapes and physical abilities, all ages, all races and ethnicities? All of them need to be encouraged to feel good about themselves, to feel beautiful, to indulge their hungers and needs as human beings.

Can we finally reject size discrimination, and other prejudices, so all women feel the freedom to be themselves as we move into the 21st century? It can happen now.

"I don't know how things will change, but it's clear that our culture needs to learn a new way of valuing women," says Susan Wooley, PhD, professor emeritus, Cincinnati Medical College. "Reducing women to appearances is a terrible waste. Our sensibilities, intuition, caring and openness are assets in every aspect of life. It's more than a way of being, it's a set of values of what it means to be human."[4]

Role models

A few large women are providing shining examples of the kind of competent and confident role models our size-focused society needs today.

"This is for all the fat girls!" proclaimed actress Camryn Manheim, to thunderous applause, as she held aloft the Emmy she won in 1998 for her role as Eleanor Frutt in ABC's "The Practice." It was a memorable moment for women and girls all over the globe.[5]

Talk-show host Rosie O'Donnell is popular, as is actress and talk-show host Oprah Winfrey, who is admired despite her very public up and down struggles with weight. Interestingly, Winfrey seems to gain popularity when she gains weight, and loses popularity when she loses weight. What is her audience trying to tell Oprah? That they like her better larger? Or that she comes across as a nicer person when well-nourished?

The barrier to casting a large actor or actress as a romantic lead was broken by Manheim, perhaps the first woman her size to be romantically kissed on television. Manheim had the vision and power to insist her romantic partner on The Practice be good looking and of an ordinary size, not a "big guy."

It is perfectly normal for people of all sizes to feel romantic about other people of any size. It's okay. Some people prefer larger partners, and it's unfair to suggest they should not. Yet some have suffered social pressure and self-doubt because they wanted to date and make a commitment to a larger person. It is time to allow both men and women to freely express their preference for people of any size.[6]

Manheim promotes well her message that large women need to be seen as beautiful, vital, intelligent, and passionate. After all, a leading sex symbol at the turn of the century was Lillian Russell, who weighed over 200 pounds. Another was Mae West.

So look in the mirror, smile at that woman looking back, and tell her she's beautiful. Tell her she's funny, intelligent, worthy of anyone's time and attention. Good health, love and friendship, and other facets of good lives can come her way, regardless of size or size prejudice.

Benefits of being large

There are benefits to being large, although we don't often hear about them.

In a chapter she wrote for *Overcoming Fear of Fat*, Angela Barron McBride uses warm words to describe large women. Many of these images came from her childhood, including large-hearted, bounteous, hospitable, indulgent, nurturing, maternal, warm, lavish, hearty, effusive, emotional, unconstrained, hearty, great, substantial, benevolent, strong, superior, healthy, generous, profound, towering, powerful, remarkable, eminent, and calling to mind fecundity, prosperity, and expansiveness. She points out that *thin,* on the other hand, is often associated with lean times, being insubstantial, frail, and insufficient.[7]

McBride values nurses highly, and she observes that many nurses are large, strong, maternal, comfortable and patient. Since they are well-rounded and pleasant it seems right that they are themselves rounded with soft edges, she says.

She admires Miss Piggy on the Muppet Show. "She is bright, strong, and does not suffer fools easily. Bedecked in lavender satins with her long blonde curls swishing about her, she is my kind of modern woman — one who has a taste both for jewels from admirers and for independence. It is not surprising to me that Miss Piggy is the only female character on the Muppet Show to achieve star status. In many situations, only a substantial woman may be viewed as having substance. Miss Piggy enjoys throwing her weight around, but doesn't she have to have weight even to be noticed and taken seriously?"

Children often find large women warm and nurturing. One director of a child care facility told me she prefers to hire larger women because they are especially good with children.

Gina Lee writing in *Radiance,* recalls that as a child, "There was always some large woman in charge of school or church activities; someone with stars in her eyes, a ready smile, and a lap where there was always room for one more. It was okay not to be perfect around her — she accepted you even if you were being bratty. They all had different faces, but their great size offered a haven of rest and comfort for all children."[8]

Large women have fewer wrinkles as they grow older. The bloom of a teenager may still be on an older, larger woman's cheeks. Plastic surgeons inject fat into the face to erase wrinkles, but perhaps natural fat does it better. A funeral director once described to me the smooth, unwrinkled beauty on the face of a 300-pound woman he had prepared for burial. She was 83. "It was amazing how beautiful her complexion was. Just like a young girl," he marveled.

Large women can have breasts, unlike many of today's macabre fashion models. Breasts are largely made up of fat tissue, so they don't need the surgical implants and special enhancements required to provide feminine curves for hollow-cheeked celebrities.

In many cultures fat is considered a sign of sexual maturity, of prosperity, of health, strength and wisdom.

On the health side, larger women have less risk of some cancers, including lower breast cancer rates before menopause. Bone studies consistently show stronger bones for larger women, less osteoporosis, and fewer broken bones. And they sleep better, with fewer disturbed periods during the night.

Even WIN, the official Weight-control Information Network of the National Institute of Diabetes and Digestive and Kidney Diseases is producing a physical activity booklet for "supersize people" that avoids any recommendation to lose weight. *Fit at Any Size!* is a great resource that owes much to the patient and persistent efforts of size-activist Lynn McAfee in educating federal health officials on the need to help large people get healthy, rather than continuing to focus on trying to change their weight.

Don't postpone life

Many large women have developed the mental habit of putting their lives on hold, waiting to be thin. It's a self-destructive mind-set that needs to be overcome.

"Picking a number on the scale and postponing our lives until we reach that number is never going to work," write Pat Lyons and Debby Burgard in *Great Shape*. "What we really want is a good life, full of friends, enjoyment, and self-respect. ... Quite simply, a way of living that feels good. And we can have it — now and forever. It is a good life that is possible."[9]

Deciding to accept ourselves as we are is not giving up, Carol Johnson says. It's taking charge of our lives, our bodies, our self-images, of this unique being that is ours and ours alone. It's focusing on being the best we can be in the bodies we have right now.

Describing how she finally stopped waiting to be thin, actress Manheim recalls thinking, "This is my body. I live in it, I play in it. I can't deny it anymore. This is my fat body. I'm standing at the corner of Life and You Better Get Going. I can either cross the street or just keep waiting — I stepped off the curb and never looked back."

"Hoping to be thin is not hope. It's hatred. Life is too short for self-hatred and celery sticks," says Marilyn Wann.

Yet giving up the dream can be painful. Some have compared it to accepting the idea of death. Lyons and Burgard urge women to move through this grieving process. "To accept the fact of being fat forever can be very difficult and can create panic and deep resistance. Rather than being consoled by the facts, you may instead hope against hope that all of the research on genetic causes of fat and the failure of diets is wrong. ... Acceptance of yourself as a self-respecting fat woman eager to get on with your life is a process that will be gradual."

It helps to share your feelings about this struggle with others.

Accept happiness

Whatever size you are, have a wonderful life, advises Barbara Bruno.

"The first step to having a happier life is to choose one. The next step is to find specific ways to bring more happiness into your life. The choice is completely yours. ... If we think we cannot be happy unless we are thin, we are left with a life choice of perpetual weight-loss attempts or misery. ... You can have a happy life and great relation-ships."

Focus on what is possible and can be changed. Large women can have the lives they want regardless of whether weight changes or not. What is the first thing you would do right now, if you were living the life you really wanted? Why not do it now?

Bruno says that for people to change, they should act as if the change has already happened. Act as you would like to if you were at your desired weight. "While there may be little you can do to perma-nently reduce your weight, there is plenty you can do to eliminate your weight or eating problem and have a wonderful life."

She urges women to silence the "peanut gallery," the negative tapes that run in their heads. "One kind of weight loss I highly recommend is to clean out the people in your life who don't support you." The next step is to fill that peanut gallery with supporters, positive thinkers, and affirmations, she says.

Friends who don't support you can be eased out of the center of your life. Therapist L. Niquie Dworkin, PhD, advises bluntly, "Begin to examine friendships with people who have negative relationships with their own bodies or who are critical of yours. If you have lovers who make negative comments about your appearance, consider ending these relationships."[10]

She says, "Focus on what your body can do, not what it looks like. Remember to appreciate all it does, such as walking, lifting, dancing, nursing, making love. Engage in physical activities that increase your awareness of your body's strength and capabilities such as dance, martial arts, yoga and sports you enjoy."

It's okay to be just ordinary you, as everyone else is ordinary.

"Celebrate being ordinary. You can do it! Be average. Be ordinary. Be amazingly you!" says Janet Garcia, MA.[11]

A metaphor often used by Bruno, who treats food and weight problems through her Weight Release program, is that of "deliciousness." She says it seems at first strange to people who have struggled with deprivation and dieting. Wait till you're hungry, and then eat "only delicious food." Deliciousness applies to body movement and other aspects of life. It reinforces the idea that satisfaction is important in relationships, activities and work.

Dress for success

In celebrating your new, size-accepting self, wear clothes you like, that fit comfortably now and allow you to move as you like, not clothes to hide, or that will fit better when you've lost a few pounds.

Carol Johnson tells a story about her husband once asking why he had never seen her wear many of the clothes hanging in her closet (some still with price tags). When she explained these were for six months later when she would weigh 60 pounds less, he proposed that she go out and buy some clothes that fit.

She did, and "It didn't take me long to realize that this was infinitely more fun."

Johnson finds many women in her Largely Positive support groups do just as she did. They buy cheaper, less attractive clothes they can wear immediately, and nicer clothes for later when they lose weight. Sometimes it's as an incentive, sometimes because they don't want to waste money on that "temporary" larger size.

Changing attitudes bring remarks like this: "Now my closet is filled with happy clothes that get worn with pleasure and pride," and "People are going to notice me one way or another, so I might as well look smashing."

The plus-size fashion industry has grown and all major designers now have larger sizes. Great looks are available from Saks Fifth Avenue to Target. And don't forget that large people do wear shorts and swim suits, and it's okay.

Activity you enjoy

If one key to happiness is accepting the way we are, the other is to take pleasure in the activities and sports that we enjoy. And not for weight loss, which may not happen, but for health and the sheer pleasure of it. At first, we may feel self-conscious, but doing the things we like gets easier each time we do them. It's ironic, say size activists, that the world screams at large women to exercise, but when they do go out they need to prepare themselves for the possibility of insults.

Yet this is no reason to give up. Exercising indoors is always an option. But the more large women are out there being active, the more it is accepted, and the more support they will get.

It's a way of blazing a trail for our daughters, says Pat Lyons.

"Strangers often offer smiles of greeting and encouragement. And you can often initiate this response by offering a smile yourself first. But even when crummy incidents do occur, they should not be allowed to deprive us of our right to live with respect in the world. We have a right to take up space, live fully in our bodies and fully in our lives. By dealing with our feelings honestly and supporting one another in this right, we make it easier for ourselves and for those who follow in our footsteps."

Lyons and Burgard have both taught dance exercise classes for large women, and are enthusiastic about them.

"Envision a room filled with happy, healthy, dancing women. They twirl and swirl, stretch with catlike grace, and then they get down, honey, and boogie to the beat. They revive dances from the fifties and sixties — they stroll, pony, boogaloo, mashed potatoes — and make up steps of their own. After dancing themselves into a drenching sweat of pleasure, they cool down, slow down, relax, feel the flush in their cheeks, and luxuriate in the warmth of their bodies. This feels go-o-o-od deep down. Now envision that all these healthy women weigh over two hundred pounds. Ooops. Fat and fit? Did you find yourself mouthing the words impossible, ridiculous? Or did you say, 'Hot damn, it's about time!'"

Water sports are especially enjoyable for larger women. Water gives buoyancy and helps improve flexibility.

Support groups sometimes rent time at local pools and set up regular swim sessions for the exclusive use of large women. This creates a safe place, where all feel welcome, comfortable, and free to be themselves. All it takes is one or two women who want to make it happen. If there are not enough women, Lyons advises publicizing these events with eye-catching fliers distributed to friends to pass out and post in the local area.

Dworkin tells people when they exercise to avoid a focus on losing weight or changing their appearance, and to stay away from health clubs that feature mirror views. "You want to get in touch with your body from the inside and try to forget about how it may or may not look."

Rich lore of literature, theater

Large people today have a wealth of helpful materials in the form of books, magazines, and Internet sources to assist them on their journey to a richer life of acceptance and fulfillment. For the most part, these were not available five or 10 years ago.

There are the highly positive writings, like Carol Johnson's self-esteem book, which radiates warmth, vitality, and confidence. It's all about accepting one's unique traits, enjoying life every day and every holiday, taking risks, creating personal affirmations, enjoying humor and laughter, living in healthy ways and dealing assertively with problems.

Johnson helps people feel good about themselves. She expands the definition of beauty and tells readers how to look good and feel good by creating a personal style: "Liking yourself is the first step to a healthy lifestyle. You're a fine person just as you are."

She faces each issue squarely, with conviction and gentle empathy. There's no room here for bitterness or anger, only the positive response that comes naturally to this writer.

Yet, some people may need to vent their anger about the injustice and humiliation they have suffered before they are ready to move on. There are books to plumb these depths, too. W. Charisse Goodman's *The Invisible Woman: Confronting Weight Prejudice in America* can be helpful.

Still another dimension is the humorous, sassy, or in-your-face-outrageous offerings.

Lee Martindale has put together slogans that she explains as a "shooting from the rump" approach to change the way society treats large people. "Call it activism, fighting back, confrontation, or just plain standing up for yourself."

A few of her messages that show up on T-shirts, cups, and posters are: *Counting calories is NOT higher math. Over WHOSE weight? No, I don't want to hear about a great new diet! If it was good enough for Rubens, it's good enough for me. My man likes me the weigh I am — why should I care what YOU think? Fat, Forty and*

Fabulous. Never trust a skinny cook![12]

Susan Miller also has a list of "sassy comebacks," to use when strangers corner her to recommend a diet, or tell her how pretty she'd be if she'd lose some weight, or "do that shame-shame-shame gesture with their fingers" when they see her eat.

- You're kidding. I'm fat? Why didn't somebody tell me?
- You're very brave to say so. Don't most people get rather hostile when you say such things?
- A good therapist can really help you learn more socially appropriate behaviors. Would you like me to recommend one?
- You have some spinach or something between your teeth.

Then there's the book *Fat! So?* by Marilyn Wann, and her newsletter by the same name.

Wann writes, "Fat people are not, by definition, lazy or stupid. People who believe in such stereotypes, however, are."[13]

You don't have to be thin to be happy, says Wann. In fact, she has

---

Improving body image

- Identify what things you have been putting off for when you're thin. Make a list and start doing them now!

- Find creative outlets for your feelings around your body. Write about them, paint, read the writing of others, share feelings with a friend.

- Think about how you treat yourself and your body. Think of ways you can be gentle with yourself. Massages, hot baths, wearing favorite colors, fabrics and styles are all ways of pampering your body.

- Enjoy being in your body. Do activities you like: dancing, yoga, karate, swimming, biking.

- Look through books or at paintings in a gallery. Notice and appreciate images of larger women and surround yourself with images that reflect your natural body size.[1]

By Rachel Sheinin. Reprinted with permission from the National Eating Disorder Information Centre, Toronto, Ontario, Canada.

WOMEN AFRAID TO EAT 2000

gleaned thousands of survey answers to the question, "What do you like about being fat?" For example:

- It makes me strong.
- It's a built-in jerk detector.
- I'm unique, not a cookie-cutter person.
- Looking younger than my age — no wrinkles.
- People like to hug a soft person.
- I've never been mugged.
- It's taught me to think for myself and not rely on the crowd.
- It has made me more accepting of other people.

The Fat Lip Readers Theatre of San Francisco is a talented group that brings a stunning message to challenge our thin-obsessed, fat-phobic culture with scenes, dialogues, snappy answers to street taunts, poetry and song. When I first saw this talented theater group, I was amazed and troubled by their revelations of the cruelty often dealt them by everyday life in America.

One unforgettable gem of growing-up large is the poem, "Wait till next year, when I'm thin." *Nothing to Lose* is a video of this group's live theater.[14]

Moving ahead with the movement

For women and men who enjoy working for a cause, the Council on Size & Weight Discrimination and the National Association to Advance Fat Acceptance (NAAFA) offer havens of like-minded leaders and springboards for activism. These and related organizations throughout the world have done much to give visibility and support to the size-acceptance movement — but there's lots more to be done.

Networking with these leaders has taught me a great deal. In turn, it has enlightened thousands who work in health care after we started a regular feature to showcase their literature for readers of *Healthy Weight Journal.* For many it was like a light bulb going off to discover for the first time what their patients were dealing with and what they were thinking. Others felt personally vindicated. One new subscriber wrote her delight, "I am amazed that you have a size acceptance article in each issue. Over the years I have steeled myself to expect castigation from health professionals because of my weight. It is an eye-opener to read articles by health professionals who are open-minded about the issue of fat and are aware of the risks of dieting."

We now give annual Healthy Weight Week awards the third week of January to honor businesses that demonstrate an appreciation for the diversity of women and confirm that beauty, health, and strength come in all sizes.

You may enjoy being an advocate, even in a small way, or starting a support group in which large people come together to discuss intolerance they might have experienced, to celebrate their survival, and heal their spirits. The Internet offers new opportunities to join with others in chat rooms and listservs, to share your experiences, to grow and help others. Being connected to a community of like-minded people not only feels good, but having strong relationships is associated with health and longevity.

To move forward in the next century, Sally Smith, former executive director of NAAFA, says respect is the key. "We must respect ourselves as individuals, as an organization, and as a movement. The next step is to take responsibility, individually and organizationally, for ending fat oppression. No one is going to do it for us ... We have to realize that we are not victims, we are not second-class citizens. We do not have to assume the role they would create for us. We are survivors, we are strong, we are proud, we are fat and thin together fighting for justice."[15]

Boycotting and writing letters does work. Even a determined Hallmark Cards backed down after first reacting to criticism of a line of "fat humor" cards by chiding the protesters, saying humor is healthy for the spirit, and that "We intend to continue this tradition of good humor in a way we hope all our customers, including you, will find appealing."

NAAFA members refused to find the cards appealing, continued their letter-writing protest, and made plans for a boycott. This was when Hallmark gave in, agreed to stop shipping the cards to stores, and to "do our best to avoid any subject matter that might be considered insensitive to fat people."[16]

Deidra Daley, a NAAFA member, tells of going into an office super store to buy an office chair. The sales clerk informed her that the "abuse" her body would give any chair would break it and she was too heavy for their chairs. Feeling humiliated, she went home, then started to think about how she'd been treated and what she could do about it. Deciding not to give in to hurt and anger, she called the store and spoke with the sales manager, who was supportive and apologetic, and offered to have the store manager contact her the next day.

As it turned out the manager, a large man himself, told her their chairs were expected to be sturdy and invited her to return and pick something out for herself free of cost. She agreed, and suggested that while she was in, the two of them might check out the chairs and rate them for sturdiness as a guide for employees when dealing with larger-than-average customers. Together they tried out the chairs, wiggled, spun, bounced, and determined which were more comfortable for large and tall people. The manager said he would train the sales people on which to recommend for large-size customers.

"I'm proud that my experience may change a policy for a major retail establishment in their dealings with fat people. I encourage all of you to stand up for what is right — and fight what is wrong," says Daley.

Some changes only come about through legal action. This was the case with flight attendants on the airlines. Stringent weight and age regulations aimed at female flight attendants have been challenged successfully in the courts for 15 years, airline by airline, through age and sex discrimination suits. Now some airlines have abandoned the requirements entirely, and we are allowed to be served by some older and larger flight attendants.

Coping with workplace issues

On the job, women need to respect themselves and communicate the expectation that others will respect them. Insulting or harassing behavior in the workplace is wrong and no one should have to endure it.

Harassment is illegal and you can do something about it, says Joseph Dadourian, PhD, a California specialist in positive behavior in the workplace.

Fighting fat prejudice

■ Don't comment on someone's weight. Even if you compliment them on losing weight, you're still focusing on self-worth through body image, and you're giving them the message that you like them better thin.

■ Start trying to appreciate different achievements in yourself and others. Work toward the point where weight is no longer something you rate your success by.

■ Allow yourself and others to begin enjoying food for the pleasure it brings and for its nutritional value. Try to eliminate the category of "forbidden" foods from your mind.

■ Challenge common stereotypes about fat and thin in your daily life, i.e. that fat equals failure, unhealthy, lazy.[2]

Reprinted with permission from the National Eating Disorder Information Centre, Toronto, Ontario, Canada

WOMEN AFRAID TO EAT 2000

Document the harassment, including dates, times, who was there, what was said or done, and why you think it was discriminatory.

Dadourian says to clearly notify the offending person that what he or she is doing makes you feel uncomfortable and you want it to end. Be direct, saying, for example, "Whatever size I am, it's verbal harassment to make fun of my body. If you're making these comments, you're attacking me, and I want it to stop." In most instances, when people hear this, they will stop.

If direct assertive statements don't do it, he advises going to your superior with documentation. "Don't keep it to yourself, because it can always be taken to a higher authority. Be specific about dates, times, places and possible witnesses. Tell your superior, 'It's demeaning to me and interferes with my job performance.' Often a person who is harassing you in some way is doing it to others as well. Get their support and strategize, but what you don't want to do is retaliate. It will only escalate the situation."

Laurel Fishman, writing in Big Beautiful Woman (BBW), advises dealing with problems early. "Long before the problems get out of control, it's possible to stop them cold." She points out that stopping disrespectful behavior may mean expressing yourself differently, and being assertive without alienating others, because you act with grace and dignity.[17]

In job hunting, size activists say follow the advice for any good job seeker: have that resume up to date and targeted for the job you're applying for, provide good references, dress well and in a professional way, and be prepared. Be sharp, pleasant, honest and assertive in the interview.

Wann suggests being up front about size. "In a very neutral, casual tone, I would say, 'You may have certain assumptions about fat people. Let me reassure you that I don't take any more sick days than anyone else, and that I'm perfectly physically able to do this job. You can check my references to see that I'm perfectly competent. If you have any reservations based on my size, I'd like to hear about them, because I can easily allay those concerns.' I think not addressing size sends a message to the employer that avoidance is the way you deal with it."[18]

Assertiveness in health care

Getting quality health care is everyone's right, but large people cannot necessarily take it for granted. Finding a doctor you feel comfortable with and who is comfortable with you is important. You deserve and need a doctor who will give respectful care, professional concern, and good medical advice, who understands that weight loss carries risks and usually results in weight cycling. When you feel comfortable with your doctor, you can be open and receptive to discussions about your health, and willing to take steps necessary to improve it.

If you're not satisfied with how you are being treated now, you may want to consider making a change. You're the customer, so shop around. Ask for recommendations from other large people.

In setting up an appointment, you might ask if it is the health facility's policy to provide health at every size, or if they usually focus on weight loss for large people. Tell them you are a large person and request a physician who is size-accepting and willing to focus on your health, rather than your weight.

Some size activists recommend interviewing prospective doctors.

Johnson suggests calling to say you'd like to speak with the doctor briefly before making an appointment. She advises asking if he or she is comfortable treating large patients and willing to focus on measures of health rather than of size and weight. Ask if the doctor will give you the same treatment for your medical problems as a thin person would receive, and can leave the choice of being weighed up to you (unless there is a medical reason for it).

Johnson provides a sample letter to the doctor for those who feel more comfortable asking these questions in writing. As she says, if it doesn't work out with a phone call or letter, you'll have saved time and aggravation, and can look for someone else.

You have the right to complain if you are treated disrespectfully, or if gowns and equipment are too small. (Be aware that a too-tight blood pressure cuff can give a false high reading, and point this out if the one being used is too small.)

Above all, don't delay or avoid health care because of negative past experiences. Conditions only get worse because of delay. It's your health — you need to take care of it with good medical care, annual check-ups if needed, and preventive testing. Be assertive in getting the care you need, along with the respect and acceptance you deserve.

Don't allow anyone to hound you about the health risks of your weight. It may well be your healthiest weight at this time in life. Besides, it's not true that thin people are healthier — studies show fit and well-nourished people are healthier at every size. Nor are they happier.

Family and friends, as well as health providers and total strangers need to get over the mistaken notion that scolding, blaming, or humiliating large people will help them improve their health or change their size. It won't, and only makes things worse. The way many large women are treated is more likely to damage their mental and physical health than enhance it.

We all need to accept our risks, live with them, and not allow them to dominate our lives. Everyone has risk factors, the most deadly of which is growing older. So let's lighten up on ourselves and others.

Furthermore, it is not subversive to suggest that good health is not everything; it is not happiness, it is not love and caring, it is not concern or lending a hand to others. Yet, in some ways health has become a kind of religion or cult in our culture. As if it is somehow sinful not to have a healthy lifestyle. As if "good" people work hard at maintaining their bodies, while "bad" people let themselves go.

How does this play out when we consider the many large, wonderful, capable volunteer community leaders who give generously, cheerfully, and enthusiastically of their time and energy, day after day? These women may not work out at the gym or exercise their 30 minutes a day. They may even bake exuberantly, share food generously, and eat heartily themselves. So what? Our communities and families could not survive without them. Shall we allow them to be compared unfavorably with others who focus on their own health, work out daily, diet, stay slim and do nothing for anyone else? Hardly. If our culture is giving these messages, then it is badly distorting the meaning of health, wellness, wholeness and happiness.

As California nutritionist Joanne Ikeda says, "When I meet St. Peter at the Pearly Gate and he asks me what I've done with my life, I don't think he'll be very impressed if I say, 'Well, I kept my weight below a BMI of 25.'"

Let's accept that health is not of itself a worthwhile goal for living our lives. Good health is a means to a happier and easier life — but a means, not an end in itself.

Instead of worrying unnecessarily over health risks they may not even have, large people, like everyone else, will be happier and healthier if they accept themselves as they are and get on with their lives. Health providers and others need to allow them the freedom to do this, without prejudice.

And remember that good health is more than numbers on the scale. It's feeling good, having plenty of energy, knowing you can depend on your body to do the things you want to do. It's being comfortable with yourself and your natural body size.

Do-it-yourself self esteem repair

by Carol A. Johnson, MA

1. Weight is not a measure of self-worth. Why should it be? Your self-worth is your view of yourself as a total person— how you treat others; how you treat yourself; the contributions you make to your family, your friends, your community, and society in general. Your weight is just your weight. Don't give it any more importance than that.

2. List your assets, talents, and accomplishments and review that list often. Add to your list daily.

3. Focus on the positive aspects of your life — a job you like, good friends, a nice home.

4. Stop criticizing yourself. The inner voice that's telling you you're no good is a liar. View the voice as an unwelcome intruder and show it the door!

5. Avoid "globalizing." Instead of saying "I'm such a failure," say: "I didn't do that one little thing quite right, but I do most things right."

6. Let go of perfectionism, particularly in terms of food. You probably eat pretty healthily a lot of the time. Stop rebuking yourself for the occasional indulgence. Quit thinking of foods as "good" and "bad." Instead, use such terms as "a good thing to eat frequently" or " a good thing to eat occasionally."

7. Develop mastery. What are you good at? Capitalize on these things. Seek further education or training. It's fun to have things we do well.

8. Develop a more positive body image by appreciating your body's functional nature. Thank your legs for carrying you around. Thank your arms for being able to embrace someone.

9. Educate yourself (and those around you) about obesity. What the research really says about obesity and what most people believe are two different things. You are not to blame for something science doesn't fully understand.

10. Subscribe to magazines that show larger women in a positive light, such as Radiance and BBW. Surround yourself with positive images of large women.

11. Don't become preoccupied with thoughts of food and weight. Dieting can cause this. Plan what you're going to eat and then forget it.

12. Put nothing on hold as a reward for weight loss. Make a list of things you've always wanted to do and start doing them now. Being thin is not a prerequisite for living life.

13. Remember that society is not always right about things. Just because we have a cultural obsession with thinness doesn't make it right. Like human beings, societies are imperfect and make mistakes.

14. Develop a personal style that announces to the world: "I like me!" How you feel about yourself is reflected in the way you carry yourself, your grooming, your clothes, your smile, the way you speak.

15. Dress comfortably. This may sound silly, but comfortable, properly fitting clothes will improve your whole mental outlook. Tight clothes will make you feel miserable and unhappy.

16. Surround yourself with positive, supportive people. If they're not, tell them that you've stopped measuring your self-worth on the basis of your weight and you hope they'll follow suit. If they won't, there are plenty of people who will.

17. List the positive aspects of being a larger person. Has being large made you more tolerant, kinder, stronger?

18. Do not buy into the notion that there is one ideal image or shape every woman needs to conform to. That is nonsense. People come in all colors, sizes, and shapes, and that should be the beauty of the human race. We do not have "figure flaws." We simply have "diverse shapes."

19. Let go of constant comparison and competition. You don't need to be or "do" better than anyone else to be a worthwhile person.

20. You do not deserve to be harassed publicly about your weight. Decide in advance how you want to handle such situations. And remember that insults are almost always born of ignorance.

21. Concentrate on developing a healthy lifestyle, not losing weight. Developing a healthy lifestyle is a positive activity, while losing weight usually is based on a negative self-image.

22. Look into your past for sources of low self-esteem. Think about messages you were given as a child and refute them. Once you understand how you were taught to have low self-esteem, it is easier to change.

23. Put weight in its proper perspective and focus on what's really important in life. Do you want people to remember you for the shape of your body or the shape of your character and soul?[3]

Reprinted with permission from Self-Esteem Comes in All Sizes, by Carol A. Johnson, 1995. Doubleday, NY.

CHAPTER 16

Creating a
more nurturing culture

■

We can no longer allow advertisers to set the standards by which people are judged. Will you refuse to buy any product that exploits body dissatisfaction in its advertising? Will you tell others? Will you refuse to participate in promoting the thin stereotype?

Can we change a culture that attacks people for being different sizes? Can we change a culture that requires women to live up to narrow beauty standards and starve themselves? That on its darker side has become "dangerous, sexualized, and media-saturated"?[1]

Shifting culture is a monumental task. Strong forces have molded today's society, and change won't be easy, nor will it happen overnight. But it is possible.

If we want the media to reflect to us images of healthy women and men in a variety of sizes, then we can work toward that. If we want our young women, who are afraid to eat, to shift to eating normally and making healthy lifestyle choices, then we can support these choices.

Each of us can make a difference, beginning right now.

I like the story of the man on the beach who is throwing stranded starfish back into the ocean. Someone comes walking along the shore that is littered with starfish, and scoffs, "You can't make a difference here."

The man tosses another starfish into the water. "Made a difference to that one," he says, and reaches for another.

Moving toward a health at any size revolution

There are signs people are ready for a change.

The mood of the nation is swinging toward a yearning for stronger family values, for safer and more nurturing communities. Leaders everywhere are taking up the cause of strengthening the family and lessening the impact of destructive elements. Worldwide, there is backlash against fashion's severe excesses in portraying malnutrition as glamorous, although the industry's resistance to change is strong.

People are fed up with dieting, and while some diet companies have cleverly repackaged their diet message and misrepresent it as nondiet, this is not what people want. They may not yet be aware of the alternatives, but when they understand they make informed choices.

Canadian dietitian Linda Omichinski reports that she has found a real breakthrough in readiness to hear and receive the true nondiet message and most importantly, to speak out and act on this message. The time has come to move forward. People are hungry for this message of body acceptance, self-trust, normalized eating, vitality, balance, freedom from dieting, health at any size, and getting on with life. The media is also receptive and interested.

"The time is here to take all that energy and passion and together work through the process of actually starting a revolution, a health at any size revolution!" challenges Omichinski.

We have come to the point where the 100th monkey has jumped the island, as in the story of how wisdom spreads. In this story, one monkey tells another and that monkey tells another and another, each telling others until they create such momentum that the 100th monkey jumps to the next island and other islands and the message spreads rapidly.

With the magic of the Internet, island barriers disappear, and the health at any size revolution can spread with unprecedented rapidity to every corner of the earth. Effective tools we can use are: protest the negative, boycott for stronger effect, and support the positive.

Female diversity in role models

We need many more images in the popular culture that reflect the rich diversity of women in our society. It is important to provide female role models in a wide range of sizes, ages, races, and even attractiveness, so young girls who are not the most beautiful in class can feel good about themselves and how they look. We want our daughters to grow up to be strong, capable, generous, loving women — so we need to provide these kinds of role models, and take the focus off the thin, weak, vulnerable, self-absorbed models so admired today.

As women move into decision-making positions in the media, I have hoped this situation would improve. Unfortunately, this has not happened, despite the many advances made by women. Female leaders have seemed all too willing to participate in the same stereotyping.

It is time that women who are executives, producers, editors, reporters, models and actresses make this needed shift. They can have a powerful effect. Women are not objects or toys, and it is most unfortunate when they are portrayed this way and led to believe this is their role. We can liberate our young people from these false and narrow images based on appearance.

Perhaps the women's movement will become more involved in defending young girls and women from the excesses of lookism and the cult of thinness. Their leadership is much needed.

I've been encouraged by public response to women's athletic achievements, to female entertainers who don't fit the stereotype, rare as they are, such as Camryn Manheim, Rosie O'Donnell, Roseanne, and Oprah Winfrey. I also applaud female politicians like Janet Reno who, when she appears on television, doesn't look as if she's spent the last four hours in the beauty shop, but working at her desk like women everywhere.

One of my projects to encourage portrayal of women's diversity comes on Women's Healthy Weight Day. Every January, during Healthy Weight Week, which promotes health at any size, we at *Healthy Weight Journal* honor television shows, networks, magazines, advertisers and businesses that portray non-stereotypical women and confirm that beauty, health and strength come in all sizes. Some radio talk show hosts feature this event on that day, and I field questions from reporters and journalists worldwide who seem delighted with the concept. We also participate in Eating Disorders Awareness Week in February, and No Diet Day on May 6. All of these events would be stronger and have more impact with increased public support.

Boycott offensive advertisers

Taking on destructive media messages — in television, movies, books, magazines, newspapers, advertising, billboards, music — is not easy, but it can be effective. Responsible journalists and media are powerful allies.

Multinational companies advertising throughout the world have seized unprecedented power in creating body dissatisfaction and negatively impacting culture everywhere. But we don't need to accept their influences helplessly. After all, they are pleading for our money, and that's a position of weakness, not of strength. Women can refuse to play their game.

We can no longer allow advertisers to set the standards by which people are judged. The adulation of malnourished female bodies can be reversed. Will you refuse to buy any product that exploits body dissatisfaction in its advertising? Will you tell others? Will you refuse to watch television shows or movies that stereotype women — and if you do, contact producers, stations, and advertisers about your dissatisfaction? If you are in the media or a decision-maker in the media, will you refuse to participate in promoting the thin stereotype?

If so, you're part of the solution.

Regardless of difficulty, cultural changes can be made. Psychologist Mary Pipher says in *Reviving Ophelia* that we can help girls fight cultural pressures, encourage their emotional toughness and self-protection, and strengthen and guide them.[2]

"Most important, we can change our culture. We can work together to build a culture that is less complicated and more nurturing, less violent and sexualized and more growth-producing. Our daughters deserve a society in which all their gifts can be developed and appreciated."

She warns that it is critically important to change the way women are portrayed in the media, as expensive toys, the ultimate recreation, "half-clad and half-witted, often awaiting rescue by quick-thinking, fully clothed men..."

I'd like to see a great outpouring of support for positive portrayals and a boycotting of the offensive. Parents and consumer groups can be vigilant in making strong complaints against destructive stereotyping in magazines, television and advertising. Working together we can change the focus of responsible media and advertising, and deflate the power of its irresponsible fringe.

Boycotting, letter writing, phone calls, faxes, email, Internet messages, and taking other action to change attitudes of company policy makers whose advertising is exploitive can be tremendously effective in combating these destructive images. When targeting offensive advertisers, don't forget that the advertising medium shares the guilt. Magazines that print these ads and stations that air them are responsible for what they sell their audience. Editors keep a wary eye on marketing and routinely slant articles to please their advertisers, often to the detriment of the public, as in the case of smoking. They can be pressured to instead edit for what their readers demand.

On their Website, the Eating Disorder Awareness and Prevention group offers many ideas for contacting exploitive advertisers. You can be included in letters of protest and support by simply adding your name.

Their Media Advocacy Campaign protesting negative body image messages has resulted in the discontinuation of four national advertising campaigns. Avia Sportswear will no longer feature a promotion with the caption, "Although fitness trainers gave advice, the mirror was her dedicated coach," and offered to involve EDAP in the early planning stages of future marketing programs. Nicole Shoes apologized for claiming, "The pair you wear to your cooking class will also look fabulous at your weight loss seminar." A spokesman wrote, "We admit a mistake was made ... and will follow the guidelines and principles you have outlined in your pamphlet for future advertising endeavours."[3]

Boycotting worked for a Boston-based consumer group that calls itself "BAM" (Boycott Anorexic Marketing). BAM forced the cancellation of Diet Sprite ads that depicted a bony, apathetic girl sipping a diet drink whose nickname was "Skeleton." BAM's Diet Sprite boycott was picked up on national news and Coca Cola hastily pulled the Diet Sprite ads.

On a more impulsive note, vigilantes are striking at offensive displays on billboards and buses by scrawling graffiti over thin women's bodies.

"I'm So Hungry," lamented the caption on one gaunt model.

"Please Give Me a Cheeseburger," another pleaded.

We can educate the public and students on how to evaluate advertising and the media.

Gail Huon, a psychologist at the University of South Wales in Sydney, Australia, says girls must be taught to critically review the media images, articles and advertising not only for female thinness, but also for passiveness and submissiveness. They need to examine how women are portrayed in advertising as "property," and as waiting, receptive, ready to contribute to someone else's life.[4]

Perhaps one reason education on the destructive elements of advertising has not gone forward is because we are a capitalistic society, and want to support small and large businesses. Perhaps it has seemed subversive to critique their advertising. Yet, when businesses are damaging our culture, we cannot stand helplessly by. We can support capitalism and, at the same time, protect ourselves from its excesses.

It is my hope that readers of this book will be inspired to initiate changes aimed at respecting the diversity of women. You can't do everything, but if you are concerned with these issues, you can choose one or two ideas to work on personally or professionally. I believe each of us can make a difference, and together two or three can make that miracle.

As Margaret Mead assures us, we can change the world. "Indeed, it's the only thing that ever has," she said.

Target women's magazines for change

Even magazines can be boycotted. If you read them at all, consider backing away from fashion and women's magazines that exploit thinness, and tell your friends. Many are little more than expensive catalogs. Evidence confirms that the thin images they portray do lower women's self-esteem. Skimming through one magazine does it for many women, at least short-term, and those gaunt images may stick for a long time in the mind of a vulnerable woman.[5]

Women's and teen girl's magazines that once supported readers in improving their lives, but now seem aimed only at delivering them to advertisers, will either return to more ethical purposes or disappear — if you as a reader stop buying, and explain why.

If a few leading teen and women's magazines will begin to depict girls and women of all sizes in both editorial and advertising pages, then I believe the unhealthy media stereotypes can change rapidly. Can you imagine how stunned other editors, television producers, and Hollywood itself would be to discover the beauty, charm and unique talents of real women in all their diversity?

Another downer you might consider rejecting are publications that exploit women like the twice-yearly *Sports Illustrated* swimsuit fantasy; since they fail to show the sport of swimming, what's the rationale, other than greed?

The magic of the Internet

A positive influence can be the new freedom of exchange offered by the Internet, in which communication counts most and appearance is irrelevant. This medium is already helping to break through rigid stereotypes.

The instant and broad communication offered gives consumers unprecedented power in zeroing in on unscrupulous advertising and spreading the word to effect change. Ordinary people can now get information out fast and at low cost. An Internet campaign against an advertiser that exploits young people can have a powerful effect. The threat of an Internet campaign may be enough.

Not always will this be well-informed, unfortunately, but on balance I believe it will work successfully against harmful elements in society.

Protecting our children

Our pop and media-focused culture is having severe effects on children and teenagers. How can schools and families protect youth from a culture that fails to nurture them in so many ways?

Working to resolve these problems is beyond the scope of this book.

However, most women are mothers or are influential in the lives of children. When important women in a child's life model positive eating, and healthy relationships with their bodies, it goes a long way toward helping that child feel secure about her own body. Parents cannot forget that little ears are listening when Mom bemoans her hips or Dad criticizes the woman next door for "letting herself go."

If we want our children to grow up in families that love and talk to each other, we can work to provide them. If we want our youth to grow up with solid, positive self respect and body images, we can work to encourage them. If we want girls to grow up free from sexual harassment and abuse, then we can stop it.

Wherever I go, in conferences and speaking engagements, these themes strike a chord with parents, teachers, counselors, and nutritionists. They are deeply concerned with cultural and body image issues as they are affecting children today.

Briefly, these are ways that families and schools can shift toward healthier attitudes and behavior for children.

In the family:
- Promote normal eating; avoid dieting
- Avoid a weight or shape focus; promote acceptance, tolerance and respect
- Eat at least one family meal a day together, if possible, and with television off
- Promote communication and sharing of feelings
- Teach positive self-talk, praise and support for each other
- Be active together
- Help children develop interests and skills that lead to success, pleasure and fulfillment without emphasis on appearance
- Promote family assets of caring neighbors and other adults

In the schools:
- Educate faculty and staff in healthy attitudes
- Stress prevention of eating and weight problems; do no harm
- Provide counseling for eating and weight problems
- Develop support groups
- Require nutrition classes
- Require health and physical education classes
- Teach evaluation of advertising and media
- Promote healthy school environment
- Coordinate food service
- Establish zero tolerance for size discrimination
- Involve parents and community

In both family and school we can teach and protect children from unscrupulous advertising and the harmful effects of pop culture. Children and teens are highly targeted today as new, moneyed, easily influenced consumers. Our children do not have to be pawns in this game. Even young children can understand an advertiser's self-interest in creating body dissatisfaction to sell products.

We can strengthen the positive effects of our culture through strong, loving families that help children grow up with healthy self-concepts, healthy attitudes, and healthy lifestyles. If you'd like more information on helping youth, these issues are addressed in *Afraid to Eat: Helping Children and Teens in Today's Weight Crisis.*

Stop fear mongering

Reducing our culture's confusion and fears over health and food issues would help people eat normally again.

Elizabeth Whelan, president of the American Council on Science and Health, calls on scientists, policy makers, the media and consumers to stop the fear-mongering and "food terrorism" in the press, and implement these changes:[6]

- Emphasize that our food supply is safe. Keep reassuring the press and public of the truth: that America has the safest, healthiest, most enviable food supply in the world. The rarity of adverse incidents should be used to prove, rather than dispute, this fact.

- Return to mainstream science that defends reason and rationality. Many scientists don't want to get involved, and yet they must, in easily understandable terms that make the relative risks clear.

- Emphasize healthy nutrition messages and insist on balance. Restore acceptance of the basic principle that health depends on the total diet, not on a few special components. Convey the message that all foods can fit into a healthy diet.

- Diffuse the power to grab headlines of "health terrorists" and "food terrorists," whether these are ill-informed consumer groups, journalists on a "politically correct" mission, talk show hosts seeking higher ratings, radical animal rights groups, or scientists shoring up their grant funding. Whelan calls them spokesmen from the "Chicken Little School of Environmental Hyperbole."

- Expose the corruption of "politically correct science." This trendy ideology makes environmentalism and consumerism the new religion, says Whelan. It is takes a stand against industry, technology, and free enterprise, and discounts science, reason and rationality. It has infused the press with false notions that American health is at exaggerated risk from additives, preservatives and substances used to increase food production.

● Reduce the influence of the tobacco industry in silencing criticism and diverting attention from the real health risks. When over 1,300 Americans die prematurely every day from tobacco, and some 300 die of the affects of alcohol every day, she says it is almost ludicrous that nonrisks get the major headlines; tobacco has privileged status which needs to be stripped.

Preventing sexual abuse

Eating disorders and other disturbed eating patterns often begin as ways of coping with the sexual abuse, sexual harassment, physical abuse, violence, bullying and stigmatization that is so pervasive in our culture — and sometimes is glamorized in the media.

Mary Pipher charges that the incidence of rape is increasing because of our culture's increasingly destructive messages about sexuality. "Sex is currently associated with violence, power, domination and status."

As a responsible society, ours needs to be doing more prevent this and to protect young people and women from sexual violations. Sexual abuse is the responsibility of adults, and concerned adults must find ways to stop these abuses which cause so much shame and disruption. It's not enough to teach potential victims to protect themselves. The spotlight needs to be turned on the perpetrators.

"Young men need to be socialized in such a way that rape is as unthinkable to them as cannibalism," says Pipher.

Some experts advise airing public service messages like these:

● Sexual molestation of children is a crime.
● A child is unable to give consent.
● Sexual molestation of children involves an abuse of power and trust that is based on coercion and intimidation.
● Sexual molestation is damaging to children.
● Preventing sexual abuse is the exclusive responsibility of adults.

Society now recognizes its responsibility in separating the sexual criminal from potential victims, and informing communities of convicted offenders in their midst. Stronger treatment programs need to be considered, perhaps including drugs or surgery, to help offenders understand the impact of their abusive behavior and develop appropriate alternative behaviors.

Potential abusers need to understand the consequences clearly, perhaps as young as in junior high school. Being convicted of this crime can mean, in addition to serving prison time (as the least popular of prisoners), having one's whereabouts exposed by police, perhaps for life.

We need to acknowledge the high rates of sexual abuse of women and children. Perhaps more and more women will break their silence, reveal their stories, and refuse to protect those who have abused them.

Abuse may occur where least expected. Stermac, Piran and Sheridan advise informing first-time parents of the high incidence of sexual abuse within the family or by close relatives, the tendency to deny abuse, and how to build a protective environment for their children. They warn of incest, and recommend that new parents be targeted for intervention, informed about appropriate and inappropriate touching, and how to detect in oneself and one's mate the inclination toward inappropriate touching and what to do about it. Discussing healthy sexuality with children in a positive context may provide opportunities to identify abnormal and destructive sexual situations.

Prevention efforts will also address the cultural structures that promote sexual exploitation and the manipulation of children's and women's bodies.

But above all, we need to respect and appreciate each other as human beings.

Federal policy impacts culture

National policy greatly influences how the media reports health issues, and how the public and health community respond. It sets the agenda for what happens throughout the country. Unfortunately, national leaders are still continuing their course of ignoring or minimizing the risks of eating disorders, disturbed eating, hazardous weight loss, and malnutrition, while exaggerating the risks of obesity.

Why does our culture ignore the deaths of so many women from weight loss programs and eating disorders? Why is there no public outcry about the nutrient deficiencies and malnutrition that haunt young girls today?

Federal health officials and the National Institutes of Health need to take a more responsible role. They have spent a quarter of a century and millions of tax dollars on the failed quest to make fat people thin. Certainly it is time to begin research on how to help them be healthier, to develop ways to improve their health independent of weight loss. These policy changes are needed now:

- Include eating disorders prevention, awareness, and treatment in national health initiatives, especially the Women's Health Initiative and the nutrition objectives of Healthy People 2010. As related issues, dysfunctional eating, undernutrition, malnutrition, hazardous weight loss efforts, and body image concerns will naturally be a part of this.

- Direct the National Center for Health Statistics to gather baseline data on eating disorder prevalence, morbidity and mortality.

- Appoint an independent panel to determine who serves on all national advisory groups dealing with obesity. Include consumers who are affected most on the advisory groups, and set a firm policy against having members with vested interests.

- Drop the fiction that weight loss treatments are effective. Stop spending tax dollars on industry-serving reports like the 1998 NHLBI Guidelines on treating obesity. Stop pressuring for health insurance coverage of unsound weight loss treatment. Do no harm.

- Replace the NHLBI Guidelines that define overweight and at risk as a body mass index of 25, with a more realistic metabolic fitness definition. Metabolic fitness defines health at any size, depending on known risk factors, which is far more useful. If BMI is part of the definition, it needs to be in a much broader range, and adjusted for age and ethnicity.

- Require that five-year safety, effectiveness, and health-outcome data be provided on weight loss treatment programs, products and drugs before being used, except on experimental patients, or marketed to the public.

- Require weight-loss programs to track and publish outcomes in ways that are verifiable, giving any complications, short- and long-term weight loss results and fat loss relative to lean mass loss. Consider a requirement to track changes in eating behavior.

- Regulate the weight loss industry as other health-related industries are regulated.

- Establish a federal reporting process for deaths and injuries related to weight loss treatment.

These problems are not simple, but unnecessary barriers are adding to the difficulty in solving them. Eating disorder prevention efforts are stalled because of deep resistance at federal levels. Some fear that addressing eating issues will set back anti-obesity efforts. Others dismiss eating problems as women's issues, affecting only a few.

Nevertheless, I believe eating disorders are the key to bringing about a healthy change in federal policy. If eating disorders are considered important, then obesity will need to be approached very differently, so as not to exacerbate eating problems. A health-centered approach is the logical outcome.

The answer is new leadership, especially knowledgeable and visionary female leadership. And yes, there is some progress as women move into leadership positions. For the first time ever, in July 1997, a congressional briefing focused on the problems of eating disorders, brought together by two women legislators, New York representatives Louise Slaughter and Nita Lowey.[7]

The time has come to move forward. Visionary women and men working in federal policy and professional groups can bring about these changes. Consumers can demand changes in national policy, and in advertising and the media. If we do, it will happen.

By taking action now, we can change our culture in positive ways.

Letter of Protest to Keds

May 1998

We are writing to voice our concern and disappointment about your television advertisement for Keds Relaxed Fit™ which shows a woman on the scale at the doctor's office. As she removes her jewelry, her barrette, and her extra padded Keds, she looks expectantly at the scale in hopes that the number staring back at her has lessened. The voice-over refers to her Keds as having something women don't want on their hips — A little extra padding.

Eating Disorders Awareness and Prevention, Inc. (EDAP) is a national non-profit organization dedicated to increasing the awareness and prevention of eating disorders. As health professionals, (psychologists, physicians, dietitians, counselors, nurses, health educators, etc.), as people recovering from eating disorders, and as parents, we feel it is our responsibility, as well as your company's, to take an active voice in promoting healthy self-esteem and body image in the many communities reached by your advertising.

Your market research may have indicated that women respond to advertisements which address some of their most pressing concerns — fat and weight loss. Unfortunately, this information is accurate. What your market research may not have shown, however, is that 5-10% of American women — that's 5-10 million women across our country — have active, destructive eating disorders, including anorexia nervosa, bulimia nervosa, and/or binge eating disorder.

For many women, a scenario such as that in your commercial is a daily occurrence, and the number staring back will determine what kind of day it will be — a day to spend appreciating themselves for being "good", or a day to spend berating themselves for being "bad".

Through the years, Keds has provided consistently positive advertising which has recognized and celebrated women's and girls' strengths and accomplishments. Keds is the first to commend itself as holding a place in people's hearts "like a trusted friend, both familiar and genuine, a friend you can be yourself with." It is especially disappointing when a company highly regarded for sending positive messages to America's women and girls — a company we can be ourselves with — has succumbed to the pressure in advertising to play on women's fears and body dissatisfaction, rather than on their strengths.

Research has shown that the pervasive presence of thinner and thinner body ideals is associated with an increased prevalence of body dissatisfaction and eating disorders. While we certainly don't mean to accuse your ad of causing eating disorders, the message in the ad contributes to the weight-conscious context within which eating disorders, widespread negative body image, unnecessary restrictive dieting, and other unhealthy patterns thrive.

Your advertisement perpetuates a climate in which women's obsession with weight-loss is not only acceptable and expected, but completely normal and humorous.

We request that you discontinue this advertisement immediately, before it causes more harm.

As critical viewers of the media and caring members of the community, we trust that you will pass this letter along to the appropriate marketing executives and advertising agencies. We also trust that you and your colleagues at Stride Rite/Keds will consider ways in which you can serve as a role model to other major corporations by sponsoring media which promote acceptance of the diversity of sizes and shapes in people.

If your organization would like to discuss this issue with us, or would like specialized advice from a dietitian, psychologist, nurse, etc., please contact the Eating Disorders Awareness and Prevention, Inc.

To join EDAP's Media Advocacy Campaign, or to add your name to letters expressing concerns and praise for current media advertisements, or to become a Media Watchdog, contact EDAP at their website: Eating Disorders Awareness and Prevention, Inc.
at http://members.aol.com/edapinc/home.html
http://www.edap.net. (1-800-931-2237).

CHAPTER 17

Prevention and treatment

■

Health-centered nondiet programs will encourage
health at any size, normal eating and active living,
and not cause harm.

Efforts to prevent eating and weight problems have proceeded slowly, with a few false starts and wrong turns. With current research, they may now be ready to take off.

"Prevention is neither a luxury nor a fantasy, but a necessity," says Michael Levine, PhD, Professor of psychology, Kenyon College, and president of the board of directors of EDAP (Eating Disorders Awareness & Prevention, Inc.).

Levine notes that prevention work is challenging, and at the same time controversial because it promotes changes in education, mass media, public health and politics.[1]

It is now clear that these efforts must start early, focus on changing behavior rather than attitudes and knowledge, and must be a sustained effort.

"Prevention is a marathon, not a sprint," says Linda Johnson, MS, director of School Health Programs for the North Dakota Department of Public Instruction. "Many prevention programs have fallen short because our approach has been single-pronged and of short duration. Often what is convenient, easy and cheap does not benefit youth."

Johnson says that a successful prevention program will:

- Develop a needs assessment
- Build in measurable goals and objectives

- Use programs that are researched and theory based, and proven effective
- Deal with problems in a comprehensive way
- Work with an active advisory council
- Include ongoing evaluations[2]

A comprehensive effort that includes school, community and families is most likely to bring about actual change, she says.

Prevention programs also must do no harm to vulnerable individuals. Experts caution that the wrong kind of prevention is useless and can make matters worse.

What does not work are one-shot programs or pre-packaged events used in isolation, with no long-term effort. Information-only programs that change knowledge, but do not teach skills or change behavior, do not make people healthier. Scare tactics don't make them safer. It is illogical to spend time, money, and energy on untested programs or efforts that will not be sustained over time, experts say.

Unfortunately, most eating disorder prevention efforts have been of this nature. There is much criticism that they have come too late, and offered too little. Much time has been wasted. Too often prevention has missed its mark with efforts that began in high school, or showcased speakers who inadvertently glamorized their eating disorder experience, or even imparted purging information that listeners put to use.

Obesity prevention efforts, too, have mostly been sporadic and unhelpful, sometimes singling out and stigmatizing certain students, and stirring up size prejudice.

In the new paradigm, prevention of eating and weight problems are addressed together in integrated, comprehensive ways that do no harm. The new programs address the needs of persons at either end of the weight scale, and any extreme of eating behavior. This bridges the barrier of contradictions that some have seen between eating disorder prevention and obesity prevention.[3]

Prevention at three levels

Prevention involves intervention at three levels:

1. Primary, aimed at preventing eating and weight problems in the general population
2. Secondary, helping high-risk individuals or those who have early stage problems
3. Tertiary, treating people with eating disorders or weight problems[4]

Currently, eating disorder prevention and treatment is more developed at the third level, than the other two. The most effective and long-lasting treatment includes some form of psychotherapy or psychological counseling integrated with nutritional and medical care. Many patients respond well to outpatient therapy; for others, inpatient care at a hospital or residential center is needed. Treatment succeeds or results in improvement for the majority of cases, however, recovery is not easy. Advanced cases end in death in alarmingly high numbers. Obesity has been treated, however unsuccessfully, for many decades, as described elsewhere in this book. Primary prevention for both is in its infancy.

An example of a comprehensive program that addresses all three levels and includes both eating disorders and obesity comes from a kibbutz in northern Israel. Launched through the community clinic, the program shows two-year success in reducing disturbed eating and eating disorders in a population of 680 persons,

Targeted for individual attention were all the 38 girls, age 12 to 17, and their parents, teachers and significant other adults. Three of the girls were diagnosed with anorexia nervosa and another at high risk, and were referred to a specialist. Twelve were referred with eating problems and received individual counseling in a non-judgmental, supportive, empathetic approach for both teenagers and parents. Six girls with weight problems, who said they wanted to lose weight, were assessed as to eating issues, and followed a program of individualized nondiet counseling.

In all, 23 girls and women and five boys and men received special help. Expenses were kept low, using resources already in place.

Results showed that after two years, at the tertiary level, two of the girls with anorexia recovered and the third was much improved. The high-risk girl developed anorexia nervosa, was diagnosed early and recovered within one year. For others, there was marked improvement in condition and behavior, greater sense of well-being, and greater willingness to ask for help for friends.

Interestingly, a big change occurred in the attitudes of clinic team members as the intervention progressed. In two years they made a paradigm shift from a focus on calories and weight to the broader aspects of eating behavior, internal regulation, feelings, self-image and coping with social pressures. Through all this, the highly committed team gave strong support to both youth and parents, and now helps train teams in other communities.[5]

Primary prevention

Because treatment of both eating disorders and obesity is so difficult, primary prevention is even more urgent. The sooner successful programs can be put in place, along with strong secondary care, the less need there will be for treatment.

There are two major models for primary prevention, say Levine and Niva Piran, PhD, of the University of Toronto. The first is what they call Top-Down or leader driven. Patterned after drug and smoking prevention programs, it aims to give girls the knowledge, skills and encouragement needed to reduce their risk factors and increase their strengths. It decreases negative body image, dieting and other stresses, and improves communication, problem-solving, decision-making, healthy lifestyle and other competencies. The second method is the Feminist-Empowerment-Relational model, developed by Piran for reducing eating disorders in high-risk students in an elite ballet company. Her method empowers girls and women to change themselves and their environments through group dialogue, similar to that in a consciousness-raising group, fostering respectful discussion about issues that are often silenced or felt to be shameful, and working with systems to bring about favorable changes.[6] It encourages girls and women to work individually and together to change what they as a group have identified as unhealthy and unfair influences in their lives.

Piran was asked to help curb the high rate of disturbed eating and eating disorders at a Toronto ballet school, which was recording nearly two new cases of anorexia or bulimia nervosa every year, or about 10 percent of the girls age 10 to 18. Piran met with all students two to six times in small focus groups and used their knowledge and experience to guide action and changes in the system. All staff were included in exploration and education.

During 10 years of intervention only one case of anorexia and none of bulimia has developed at the school. Positive scores on eating disorder screening tests dropped from 50 percent in 1987 to about 15 percent. Surveys showed similar decreases in body dissatisfaction and the percent of students who binged, vomited, used laxatives, went on diets or skipped meals. Furthermore, students are strongly demanding safe and respectful treatment of their bodies by school staff and peers.[7]

Levine and Piran advocate combining these two prevention models.

They suggest that preventive programs include these four components:

- Media literacy and other ways of analyzing the culture
- Student discussion of the impact of culture
- Nutrition education that challenges dieting and promotes healthy eating
- Ways of developing personal competencies

At the same time, there is a great need to support teen girls by increasing social support and mentoring, reducing environmental stressors like sexual harassment and teasing, transforming girls' lives by reducing the importance of appearance, and changing institutions such as the mass media that disempower them. A variety of techniques and ways of resisting negative influences are included in successful prevention efforts.

In addition, Levine and Piran say that comprehensive preventive programs for change need somehow to address boys and men, their power, their fears, their dreams, and their capacity to care for themselves and others.[8]

Media literacy

Training in media literacy promotes the ability to question, evaluate, understand and respond thoughtfully to the media. It helps students ask the necessary questions: Is this a realistic portrayal? If so, am I or my experience similar to this person? If so, then do I want to act or be like this person?

Media literacy also helps students learn how to use the media for positive change.

GO GIRLS! (Giving Our Girls Inspiration and Resources for Lasting Self-esteem!) from EDAP is an action oriented prevention program that combines media awareness and analysis with media activism and advocacy. It is designed to help teenage girls develop critical thinking skills to learn about and challenge the media images of women, and how they promote negative body image and damage the spirits of many women.

Technology will play an increasingly important role in prevention. The Internet offers a wealth of evolving possibilities, including various forms of multimedia, and interactive, health-related educational opportunities. It provides a wealth of health information, and a way of exchanging treatment and prevention information between professionals around the world. Increasingly, it will be an important resource for engaging students in both the analysis of media and the creation of their own preventive education sites. At the same time, it has destructive elements, and we will need to learn to deal with the current explosion of exploitive marketing and false information.

Prevention in schools

Teachers are telling me they get no training in eating disorders, there seems to be no discussion of the risks, and that their training in eating disorders was like a fad about 10 years ago that has faded from sight. Yet invariably, these same teachers say they are seeing more problems than ever before that look like eating disorders at every grade level.

Preventive programs are most promising when they have assessed the need for prevention, then deliver the program one year before the age of specific need, before the behavior starts. Research-based, theory driven (such as social learning theory, or behavior change theory) curricula are most effective. Comprehensive programs will be integrated throughout the school — with classroom studies (in health, nutrition, physical education), counseling, food service, staff training, healthful changes in the environment — and involve home and community.

What I'd most like to see is a coordinator or designated point person in each school who is committed to the health at any size paradigm and trained in nutrition and eating and weight issues. She would be a team leader in developing a network of teachers, coaches, counselors and staff working together to prevent eating and weight problems and identify and help youth at early stages. She could coordinate classroom curricula at all grade levels, work with individual students and parents, develop support groups, and extend team efforts into the community. Zero tolerance would be established for size prejudice, sexual harassment and bullying.

Evaluation of eating disorder prevention programs in schools show they need to begin early, by fifth or sixth grade, with body acceptance issues being addressed much earlier. Three recommended curricula are:

- Healthy Body Image — Teaching Kids to Eat and Love Their Bodies Too, by Kathy Kater, LICSW, for grades 4 to 6 (EDAP).
- A 5-Day Lesson Plan on Eating Disorders: Grades 7 to 12, by Michael Levine, PhD, and Laura Hill, PhD, (EDAP).
- Teens and Diets — No Weigh, by Linda Omichinski, RD, age 12 to 17 (www.hugs.com).

It is important for teachers to understand, and perhaps improve, the process of referral and parent notification in their schools. Currently, it can be difficult to get any help for students at early stages of eating problems.

We sorely need support groups in college, high school, and even junior high for students who struggle with eating, weight and body image issues, or who deprive themselves of food, so that problems can be resolved before reaching a more severe level. There is an urgent need for colleges to address the current situation of sending out young professionals in health, nutrition and education fields who have not resolved serious eating issues.

A college class that shows promise of changing behaviors even though not directed toward personal change is *Body Traps: Perspectives on Body Image*. This Stanford University class includes multimedia presentations and discussions on body image, media and advertising, history of beauty, and disordered eating patterns. Students are required each week to write a two to three page reaction paper expressing their thoughts, feelings and criticisms from assigned readings. Focus is on impersonally and critically evaluating the issues, not on personal change. Yet results show significant improvement in body image, eating attitudes and eating behaviors for class members as compared with a control group.[9]

Developing support groups

Consciousness-raising support groups can be empowering in healing body shame and body dissatisfaction, say Carla Rice and Vanessa Russell, Toronto, women's studies specialists at the Ontario Institute for Studies in Education.[10] As they uncovered sexual harassment issues in teenage focus groups, Rice and Russell report that the girls felt relief when they found the courage to share their experiences and realized they were not alone. At first, no one wanted to talk, then one would cautiously tell an incident she thought might be sexual harassment. Others agreed the same thing had happened to them, "and then the stories flowed."

As they connected the shame they felt about their bodies to incidents of violence or harassment, the girls grew outraged. Each had endured her humiliation in secret, ashamed to tell anyone, because she feared she either deserved or had provoked the hurtful comments. As they shared their experiences, the girls grew more affirming and appreciative of each other, and became a force to be reckoned with. Their shame turned to anger and their self-loathing to acceptance as they realized most other girls had the same experiences with harassment. This transition from "I deserve to be violated," to "I have been violated," to "I do not deserve and will not tolerate violation," can be a key to empowerment, Rice and Russell suggest.

In organizing support groups for women and girls with eating issues, it is important to note that these groups will need the guiding hand of a professional. There are risks that such groups can perpetuate distorted thinking about eating, exercise and women's bodies.

Medical care in the new paradigm

Health providers who are committed to providing quality health care at every size know that people who feel good about themselves, and are supported by the health care system, are more empowered to make healthy changes in their lives. They recognize that much harm has been done by health providers in harassing and shaming of obese patients, and by prescribing weight loss treatments that were neither safe nor effective.

In California, a state-wide training program, *Children and Weight:*

What Health Professionals Can Do About It, is helping physicians and others shift toward a health-centered perspective in dealing with obesity. The goal is to help them deal with pediatric overweight in helpful ways, and motivate health professionals to work with parents, schools, and their communities to create environments that promote optimal health in children.

In assessing the initial pilot program, Joanne Ikeda, MA, RD, nutrition education specialist with Cooperative Extension, of the University of California Berkeley, reports that after a one-day training seminar all health practitioners said they would be making positive rather than negative comments about a child's body during physical exams, would describe body changes that come with growth, especially puberty, assess the child's eating and exercise habits, and focus on improving these rather than changing body size.[11]

A rural medical center I work with has designated a Health at Any Size Task Force to address the issues of size sensitivity and ensure that the hospital and its nine satellite clinics offer comfortable, accepting and

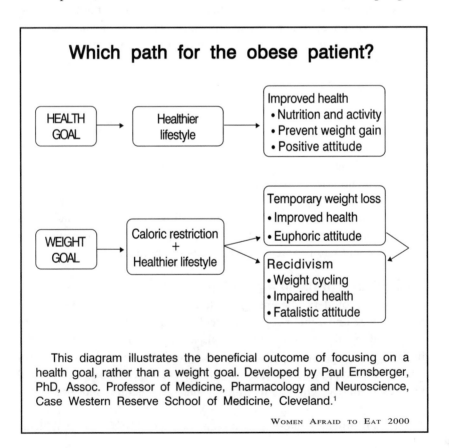

Which path for the obese patient?

HEALTH GOAL → Healthier lifestyle → Improved health
• Nutrition and activity
• Prevent weight gain
• Positive attitude

WEIGHT GOAL → Caloric restriction + Healthier lifestyle →

Temporary weight loss
• Improved health
• Euphoric attitude

Recidivism
• Weight cycling
• Impaired health
• Fatalistic attitude

This diagram illustrates the beneficial outcome of focusing on a health goal, rather than a weight goal. Developed by Paul Ernsberger, PhD, Assoc. Professor of Medicine, Pharmacology and Neuroscience, Case Western Reserve School of Medicine, Cleveland.[1]

WOMEN AFRAID TO EAT 2000

respectful environments for large patients, a population that may be underserved.

An advisory group of people familiar with size needs in their local communities is assessing positive and negative experiences, and making recommendations. The program will address staff attitudes and relationships with patients, the physical environment (size of equipment, gowns, beds, weighing procedures), and empowering patients to participate in their own health care. A consciousness-raising support group may be included to explore wider issues, promote self-esteem, size acceptance and healthy lifestyles. The Health at Any Size Task Force will also address eating disorder prevention and care in this large area of over 18,000 square miles served by the West River Regional Medical Center, Hettinger, N.D, and its staff of 16 physicians, dedicated to the principle that rural people deserve the same quality care as urban residents.

Ideally physicians diagnose and treat large patients as they do any

---

What doctors need to know about weight loss —

1. Weight loss programs only weight cycle most people. Failure rates are 95 to 97 percent.[2] Moreover, people often lose weight, then regain more than they lost. Weight cycling increases risk of death from all causes and from coronary heart disease, in the Framingham Heart Study, Harvard Alumni Study and others.[3]

2. Even when successful, weight loss may not benefit long-term health. Weight loss is associated with higher overall mortality, as seen in the long-term Framingham and Harvard Alumni studies, MRFIT, and others.[4] Recent analysis of the Framingham and Tecumseh studies suggests that the reason for higher mortality with weight loss may be that on average the beneficial effects of fat loss are outweighed by the harmful effects of lean body mass loss (including muscle, bone and organ tissue).[5]

3. It is recommended that health providers discourage behavior that causes weight cycling and encourage healthy lifestyles for patients of all sizes. Helping people to eat well, live actively and feel good about themselves and others can empower them to take charge of their own health.

WOMEN AFRAID TO EAT 2000

others, offering the same testing and treatment when appropriate. They recognize that large people may have special health needs, while not assuming this. They help large patients feel comfortable by treating them with sensitivity, giving them a better understanding of their health and medical conditions, and offering them the best care possible.[12]

Addressing the health care needs of large persons in a realistic, health-centered, sensitive way in medical schools and continuing education courses is needed.

If you are a physician or other health provider, how can you best help your large patients?

Will you urge them to lose weight or prescribe a weight loss pill? (Do you really want to prescribe medication long-term that will keep off less than 10 pounds, and is approved for only one year?) Or will you help them make lifestyle changes that can have a lasting impact on their health and quality of life?

The physician concerned about these issues will recognize that it may be time to stop asking, "How can I help this woman lose weight?" and instead focus on, "How can I help this woman be healthier?"

Paul Ernsberger, PhD, of Case Western Reserve School of Medicine, Cleveland, has developed the diagram *Which path for the obese patient?* that can be helpful for health providers. It illustrates clearly that choosing a health goal moves the patient toward improved health, while choosing a weight goal only causes more weight cycling and perhaps long-term harm.

In light of the new research that suggests injury from loss of lean body mass, weight loss treatments will need to demonstrate an acceptable ratio of fat loss to lean loss. They also need to show long-term health benefits and that they are not associated with higher mortality.

I would urge physicians to stop the weight cycling of patients, and to discourage their patients from behavior that results in weight cycling. It seems unfair to advise patients to lose weight without giving them clear guidelines on how to do this in a way that is proven safe and long-term effective. No such method currently exists. Our best option is to promote healthy lifestyles — health at any size.

Physicians moving into the new paradigm will learn all they can about eating disturbances, eating disorders, the effects of undernutrition and malnutrition, the high-risk periods of early and late adolescence, and how these problems are affecting girls and women today. They will resist oversimplification of these complex issues. And they will seek collaboration between health professionals, teachers and parents in dealing with them.[13]

In diagnosing depression physicians will take time to investigate the female patient's nutrition status and eating patterns, not assume a mental problem that needs medication. Depression is often related to undernutrition and malnutrition. Thus, medication may not be the answer, but rather, food.

Eating disorders screening

The annual National Eating Disorders Screening Program has shown remarkable success in getting help for individuals who are often reluctant to seek treatment. In February 1998, during Eating Disorders Awareness and Prevention Week, 35,897 people were screened at 1,083 sites. They first took the screening test, then attended informational sessions. Those who met the criteria were given referrals for further evaluation.

Results from a follow-up interview showed over one-third tested positive, having a score that indicates symptoms or concerns consistent with an eating disorder. Ninety percent of these were not in treatment. Nearly half of them followed through and saw a clinician. Over three-fourths of those who saw a clinician continued for further treatment. Many reported that the screening experience had helped them improve their eating behaviors, and 82 percent felt it had been helpful in some way, including for friends and family members.[14]

Eating disorder screening is an ongoing program that could be conducted much more widely, perhaps in all communities and schools every February. It is possible that varied degrees of dysfunctional eating could be assessed at the same time for possible secondary prevention treatment

Moving ahead with eating disorder awareness and prevention, EDAP is bringing together and training teams from around the country for Eating Disorder Awareness and Prevention Week, which is celebrated in February in all 50 states and Canada. Every year these teams grow stronger in developing comprehensive programs in their communities that can continue through the year, highlighted by workshops, seminars, theater events, art and puppet shows and media promotions.

In Montana, active teams are working state-wide in schools, community, and health care institutions in a systematic attempt to change the circumstances that promote, sustain, and intensify eating and weight problems. Called *Pathways to Health: Preventing eating disorders,* the program targets intervention at all three levels: to help prevent eating disorders from occurring, identify problems early, and provide the best treatment possible when someone is diagnosed with an eating disorder, says Lynn Paul, EdD, RD, Montana State University Extension nutrition specialist, Bozeman.[15]

Developing new programs: nondiet weight counseling

Healthy lifestyle programs based on nondieting and health at any size offer a fresh approach that is flexible, open, accepting, individualized and family-centered. They focus on the mental and physical well-being of each individual within the context of what is doable and appropriate in her life, her wellness and wholeness. Leaders in the new programs recognize that people are confused and shaken by today's conflicting health messages and need to trust themselves again.

The HUGS program developed by Linda Omichinski, RD, of Portage la Prairie, Manitoba, Canada, is a classic in this field. This program is franchised and facilitated by dietitians and other health professionals throughout the world.[16] Other healthy lifestyle programs based on these principles are being offered by dietitians in private practice and hospital-based programs.

In implementing health-centered programs in the new paradigm, facilitators can use a variety of approaches. They may focus on healthy lifestyle, healthy weight management, or improving body image and self-esteem. They may involve individual counseling, group training, or support and consciousness-raising groups. They may develop in schools, community, or health-care settings.

Yet, at the core they will be consistent and comprehensive, shifting emphasis away from weight, and toward self trust, empowerment, self-acceptance, and the prevention of problems. They will encourage people to eat and move and in normal, pleasurable ways, working with their natural regulatory abilities. Physical activity is an integral part of the health at any size approach. When people are comfortably active, they can eat more and be fully nourished. Appetite and hunger are more responsive, and more likely to be synchronized in rhythm with other natural body processes.

In the new programs, participants focus on how they can help themselves be healthier by changing habits in a gradual way, how they can feel better physically and mentally, and learn worthwhile family patterns. The facilitator will ask: Does this person want to change some habits, and what is she willing or able to change? Looking at the whole person, what might work in her particular situation? What makes sense in the context of her life?

A goal is to help people stabilize at what seems their natural weight, a weight at which they are healthy and well nourished. We can help people understand that keeping a stable weight is a worthy goal, since most people gain weight as they grow older (while accepting that women will typically gain some weight at midlife).

When they gradually change lifestyle habits, some people will lose weight, and if lost this way, it will likely stay off. However, we can't promise weight loss. Some will not lose weight. Others who have kept their weight unnaturally low may gain weight, and we can help them appreciate the benefits of maintaining a more natural weight around their setpoint.

Nondiet has become something of a popular term for diet promoters today, since consumers have learned that diets don't work. Therefore, some diet centers have cleverly disguised the controlling, restrictive, dieting message by telling people their programs are nondiet and clients can eat whatever they want. They may have moved away from counting calories, away from exchanges or fat grams, but only moved on to other ways of counting that keep clients preoccupied with their weight and prevent them from the enjoyment of eating in natural ways. They continue to reinforce unhealthy eating patterns.

Health-centered nondiet weight management programs will:

- Encourage health at any size
- Emphasize active living and normal eating with reliance on hunger and satiety (and will not disrupt normal eating patterns)
- Promote habit change goals, not set weight loss goals or promise weight loss
- Not cause harm or have the potential for harm
- Benefit the individual even if weight is not lost or is regained, through increased self-esteem, self-acceptance, and sense of well-being, as well as improved lifestyle changes in eating, activity and stress management
- Promote family lifestyles that are preventive of eating and weight problems

The traditional lure of such programs has been the promise of weight loss. Thus, expectations of both leaders and participants will need to change. How will we emphasize and help people appreciate the true benefits?

Nondieting programs help people to be healthier, better nourished, and have more energy and fun in their lives. We can assure participants of all these positives.

The new programs will not create eating or weight problems, nor obsession with exercise. Neither will they set up competitions. Everyone should feel good about progressing in her own way, at her own rate.

Programs in the new paradigm will appreciate ethnic culture and local values. People are assured they can trust their family heritage, that traditional foods and ways of celebrating with food are valuable to pass down through the generations, shaped and expressed in modern ways as they may be, yet honoring the past. Participants learn to trust their own judgment and feel confident that they and their children can make good decisions.

Improved attitudes at health clubs

New approaches in some health and fitness centers promote comfort for people of all sizes. Fitness centers have been criticized for taking all the fun out of being active — and adding plenty of anxiety. First the instructor — thin, with chiseled muscles, wearing stunning spandex — takes the new client through fitness testing and goal setting, explaining complex numbers in scientific, authoritative language. A rapid 10-week program is said to get her up to speed, working out on various machines, keeping heart rate between 60 and 80 percent for 30 minutes, burning calories.

These methods don't have a good record of success. Dropout rates at fitness centers are notoriously high with a reported half of all clients dropping out by the second week, and over 70 percent in the first year. For large women, it takes a good deal of courage just to begin.

In contrast, large women stick with the program at the Women's Exercise Research Center at George Washington University Medical Center in Washington, DC, say Jolie Glass, director, and Wayne Miller, exercise science professor. Most continue their exercising for months and years after they complete the 14-week program.

The most important reason? They feel safe.

"Surprisingly, they don't mean physically safe, they mean emotionally safe. These women love to come to a place where there are no men, where the health club atmosphere and attitude is absent, where they can exercise at their own level without feeling intimidated." says Glass.[17]

The women also rank the caring atmosphere high on their priority list, and a staff that is knowledgeable and sensitive to women's issues of body size and acceptance.

"Many of our women need to talk about how their exercise is affecting them emotionally, spiritually, and psychologically, in addition to how it is affecting them physiologically," says Glass. "These factors, along with the social aspects many women desire, help them change their attitude from an angry and determined 'I can exercise' to a pleasant and satisfying 'I like to exercise.'"

The first question most women ask is, "How much weight will I lose and how fast?"

Trainers work hard to change this attitude. They emphasize that whether weight is lost or not, there are improvements in aerobic fitness, strength and flexibility, blood pressure and cholesterol profile, and lowered risk for diabetes, cardiovascular disease, osteoporosis and premature death. They point out that not all overweight women will reduce weight in an exercise training program.

Once sold on this idea, the women's attitudes change, and they become enthusiasts who keep up their exercising in a lasting way.

For the health professional, Miller recommends individualizing a physical activity program based on what a woman finds enjoyable, is easily accessible for her, and within her capability. Her progress should be monitored in terms of strength, flexibility and endurance, not weight.[18]

Miller gives these recommendations for the health or fitness provider:

1. Perform an exercise evaluation. Testing for strength, flexibility and endurance provides valuable information that can be used to individualize the exercise prescription (instead of body weight).
2. Select exercises or activities that are enjoyable, easily accessible, and within the functional capacity of the individual. This will help ensure safety and adherence to the program.
3. Set the exercise intensity according to what is most relevant to the individual. In general, low intensity exercise of long duration will provide the most fat to the fuel mix as well as increase the total caloric expenditure (40 to 60 percent of maximal aerobic capacity or heart rate range).
4. Add strength and flexibility training. Strength training will help maintain lean body mass as well as metabolic rate. Flexibility training will help maintain functional capacity and may prevent injury.
5. Focus the activity plan on improvement of overall health and quality of life. If a reduction in body weight occurs, this should be viewed as a side benefit of lifestyle change, not the end product.

"We have been applying these recommendations to hundreds of clients in our clinical exercise programs for over 10 years and have witnessed only a few injuries, seen modest weight losses, shown significant decreases in disease risks and symptoms, and have a high adherence ratios," says Miller.

Monitor obsessive activity

At the same time they promote fitness, trainers need to monitor clients closely for signs of overtraining or activity disorder, such as fatigue, injury, loss of emotional vigor, and increased compulsivity. Compulsive exercise can be most harmful when combined with calorie restriction, as often happens for female athletes.

For women with eating disorders, exercise should not be recommended until eating behaviors are relatively stable. Then professionals might prescribe low intensity, low duration aerobic exercise as well as strength training to increase strength, muscle mass and possibly prevent bone loss. For patients with a history of eating or activity disorders, Glass recommends:

- Educate the patient concerning the potential health benefits and risks of exercise.
- Create a written agreement with the patient that specifically details the exercise program and eating plan.
- Require the patient to keep exercise records and review these regularly for signs of activity disorder.
- Require the patient to consume a calorie-containing sport drink during the exercise session.
- Monitor body weight and reduce exercise activities if weight begins to drop.[19]

Take a personal inventory

As professionals turning to the health at any size paradigm, we each need to examine ourselves. Where are you in all this? How do your personal issues affect your work? What happens if you as a professional are intellectually size accepting and sincerely teaching the health at any size approach — but before trusting your own body you *need* to go on one more diet and lose 10 pounds? What kind of conflict does this create? Will you give out mixed messages?

Educators, health providers and athletic trainers are caught up in all this as much as anyone else — it's part of our culture, and we can hardly escape it. Yet, we can shift from a weight-centered to a health-centered focus. If you are struggling with self-acceptance and body dissatisfaction, I'd suggest re-reading some of the early sections of this book that apply to you. Then reconnect with guidelines in the second part that seem most helpful, such as the self-acceptance issues in Chapter 12: *It's about you.*

Once you fully accept health at any size, it's unlikely you'll ever go back. You will be empowered personally and professionally.

CHAPTER 18

Call to action

■

How can we reach a shared vision and effectively communicate that vision? How can we promote wellness and wholeness in positive ways for people of any size?

It's time to move forward with vision. This is an urgent challenge for America and countries around the world. We need to deal with the current weight and eating crisis in healthy ways — ways that don't repeat the mistakes of the past.

The new health at any size paradigm recognizes the interrelatedness of the four major problems: dysfunctional eating, eating disorders, overweight and size prejudice. It promotes healthy growth and development of the whole person in mind, body and spirit, and it includes people of all sizes.

The process of furthering this vision needs to involve experts and lay people, teachers and parents, health care providers and community leaders — people of insight and integrity, with an understanding of the needs and concerns of women and minorities.[1]

How can we reach a shared vision and effectively communicate that vision? How can we promote wellness and wholeness in positive ways for people of all sizes?

Health at any size — the integrated health-centered paradigm — challenges us to make changes in these five areas: attitude, lifestyle, prevention, health care, and knowledge.

1. Attitude shift
The new approach advocates a shift in attitudes toward:

- Wider awareness and concern for weight and eating issues, for their inter-relatedness, and their importance to health and well-being.
- Greater appreciation for healthy lifestyles and balanced living (versus being thin) to help people feel encouraged to make healthy changes in their lives. Appreciation of the pleasurable aspects and healthful benefits of healthy lifestyle.
- Less focus on appearance and more on the worth of the individual, on character, responsibility, talent, achievement, and relationships with family and community. Conveying to girls and women who may be fixated on appearance that when well nourished they can live richer, more interesting lives.
- Acceptance of a wider range of sizes, more respect, tolerance of differences, appreciation of diversity, and recognition that beauty comes in all shapes and sizes. Rejection of extreme thinness (or any size or shape) as the ideal female body type.
- Stronger sense of outrage over violations against persons, such as harassment, stigmatization, bullying and mental, physical and sexual abuse.
- Increased determination to deal effectively with negative aspects of the media, and to use the media as a powerful instrument for positive change.

2. Healthy lifestyles

The new approach promotes healthy lifestyles which embrace:

- Pleasurable, normal eating and a moderate, varied, balanced nutrition, moderately low in fat, avoiding extremes.
- Active living. Improving physical education programs in schools and motivating people to continue being active through life. Encouraging active living through national public health programs.
- Promoting the attainment and maintenance of genetically favorable weights for growing children, and natural, stable weights for adults. Stopping dieting and ineffective, unsafe weight loss practices.
- Managing stress levels. Promoting effective ways to reduce and manage stress. Enhancing self-respect, self-acceptance, feelings of being needed, and positive relations with family, friends, community. Focusing on balance, moderation and contentment with life. Avoiding extremes.
- Reducing violence, sexual abuse, harassment and stigmatization, particularly against children, teenage girls and women. Finding effective ways to protect girls from aggressive men. Providing

more counseling accessibility and support for victims. Increasing law enforcement and incarceration to separate abusers from potential victims.

- Promoting environments that support being active, eating well, reducing stress and appreciating size diversity through schools, health care providers, the community, media and home. Communities can do much to encourage active living: developing safe, well-lighted playgrounds, parks, swimming pools, skating rinks, and trails for walking, bicycling and cross-country skiing. They can open school gymnasiums to the public, provide recreation centers, and organize community fitness campaigns and events.

3. Prevention focus

The health-centered approach to preventing eating and weight problems will:

- Promote prevention at three levels: primary, aimed at reducing problems in the general population; secondary, helping high-risk individuals or those who have early stage problems; tertiary, treating people with eating disorders or weight problems.
- Integrate eating disorder prevention and obesity prevention in establishing a sound foundation for comprehensive programs.
- Continue to develop, test and evaluate comprehensive preventive programs for use in schools, college, community, and health care. Recognize the concerns about adopting preventive programs prematurely, without adequate research into safety and effectiveness.
- Move forward with programs that are tested effective and safe. Integrate a needs assessment and measurable goals and objectives. Work with an active advisory council. Sustained, comprehensive efforts that encompass school, community and families will be most effective. Continue to test, evaluate and fine-tune programs.
- Expand the National Eating Disorders Screening Program to more schools, colleges and communities. Follow up with participants needing or requesting help, especially at secondary prevention levels.
- Increase the impact of Eating Disorders Awareness and Prevention Week in February. Support and expand the work of EDAP-trained coordinators and teams.
- Develop consciousness-raising and support groups to deal with weight and eating concerns.
- Teach body image curricula, including puberty changes, from

fourth grade through junior high.

- Teach media literacy at all school levels, from elementary school through college classes in marketing, psychology, health and nutrition. Promote the ability to question, evaluate, understand and respond to negative influences.

- Enlist and support the media in promoting positive images. Strong, talented, intelligent women of diverse sizes, ages and ethnicity need to be much more visible in the media, entertainment industries and public life.

- Promote more responsible reporting of health news, keeping risks in perspective, not sensationalizing them. Expose "health terrorists" and unsound "politically correct" views.

4. Health care changes

A health promoting shift in national policy and local health care services will:

- Ensure that health professionals consistently promote healthy lifestyles and being healthy at any size. Focus on improving the health of large individuals, not on ineffective weight loss.

- Reduce size prejudice in health care. Many health care providers need to be aware of and work to overcome their size biases, so that large patients can come to them with assurance of sensitive and respectful treatment.

- Provide more training for health providers in medical school and continuing education on eating and weight issues, eating disorders, the effects of undernutrition and malnutrition in girls and young women, the need for respectful, sensitive care of large people.

- Identify and treat dysfunctional eating at early stages, instead of waiting for clinical eating disorder diagnoses.

- Improve access to qualified services for high-risk populations.

- Call a moratorium on weight loss treatment — especially diets, drugs and surgery — until there is reasonable proof of long-term (five year) safety and effectiveness. It's time to up the ante and also insist on documentation of an optimal fat to lean loss ratio and an improvement in long-term health (or at least the absence of harm).

- Regulate obesity treatment. Require full disclosure and accountability, reporting of weight loss and fat loss results, adverse effects, morbidity and mortality. Require adequate safety and effectiveness studies before going ahead with treatment (preferably five-year data as in American Heart Association guidelines). See

Connecticut law for model regulations.[2]

- Add eating disorders, undernutrition, and hazardous weight loss to the nutrition priorities in updates of Healthy People 2010, establishing objectives, baselines and measurable targets.

- Develop a sound policy on use of weight loss drugs, since the potential for abuse now and in the future is high. Require credible studies demonstrating long-term safety and effectiveness (five year data), not one-year studies, as today. Begin dialogue on ethical use of drugs: When more effective drugs do become available will it be ethical to prescribe them widely, for children as well as adults? Should they be available without prescription?[3]

5. Knowledge expansion

The comprehensive health-centered approach, in meeting challenges for research and information, will:

- Encourage dietetics and nutrition schools to develop programs and support groups to deal effectively with the high levels of dysfunctional eating now found among college students, including students in their own departments. Develop more extensive courses in weight and eating issues at undergraduate and graduate levels.

- Encourage medical schools to require basic studies in nutrition, obesity and eating disorders. At the same time, promote more reliance by doctors on nutritionists and others with special training in these areas, and the referring of patients to specialists.

- Consolidate eating and weight studies into one academic department within a field such as nutrition or health, developing graduate programs to train specialists. This will move the field ahead more rapidly. Bringing these now-fragmented specialties together into a respected field of study will mean the information is researched, analyzed and used in more comprehensive ways. Also, the power of vested interests will be lessened.

- Communicate and disseminate research and information in more comprehensive, health-promoting ways to health providers and consumers.

- Encourage women researchers to take more leadership positions, report at conferences, and publish in scientific literature. This will more quickly move forward women's health care and concerns, such as eating disorders, dysfunctional eating, undernutrition and malnutrition of teenage girls, and sexual abuse.

- Raise ethical standards. Require full disclosure of funding and commercial relationships at scientific conferences, on journal editorial boards and in public policy, to reduce the influence of vested interests, particularly by the weight loss industry. (Obesity research and federal policy on obesity has been particularly vulnerable to vested interests.) Expose dishonest research reporting, in the public's best interest, and drop the fiction that current obesity treatments are safe and effective.

- Increase research study of the four major problems (dysfunctional eating, eating disorders, overweight, size prejudice), their etiology, causes, treatment and prevention. Extend study on normal eating; body regulation of weight, hunger, appetite and satiety; the physical and mental effects of starvation and semistarvation; the nature of the "thrifty gene" and how it impacts populations undergoing cultural change.

If we can pull together to do these things, we'll create a new world where women are healthy at any size and no longer afraid to eat.

APPENDIX

Body Mass Index for Selected Weight and Stature

Stature meters (inches)

Weight kg	lb	1.47	1.50	1.52	1.55	1.57	1.60	1.63	1.65	1.68	1.70	1.73	1.75	1.78	1.80	1.83	1.85	1.88	1.90	1.93
		58	59	60	61	62	63	64	65	66	67	68	69	70	71	72	73	74	75	76
43	95	20	19	19	18	17	17	16	16	15	15	14	14	13	13	13	12	12		
45	100	21	20	20	19	18	18	17	17	16	16	15	15	14	14	14	13	13	13	12
48	105	22	21	21	20	19	19	18	17	17	16	16	16	15	15	14	14	13	13	13
50	110	23	22	22	21	20	19	19	18	18	17	17	16	16	15	15	15	14	14	13
52	115	24	23	23	22	21	20	20	19	18	18	17	17	16	16	16	15	15	14	14
54	120	25	24	24	23	22	21	20	20	19	19	18	18	17	17	16	16	15	15	15
57	125	26	25	25	24	23	22	21	21	20	20	19	19	18	17	17	17	16	16	16
59	130	27	26	26	25	24	23	22	22	21	20	20	19	19	18	18	17	17	16	16
61	135	28	27	27	25	25	24	23	22	22	21	20	20	19	19	18	18	17	17	16
64	140	29	28	27	26	26	25	24	23	22	22	21	21	20	20	19	19	18	18	17
66	145	30	29	28	27	27	26	25	24	23	23	22	21	21	20	20	19	19	18	18
68	150	31	30	29	28	28	27	26	25	24	24	23	22	21	21	20	20	19	19	18
70	155	33	31	30	29	29	27	26	26	25	24	23	23	22	22	21	21	20	19	19
73	160	34	32	31	30	29	28	27	27	26	25	24	24	23	22	22	21	21	20	19
77	170	36	34	33	32	31	30	29	28	27	27	26	25	24	24	23	23	22	21	21
79	175	37	35	34	33	32	31	30	29	28	27	27	26	25	24	24	23	22	22	21
82	180	38	36	35	34	33	32	31	30	29	28	27	27	26	25	24	24	23	23	22
84	185	39	37	36	35	34	33	32	31	30	29	28	27	26	26	25	25	24	23	23
86	190	40	39	37	36	35	34	32	32	31	30	29	28	27	27	26	25	24	24	23
88	195	41	39	38	37	36	35	33	32	31	31	30	29	28	27	26	26	25	25	24
91	200	42	40	39	38	37	35	34	33	32	31	30	30	29	28	27	27	26	25	24
93	205	43	41	40	39	38	36	35	34	33	32	31	30	29	29	28	27	26	26	25
95	210	44	42	41	40	39	37	36	35	34	33	32	31	30	29	28	28	27	26	26
98	215	45	43	42	41	40	38	37	36	35	34	33	32	31	30	29	28	28	27	26
100	220	46	44	43	42	40	39	38	37	35	35	33	33	31	31	30	29	28	28	27
102	225	47	45	44	42	41	40	38	37	36	35	34	33	32	31	30	30	29	28	27
104	230	48	46	45	43	42	41	39	38	37	36	35	34	33	32	31	30	30	29	28
107	235	49	47	46	44	43	42	40	39	38	37	36	35	34	33	32	31	30	30	29
109	240	50	48	47	45	44	43	41	40	39	38	36	36	34	34	33	32	31	30	29
111	245		49	48	46	45	43	42	41	39	38	37	36	35	34	33	32	31	31	30
113	250		50	49	47	46	44	43	42	40	39	38	37	36	35	34	33	32	31	30
116	255			50	48	47	45	44	43	41	40	39	38	37	36	35	34	33	32	31
118	260				49	48	46	44	43	42	41	39	39	37	36	35	34	33	33	32
120	265				50	49	47	45	44	43	42	40	39	38	37	36	35	34	33	32
122	270					50	48	46	45	43	42	41	40	39	38	37	36	35	34	33
125	275						49	47	46	44	43	42	41	39	38	37	36	35	35	33
127	280						50	48	47	45	44	42	41	40	39	38	37	36	35	34
129	285						50	49	47	46	45	43	42	41	40	39	38	37	36	35
132	290							50	48	47	46	44	43	42	41	39	38	37	36	35
134	295							50	49	47	46	45	44	42	41	40	39	38	37	36
136	300								50	48	47	45	44	43	42	41	40	39	38	37

Body mass index (BMI) = weight (kg)/height (m)^2

AMERICAN MEDICAL ASSOCIATION 1995

Assessing size attitudes

This behavior assessment can be used to evaluate your support for the health and well-being of large people. Use the following scale to indicate the frequency of each behavior.

1-never   2-rarely   3-occasionally   4-frequently   5-daily

How often do you: **Never . . daily**

1. Make negative comments about your fatness   1 2 3 4 5

2. Make negative comments about someone else's fatness 1 2 3 4 5

3. Directly or indirectly support the assumption that no 1 2 3 4 5
   one should be fat

4. Disapprove of fatness (in general)   1 2 3 4 5

5. Say or assume that someone is "looking good"   1 2 3 4 5
   because s/he has lost weight

6. Say something that presumes that a fat person(s)   1 2 3 4 5
   wants to lose weight

7. Say something that presumes that fat people   1 2 3 4 5
   should lose weight

8. Say something that presumes that fat people   1 2 3 4 5
   eat too much

9. Admire or approve of someone for losing weight   1 2 3 4 5

10. Disapprove of someone for gaining weight   1 2 3 4 5

11. Assume that something is wrong when someone   1 2 3 4 5
    gains weight

12. Admire weight loss dieting   1 2 3 4 5

13. Admire rigidly controlled eating   1 2 3 4 5

14. Admire compulsive or excessive exercising   1 2 3 4 5

15. Tease or admonish someone about their eating   1 2 3 4 5
    (habits/choices)

16. Criticize someone's eating to a third person   1 2 3 4 5
    ("so-and-so eats way too much junk")

17. Discuss food in terms of "good/bad"   1 2 3 4 5

18. Talk about "being good" and "being bad" in   1 2 3 4 5
    reference to eating behavior

19. Talk about calories (in the usual dieter's fashion) 1 2 3 4 5

20. Say something that presumes being thin is better (or more attractive) than being fat — 1 2 3 4 5

21. Comment that you don't wear a certain style because "it makes you look fat" — 1 2 3 4 5

22. Comment that you love certain clothing because "it makes you look thin" — 1 2 3 4 5

23. Say something that presumes that fatness is unattractive — 1 2 3 4 5

24. Participate in a "fat joke" by telling one or laughing/smiling at one — 1 2 3 4 5

25. Support the diet industry by buying their services and/or products — 1 2 3 4 5

26. Undereat and/or exercise obsessively to maintain an unnaturally low weight — 1 2 3 4 5

27. Say something that presumes being fat is unhealthy — 1 2 3 4 5

28. Say something that presumes being thin is healthy — 1 2 3 4 5

29. Encourage someone to let go of guilt — 1 2 3 4 5

30. Encourage or admire self-acceptance and self-appreciation/love — 1 2 3 4 5

31. Encourage someone to feel good about his/her body as is — 1 2 3 4 5

32. Openly admire a fat person's appearance — 1 2 3 4 5

33. Openly admire a fat person's character, personality, or actions — 1 2 3 4 5

34. Oppose/challenge fattism verbally — 1 2 3 4 5

35. Oppose/challenge fattism in writing — 1 2 3 4 5

36. Challenge or voice disapproval of a "fat joke" — 1 2 3 4 5

37. Challenge myths about fatness and eating — 1 2 3 4 5

38. Compliment ideas, behavior, character, etc. more often than appearance — 1 2 3 4 5

39. Support organizations which advance fat acceptance (with your time or money) — 1 2 3 4 5

Behaviors 1-28 are unhelpful or harmful; look over areas which need improvement and strive to avoid these and similar behaviors in the future. Behaviors 29-38 help support size acceptance; re-read items you marked "never" (1) or "rarely" (2); make a list of realistic goals for increasing supportive behavior. Reprinted with permission as adapted by Susan Kano from her book *Making Peace With Food: Freeing Yourself from the Diet/Weight Obsession*, 1989. New York: Harper & Row.

National eating disorders screening program

Age _____   Sex _____   Height _____

Current weight _____   Highest weight _____   Lowest adult weight _____

EATING ATTITUDES TEST (EAT-26)

Please check a response for each	Always	Usually	Often	Sometimes	Rarely	Never
1. Am terrified about being overweight.	☐	☐	☐	☐	☐	☐
2. Avoid eating when I am hungry.	☐	☐	☐	☐	☐	☐
3. Find myself preoccupied with food.	☐	☐	☐	☐	☐	☐
4. Have gone on eating binges where I feel that I may not be able to stop.	☐	☐	☐	☐	☐	☐
5. Cut my food into small pieces.	☐	☐	☐	☐	☐	☐
6. Aware of the calorie content of foods that I eat.	☐	☐	☐	☐	☐	☐
7. Particularly avoid food with a high carbohydrate content; i.e. bread, rice, potatoes, etc.	☐	☐	☐	☐	☐	☐
8. Feel that others would prefer if I ate more.	☐	☐	☐	☐	☐	☐
9. Vomit after I have eaten.	☐	☐	☐	☐	☐	☐
10. Feel extremely guilty after eating.	☐	☐	☐	☐	☐	☐
11. Am preoccupied with a desire to be thinner.	☐	☐	☐	☐	☐	☐
12. Think about burning up calories when I exercise.	☐	☐	☐	☐	☐	☐
13. Other people think that I am too thin.	☐	☐	☐	☐	☐	☐
14. Am preoccupied with the thought of having fat on my body.	☐	☐	☐	☐	☐	☐
15. Take longer than others to eat my meals.	☐	☐	☐	☐	☐	☐
16. Avoid foods with sugar in them.	☐	☐	☐	☐	☐	☐
17. Eat diet foods.	☐	☐	☐	☐	☐	☐
18. Feel that food controls my life.	☐	☐	☐	☐	☐	☐
19. Display self-control around food.	☐	☐	☐	☐	☐	☐
20. Feel that others pressure me to eat.	☐	☐	☐	☐	☐	☐
21. Give too much time and thought to food.	☐	☐	☐	☐	☐	☐
22. Feel uncomfortable after eating sweets.	☐	☐	☐	☐	☐	☐
23. Engage in dieting behavior.	☐	☐	☐	☐	☐	☐
24. Like my stomach to be empty.	☐	☐	☐	☐	☐	☐
25. Have the impulse to vomit after meals.	☐	☐	☐	☐	☐	☐
26. Enjoy trying new rich foods.	☐	☐	☐	☐	☐	☐
TOTAL SCORE	__	__	__	__	__	__

BEHAVIORAL SCREENING QUESTIONS

1. Have you gone on eating binges where you feel that you may not be able to stop? (Eating much more than most people would eat under the same circumstances)

   NO   YES How many times in the last 6 months? _____

2. Have you ever made yourself sick (vomited) to control your weight or shape?

   NO   YES How many times in the last 6 months? _____

3. Have you ever used laxatives, diet pills or diuretics (water pills) to control your weight or shape?

   NO   YES How many times in the last 6 months? _____

4. Have you ever been treated for an eating disorder?

   NO   YES When? _____

5. Have you recently thought of or attempted suicide?

   NO   YES When? _____

Scoring instructions for EAT-26

Responses for items 1-25:
   always - 3; usually - 2; often - 1; sometimes, rarely, never - 0

Responses for item 26:
   always, usually, often - 0; sometimes - 1; rarely - 2; never - 3

Add to find the total EAT score.

The five criteria for referring particpants for a follow-up evaluation are:

1. a score of more than 20 on the EAT-26;
2. a "yes" to any one of the behavioral screening questions;
3. a body mass index (BMI) below 18 *(see BMI chart, page 339)*;
4. a respondent who feels that he or she has significant eating or weight concerns and therefore specifically requests a referral; or
5. the clinician, based on interview, believes that there is reason for referral.

Source: Garner DM, and Garfinkel PE. The Eating Attitudes Test: An index of the symptoms of anorexia nervosa. *Psychological Medicine* 1979:9:273-279.

Vegetarian self-test

Origin of choice

1. I ate a variety of protein products as a child, but have gradually narrowed my protein choices to a few "acceptable" items. T F

2. I avoid animal-based foods as much as possible, but find that I get cravings that turn into binges. T F

3. I feel superior to others when I eat differently than them. T F

4. I eat nut butters, avocados, seeds, and fats on a regular basis. T F

5. Sometimes I think I would like to eat a piece of meat, but I am afraid to. T F

6. I feel less guilty about myself when I eat a vegetarian diet. T F

7. I can eat meatless products that look, taste, and smell exactly like meat without discomfort. T F

8. I am willing to eat 1/3 more volume of food and add a serving of fat to my meal plan to insure that my diet has the necessary amount of fat, calories, and protein. T F

9. I feel that people who eat less meat are more "perfect" or "acceptable" than people who eat meat. T F

10. Eating meat makes me feel uncomfortable. T F

Score 1 point for each *true* answer on numbers 4, 7 and 8; score 1 point for each *false* answer on numbers 1, 2, 3, 5, 6, 9 and 10. A score of 0 indicates a high probability that the vegetarian choice is disordered in its origin, and a score of 10 indicates a low probability of disordered motivation. In-between scores indicate the degree of disordered thoughts contributing to the vegetarian decision.

Reprinted with permission. Copyright 1996, Monika M. Woolsey, MS, RD, A Better Way Health Consulting, Glendale, Arizona.

How to help a friend
with an eating disorder

If you and others have observed behaviors in your friend or roommate that are suggestive of an eating disorder, you are in a position to help.

- Make a plan to approach the person in a private place when there is no immediate stress and time to talk.

- Present in a caring but straightforward way what you have observed and what your concerns are. Tell him or her that you are worried and want to help. (Friends who are too angry with the person to talk supportively should not be a part of this discussion.)

- Give the person time to talk and encourage them to verbalize feelings. Ask clarifying questions. Listen carefully; accept what is said in a non-judgmental manner.

- Do not argue about whether there is or is not a problem — power struggles are not helpful. Perhaps you can say, "I hear what you are saying and I hope you are right that this is not a problem. But I am still very worried about what I have seen and heard, and that is not going to go away."

- Provide information about resources for treatment. Offer to go with the person and wait while they have their first appointment with a counselor, physician, or nutritionist. Ask them to consider going for one appointment before they make a decision about ongoing treatment.

- If you are concerned that the eating disorder is severe or life-threatening, enlist the help of a doctor, therapist, counseling center, relative, friend, or roommate of the person before you intervene. Present a united and supportive front with others.

- If the person denies the problem, becomes angry, or refuses treatment, understand that this is often part of the illness. Besides, they have a right to refuse treatment (unless their life is in danger). You may feel helpless, angry, and frustrated with them. You might say, "I know you can refuse to go for help, but that will not stop me from worrying about you or caring about you. I may bring this up again to you later, and maybe we can talk more about it then." Follow through on that — and on any other promise you make.

- Do not try to be a hero or a rescuer; you will probably be resented. If you do the best you can to help on several occasions and the person does not accept it, stop. Remind yourself you have done all it is reasonable to do. Eating disorders are stubborn problems, and treatment is most effective when the person is truly ready for it. You may have planted a seed that helps them get ready.

- Eating disorders are usually not emergency situations. But, if the person is suicidal or otherwise in serious danger, GET PROFESSIONAL HELP IMMEDIATELY. By Marcia Herrin and Heidi Fishman, Dartmouth College Health Service.

Median daily intake
Percent of Recommended Dietary Allowances (RDAs)
Male

Nutrient	12-15 years			16-19 years			20-59 years			≥60 years		
	NHW	NHB	MA	NHW	NHB	MA	NHW	NHB	MA	NHW	NHB	MA
Food energy	102	92	84	106	89	82	90	84	82	81	67	72
Protein	184	160	187	173	163	156	149	140	152	117	103	113
Vitamin A	85	55	70	77	55	67	78	53	62	91	55	61
Vitamin E	68*	74	67	93	92	77	90	75	80	70	51	59
Vitamin C	194	204	180	112	188	137	140	153	148	138	108	125
Thiamin	146	122	134	148	120	109	119	108	109	135	102	120
Riboflavin	169	120	147	148	120	118	129	102	116	139	108	119
Niacin	140	115	120	135	122	96	140	131	120	146	112	108
Vitamin B_6	110	92	95	104	93	83	100	89	98	89	65	67
Folate	203	133	169	140	106	132	146	114	144	141	100	122
Vitamin B_{12}	242	188	212	258	248	244	248	210	225	210	165	164
Calcium	90	60	85	103	76	79	113	74	103	90	62	82
Phosphorus	118	97	114	141	126	122	188	155	196	152	121	148
Magnesium	103	85	97	78	68	70	95	74	96	83	58	74
Iron	128	110	119	146	119	114	161	139	152	140	102	127
Zinc	77	59	70	90	82	80*	87	75	84	72	57	55
Copper	81	76	79	93	87	84	100	82	97	81	59	79
Sodium	154	137	134	194	179	134	161	151	143	128	98	118

NHW-nonHispanic white   NHB-nonHispanic black   MA-Mexican American

Shaded values indicate that median intakes are below recommended amounts (for sodium, above). Considered to be current public health issues are the intakes of food energy (calories), calcium, iron and zinc. Considered to be potential public health issues for which further study is needed are the intakes of vitamin A, vitamin C, vitamin B_6 and folate. Values represent percentage of Recommended Dietary Allowances (RDAs); for food energy, values represent percentage of the Recommended Energy Intake (NRC, 1989a). An asterisk (*) indicates a statistic that is potentially unreliable. Third Report on Nutrition Monitoring in the U.S. Vol 1, p135. 1995. USDA, HHS, NHANES III, 1988-1991. *(For female intake, see Chapter 9.)*

Dysfunctional eating
Research basis

The concepts of dysfunctional eating and the starvation syndrome are defined as such in the *Afraid to Eat* books for the first time. However, they are based on the insight and research of numerous leaders in the fields of eating disorders, eating restraint, obesity and size acceptance. Among the important sources for the foundation of these concepts are the early work on restrained eating by Janet Polivy and Peter Herman[1]; writings and presentations by Susan Wooley[2]; writings and work by Ellyn Satter on normal eating and her workshops on "Treating the dieting casualty"[3]; Linda Omichinski's nondiet leadership and program development devoted to breaking the dieting cycle[4]; the concept development on thinking about food by Dan and Kim Reiff[5]; starvation studies, including the Minnesota Experiment,[6] United Nations reports on world malnutrition,[7] and Colin Turnbull's striking portrait of *The Mountain People*[8]; national and local studies showing the high prevalence of dieting and disordered eating among children and adolescents[9]; eating disorder research showing mental and physical effects of eating disorders, and the associations of eating disorders with dieting[10]; discussions on the risks of dieting and the need to treat the chronic dieting syndrome by Arnold Andersen and Mike Bowers[11]; and the progress of No Diet Day observances, led by Mary Evans Young,[12] and Eating Disorder Awareness Week, organized by eating disorder specialists.[13]

Most of this information has been reviewed in *Healthy Weight Journal* over the past 15 years, and is discussed extensively in my 1995 book *Health Risks of Weight Loss.*[14]

1. Herman P, J Polivy. A boundary model for the regulation of eating. Eating and its disorders, edit Stunkard and Steller, 1984, 141-56. Raven Press, N.Y.
   Healthy Weight J Mar/Apr 1996;10:2:32-33.
2. Wooley S, W Wooley. Should obesity be treated at all? Eating and its Disorders, Stunkard and Steller, edits; 1984. Raven Press, N.Y.
3. Satter, Ellyn, How to get your kids to eat — but not too much, Bull Publ, Palo Alto, Calif.
   Workshops, "Treating the dieting casualty," Satter Assoc., Madison, Wis.
4. Omichinski L, You Count, Calories Don't, 1992; HUGS facilitator programs, HUGS International, Box 102A, Rt 3, Portage la Prairie, Manitoba, R1N 3A3, Canada; Teens & Diets — No Weigh, Healthy Weight J 1996;10:3:49-52; Berg F, Nondiet movement gains strength HWJ/Obesity & Health Sep/Oct 1992;6:5:82-90.
5. Reiff D, KK Lampson Reiff, Eating Disorders: Nutrition Therapy in the Recovery Process, 1992. Aspen, Gaithersburg, MD; Personal communication with Dan Reiff, 1996.
6. Keys A, et al. Biology of human starvation, 1950. U of Minn Press, Minneapolis, Minn.
   Berg F, Starvation stages in weight loss patients similar to famine victims, HWJ/Obesity & Health Apr 1989;3:4:27-30.
7. Body Mass Index. FAO, A measure of chronic energy deficiency in adults, 1994,

United Nations report.

Berg F, World starvation: weight may be best tool to measure malnutrition, Healthy Weight J May/Jun 1995;9:3:47-49.

8. Turnbull, Colin, 1972, The Mountain People. Simon and Schuster, N.Y.

9. CDC USHHS, Behavioral Risk Survey; Calorie Control Council, 1991 National Survey.

Berg F, Who is dieting in the U.S. Healthy Weight Journal/Obesity & Health 1992;6:3:48-49.

Dieting and purging behavior in black and white high school students, JADA 1992;92:3:306-312.

Adolescents dieting; JAMA 1991;266:2811-2812.

Berg F, Harmful weight loss practices among adolescents, HWJ/O&H Jul/Aug 1992;6:4:69-72.

10. Fallon P, Katzman M, Wooley S, Feminist perspectives on eating disorders 1994, Guilford Press, N.Y.

Baker D, R Sansone, Overview of eating disorders, 1994:1-10, NEDO.

Kaplan A, P Garfinkel, Medical issues and the eating disorders, 1993, Brunner/Mazel, N.Y.

Berg F, Eating disorders: physical and mental effects, Healthy Weight J Mar/Apr 1995;9:2:27-30.

Smolak L, M Levine, Toward an empirical basis for primary prevention of eating problems with elementary school children, Eat Disorders 1994;2:4:293-307

11. Andersen A. The last word, Eating Disorders 1994;2:1:81-82.

Bowers M. The last word. Eating Disorders 1994;2:4:375-377.

12. Young, Mary Evans, Diet Breaking, 1996, Hodder & Stoughton, London.

13. Biely J, Eating Disorder Awareness Week '96, EDAP Matters Winter 1996;2.

14. Berg F. Health Risks of Weight Loss, 1995. Chapter 1. General treatment risks, 14-26; Ch 7. Eating disorders, 56-62; Ch 8. Psychological risks, 63-69; Ch 9. Weight cycling, 70-79; Ch 11. Thinness: a cultural obsession, 89-99; Ch 13. To treat or not to treat, 108-113. 66:2811-2812; Berg F, Harmful weight loss practices among adolescents, HWJ/O&H Jul/Aug 1992;6:4:69.

Health-centered resources

HUGS International
Box 102A RR 3
Portage la Prairie Manitoba
Canada R1N 3A3
Tel: 204-428-3432; fax: 204-428-5072
www.hugs.com

Ellyn Satter Associates
4226 Mandan Crescent
Madison WI 53711
Te/fax: 608-271-7976
www.ellynsatter.com

OBESITY

International Association for the Study of Obesity (IASO)
Stephan Rossner, Secretary
Karolinska Hospital
Box 605000
104 01 Stockholm, Sweden
46-8-729 2000; fax: 46-8-33 0603

North American Association for the Study of Obesity (NAASO)
8630 Fenton Street #412
Silver Spring, MD 20910
301-563-6526; fax 301-587-2365
www/naaso.org

EATING DISORDERS AND PREVENTION

Eating Disorders Awareness and Prevention (EDAP)
603 Stewart St #803
Seattle WA 98101
1-800-931-2237; fax: 206-292-9890
edapinc@aol.com
www.members.aol.com/edapinc
or www.edap.org

Anorexia Nervosa and Related Eating Disorders (ANRED)
PO Box 5102
Eugene OR 97405
541-344-1144
jarinor@rio.com
www.anred.com

National Eating Disorder Information Centre
College Wing 1-211
200 Elizabeth St
Toronto Ontario
Canada M5G 2C4
416-340-4156; fax: 416-340-4736
mdpw@torhosp.toronto.on.ca
www.nedic.on.ca

National Eating Disorders Screening Program
One Washington St Ste 304
Wellesley Hills MA 02481
781-239-0071
info@nmisp.org
www.nmisp.org

EATING DISORDERS AND PREVENTION

Gurze Books
PO Box 2238
Carlsbad CA 92018
1-800-756-7533; fax: 206-292-9890
gurze@aol.com
www.gurze.com

Association of Anorexia Nervosa and Associated Disorders (ANAD)
PO Box 7
Highland Park IL 60035
847-831-3438; fax: 847-433-4632
and20@aol.com
www.members.aol.com/anad20/index.html

Academy for Eating Disorders
Division of Adolescent Medicine
Montefiore Medical Center
111 E 210th St.
Bronx, NY 10467
718-920-6782; fax: 718-920-5289

American Anorexia/Bulimia Association
165 W 46th St Ste 1108
New York NY 10036
212-575-6200; fax: 212-278-0698
info@aabainc.org
www.aabainc.org

National Eating Disorders Organization (NEDO)
6655 S Yale Ave
Tulsa OK 74136
918-481-4044; fax: 918-481-4076
lpchnedo@ionet.net
www.laureate.com

EVENTS

Healthy Weight Week. 3rd full week in January. Celebrates healthy lifestyle habits as an antidote to January dieting.

Rid the World of Fat Diets and Gimmicks Day. Tuesday of Healthy Weight Week. Exposes fraud and quackery in weight loss industry. Annual Slim Chance Awards given for the "worst" weight loss products of the year.

Women's Healthy Weight Day. Thursday of Healthy Weight Week. Celebrates size diversity in women. Women's Healthy Weight Awards given for businesses that portray size diversity in women.

Eating Disorder Awareness and Prevention Week. February. Special events, and screenings.

Fearless Friday. Friday of Eating Disorder Awareness and Prevention Week. A day to reject dieting and restricting food.

No Diet Day. May 6.

SIZE ACCEPTANCE

Council on Size & Weight Discrimination
PO Box 305
Mt Marion NY 12456
914-679-1209; fax: 914-679-1206
cswd@ulster.net
www.cswd.org

Largely Positive
Carol Johnson
PO Box 17223
Glendale WI 53217
414-299-9295; fax: 414-224-0243
positive@execpc.com

National Association to Advance Fat Acceptance (NAAFA)
PO Box 188620
Sacramento CA 95818
916-558-6880; fax: 916-558-6881
naafa@naafa.org
www.naafa.org

Body Trust
Dayle Hayes
3112 Farnam St
Billings, MT 59102
Te/fax: 406-655-9082; 406-656-0580

Radiance Magazine
PO Box 31703
Oakland CA 94604

Big Beautiful Woman (BBW)
11492 Sunrise Gold Circle, #D
Rancho Cordova, CA 95742

DietBreakers
Mary Evans Young
Church Cottage - Barford St. Michael
Banbury Oxon
England 0X15 OUA
0869-37070

Amplestuff
PO Box 116
Bearsville, NY 12409
914-679-3316; fax 914-679-1206
amplestuff@aol.com
www.amplestuff.com

Ample Opportunity
Nancy Barron
PO Box 40621
Portland OR 97240
503-245-1524

National Size Acceptance Coalition (SIZE)
Diana Pollard, Director
56 Gloucester Road, Suite 147
Kensington London
SW7 4UB England
0171 700 0509; fax: 0171 581 9213
dwm(@premier.co.uk

International Size-Acceptance Association (ISAA)
P. O. Box 82126
Austin TX 78758
Director@size-acceptance.org
www.size-acceptance.org/

Largesse, the Network for Sie Esteem
largesse@eskimo.com
www.eskimo.com/~largesse

Melpomene Institute for Women's Health Research
1010 University Avenue
St. Paul NM 55104
612-642-1951

WEBSITES

Health and weight

http://www.health.org/gpower .... Girl Power!

http://www.healthyweight.net .... Healthy Weight Network
(eating and weight research and information; quackery)

http://www.heartinfo.org .... Heart Information

http://www.hugs.com .... HUGS International

http://www.intelihealth.com .... John Hopkins University

http://www.justhink.org .... Just Think Foundation

http://www.nih.gov .... National Institutes of Health

http://www.mayohealth.org .... Mayo Clinic

http://www.igc.org/mef .... Media Education Foundation (media literacy)

http://www.ncahf.org .... National Council Against Health Fraud

http://www.niddk.nih.gov/health/nutrit/nutrit.htm — NIDDK nutrition and obesity

http://www.quackwatch.com .... Quackwatch
(guide to health fraud and quackery)

http://www.nal.usda.gov/fnic .... USDA Food and Nutrition Information Center

http://www.niddk.nih.gov/health/nutrit/win.htm — Weight Control Information Network

http://www.nhlbi.nih.gov/nhlbi/whil ... Women's Health Initiative

Eating disorders

http://www.about-face.org .... About Face

http://www.anred.com .... ANRED

http://www.members.aol.com/edapinc .. EDAP

http://www.hedc.org .... Harvard Eating Disorders Center

http://www.mirror-mirror.org/eatdis.htm Mirror Mirror Website on Eating Disorders

http://www.nmisp.org .... National Eating disorders Screening Program

http://www.nedic.on.ca .... National Eating Disorder Centre, Canada

http://something-fishy.org .... Something Fishy Website on Eating Disorders

Size acceptance

http://www.amplestuff.com .... Amplestuff

http://www.bbwmagazine.com .... BBW (Big Beautiful Woman)

http://www.naafa.org .... National Assoc. to Advance Fat Acceptance

http://www.radiancemagazine.com ..... Radiance Magazine

http://www.SizeWise.com .... Size Wise (updated catalog of resources)

References

Chapter 1

1. Berg F. Kids fear being fat early. *HWJ/ Obesity & Health* 1993;7:3:46-47. JADA 1992:92;92:7:851-53.
2. Mundy A. Weight-Loss Wars: deaths and a raft of lawsuits over diet drugs. *U.S. News & World Report* February 15, 1999.
3. National Center for Health Statistics, CDC 1992.
   Berg F. 1995. *Health Risks of Weight Loss.* p70-79. Hettinger, ND: Healthy Weight Journal.
4. Wolf N. Hunger. 1994. In *Feminist perspectives on eating disorders,* eds. P Fallon, M Katzman, and S Wooley. New York: Guilford Press.
5. *NHLBI Guidelines: Clinical Guidelines on the Identification, Evaluation, and Treatment of Overweight and Obesity in Adults: The Evidence Report.* National Institutes of Health, National Heart, Lung, and Blood Institute. Preprint June 1998. Bethesda, MD.
6. Taste, health, and the social meal. *J of Gastronomy,* Winter/Spring 1993. San Francisco: American Institute of Wine & Food.
7. Berg F. Nurses' Study garners headlines. *Healthy Weight J* 1996;10:1:16-18.
   Monson J, Willet W, et al. The Nurses' Health Study. *New Engl J Med* 1995;333:677-685.
8. NHLBI Guidelines, *see 5.*
9. *JAMA* 1996;276:1907-1915.
   Berg F. Task Force advises against diet drugs. *Healthy Weight J* 1997;11:2:27.
10. *Am J of Clinical Nutrition* 1994;60: 613-616.
11. Vitality Leader's Kit, 1994. Health Services and Promotion, Health and Welfare Canada. 4th Floor, Jeanne Mance Bldg, Ottawa, Ontario, Canada K1A 1B4 (613-957-8331).

Chapter 2

1. Hirschmann, Jane, and Munter, Carol. 1995. *When Women Stop Hating Their Bodies.* New York: Fawcett Columbine.
2. *Newsweek.* Feb 1, 1993;p64-65.
   Berg F. Gaunt idols. *HWJ/Obesity & Health* 1993;7:2:23.
3. *I J Eating Disorders* 1992;11:1:85-89.

Berg F. Thin mania turns up pressure. *HWJ/Obesity & Health* 1992;6:5:83.
Berg, *see Ch1:3:*p90.
Mustajoki M. *Ann Clin Research* 1987;19:143-146.
4. Morgan L. Why are girls obsessed with their weight? *Seventeen* Nov. 1989;118-119,145,150,154.
5. *Eating Disorders* 1993;1:2:109-114.
   Berg F. False media messages. *HWJ/ Obesity & Health* 1994;8:1:5.
6. Young, Mary Evans. 1995. *Diet Breaking: Having it all without having to diet.* p5-9. London: Hodder and Stoughton.
7. *Eating Disorders* 1993;1:1:52-61.
   Berg F. Television ads promote dieting. *HWJ/Obesity & Health* 1993;7:6:106.
8. Kilbourne J. 1994. Still killing us softly: Advertising and the obsession with thinness. In Feminist, *see Ch1:4.*
9. Fallon P, M Katzman, and S Wooley, eds. 1994. *Feminist perspectives on eating disorders.* New York: Guilford Press.
10. Larkin, Marilynn. Confessions of a former women's magazine writer. *Nutrition Forum* 1993;10:3:17-20.
11. Nichter M, Park S, and Nichter M. *Body image and weight concerns among African American and white adolescent females.* Anthro. Dept, Tucson, AZ: U of Arizona.
    Berg F. Beauty ideas are fluid. *Healthy Weight J* 1995;9:2:26.
    Berg, *see Ch1:3:p123.*
12. *Third report on nutrition monitoring in the US,* Vol 1-2, Dec 1995. National Center for Health Statistics, NHANES III. Life Sciences Research Office, Interagency Board for Nutrition Monitoring and Related Research, US Dept. of Health and Human Services, US Dept. Of Agriculture.
13. Fraser, Laura. 1994. *Losing it: America's obsession with weight and the industry that feeds on it.* p157. New York: Penguin/Dutton.
14. Wolf, Naomi. 1997. Dying to be Thin: The prevention of eating disorders and the role of Federal Policy. Testimony at Congressional Briefing, July 10, 1997.
15. Cantrell S. 10/4/98. *Milwaukee J/Sentinel.*
    Young K. The Opera: Only the Slender Need Apply. *On a Positive Note.*

1998;10:2:1.
16. *New York Times Magazine.* 10/25/98.
17. Visser, Margaret. *J of Gastronomy.* 1993;7:1.
18. Fallon, *see 9.*
19. De Garine I, and Pollock NJ. 1995. *Social Aspects of Obesity.* S. Australia: Gordon and Breach Publ.
20. Hesse-Biber, Sharlene. 1996. *Am I Thin Enough Yet?* New York: Oxford University Press.
21. Fallon, *see 9.*
    Berg, *see Ch1:3:*p89.
22. Kano Susan. 1989. *Making Peace With Food.* New York: Harper & Row.
23 Finding the inner swine. *Newsweek* 2/1/99;52-53.
24. Rothblum E. I'll die for the revolution but don't ask me not to diet. In Feminist, *see 9:*p53-76.
    Berg, *see Ch1:3:*p89, 91.
25. Larkin J, Rice C, and Russell V. Slipping through the cracks: sexual harassment, eating problems, and the problem of embodiment. *Eat Disorders* 1996; 4:1:5-26.
26. Larkin, *see 25.*
27. Pipher M. 1994. *Reviving Ophelia.* New York: Ballantine Books/Random House.
28. Levine P. President's message. *Eating Disorders Awareness and Prevention Newsletter.* Spring 1995:1-3.
29. Tolman D, and Debold E. Conflicts of body and image. In Feminist, *see Ch1:4:*p301-317.
    30. *Clin Psych Rev* 1991;11:729-780.
31. Levine P. The Last Word. *Eat Disorders.* 1995;3:1:92-95.

Chapter 3
1. Berg, *see Ch1:1.*
   JADA 1992;92;92:7:851-53.
2. Niven C, and Carroll D. 1993. *The Health psychology of women.* p115. Chur, Switzerland: Harwood Academic Publ.
3. Stunkard AJ. 1976. *The Pain of Obesity.* p77. Palo Alto, Calif.: Bull Publishing.
4. *Restaurants USA* 1994;14:18-21.
   Berg F. Customers want bigger meals. *Healthy Weight J* 1995;9:2:26.
5. Taste, *see Ch1:6.*
   Berg F. Review of special issue, J Gastronomy. *Healthy Weight J* 1994;8:3:59.

6. Kratina K, and King N. Hunger and satiety: helping clients get in touch with body signals. *Healthy Weight J* 1996;10:4:68-71.
7. Satter E. 1987. *How to Get Your Kid to Eat ... But Not Too Much.* Palo Alto, Calif.: Bull Publishing.
   - 1983. *Child of Mine: Feeding With Love and Good Sense.* Palo Alto, Calif.: Bull Publishing.
8. HUGS Club News, Jan. 1997, p6.
9. Berg F. Weight-loss programs for children and adolescents. *HWJ/Obesity & Health* 1989;3:10:78.
   Nutrition News 1988;51:2:5-7.
10. Fabrey W. Big News. *Radiance.* Fall 1995.
11. *I J Eat Disorders* 1994;16:1:83-88.
12. *See Ch2:30.*
    Berg F. Nondiet movement gains strength. *HWJ/Obesity & Health* 1992;6:5:85-90.
13. Satter, *see 7.*
14. Reiff D, and Reiff KK. 1992. *Eating Disorders: Nutrition Therapy in the Recovery Process.* p162. Gaithersburg, MD: Aspen Publishers.
15. Jewish Family and Children's Services. *Begin from Within* brochure. San Francisco.
16. National Eating Disorder Information Centre. 1996. Eating Disorder Awareness Week Kit: *Celebrating our natural sizes.* Toronto.
17. Young, *see Ch2:6:*p41-42,56-57.
18. Herman CP, and Mack D. Restrained and unrestrained eaters. *J Pers* 1975;43:647-660.
19. Stuart J. Restrained eaters rigidly control their food intake. *Healthy Weight J* 1997;11:3:49-51.
20. McCabe RE, Mills JS, and Polivy J. Exploding the myth: dieters eat less than nondieters. *Healthy Weight J* 1999;13:1:11-13.
21. White F. Treating overeating disorders. *NEDO Newsletter* 1998;32:2:1-4.
22. Saunders R, Johnson L, and Teschner J. Prevalence of eating disorders among bariatric surgery patients. *Eat Disorders.* 1998;6:4:309-317.
23. Structure House news release 10/15/96. NAASO conf 10/12-15/96.
24. McCabe RE, Mills JS, and Polivy J. Exploding the myth: Dieting makes you happier. *Healthy Weight J* 199;13:1:9-10.

25. *Diet Related to Killer Diseases,* Part 2, Obesity. 1977. Hearings before the Select Committee on Nutrition and Human Needs of the U.S. Senate, Feb. 1-2, 1977.

26. *J Health Soc Behav* 1994;35:63-78.

27. Wayler AH. Fear of food, compulsive eating, and extreme anger scar ex-liquid dieters. *HWJ/ Obesity & Health* 1992;6:3:50-51.

28. *Eat Disorders* 1995;3:3:229-236.

29. National Center, *see Ch1:3.*
    Berg, *see Ch1:3*:p70-79.

30. Pereyra L, et al. Eating attitudes, dietary intake, and dieting behaviors in college females. *J Am Diet Assoc* 1997;97(S):9:A-48.

31. Brownell K, and Rodin J. Medical, metabolic, and psychological effects of weight cycling. *Arch Intern Med* 1994;154;1325-1330.

32. Saunders, *see 22.*

33. *Weight Cycling.* Weight-Control Information Network, NIDDK, NIH, March 1995.
    JAMA 1994;272;15:1196-1202.
    Berg F. Weight loss campaign heats up. *Healthy Weight J* 1995;9:1:11-12,18-19.

34. Lissner L, Odell P, D'Agostino D, and Stoke J, et al. Variability of body weight and health outcomes in the Framingham population. *New Engl J Med* 1991;324:1839-44.

35. *Obesity in Europe 88* 1989:55-58.
    Berg F. Weight cycling. *HWJ/Obesity & Health* 1989;3:10:73.

36. Abstract, 34th Annual Conference on Cardiovascular Disease Epidemiology and Prevention, March 16-19, 1994.
    Berg F. Harvard alums risk disease by "always" dieting. *Healthy Weight J* 1994;8:3:52.

37. Lu H, et al. Long-term weight cycling in female Wistar rats. *Obes Res* 1995;3:521-530.

38. Brownell, *see 31.*

39. Brownell, *see 31.*

40. Davis KS. *Resetting the American table.* National Pork Producers Council. Presentation at Family and Consumer Science Annual Meeting, Atlanta 1998.

41. Reinhardt M. American Foodways. *SNE Communicator.* Fall 1997.

42. Allison DB, ed. 1995. *Handbook of Assessment Methods for Eating Behaviors and Weight-Related Problems: Measures, Theory, and Research.* Thousand Oaks, Calif.: Sage Publ.

Chapter 4

1. Special Report: The skinnier I got the fatter I felt. Mademoiselle March 1996.

2. Nottveit M. Battling eating disorders. *Healthy Weight J* 1997;11:4:75-76.

3. Morton, Andrew. 1997. *Diana, Her true story — in her own words.* As quoted in the Washington Post, 10/8/17.

4. Special Report, *see 1.*

5. Reiffs, *see Ch3:14*:p503.

6. Reiffs, *see Ch3:14*:p421.

7. Keys, Ancel et al. 1950. *The biology of human starvation.* School of Public Health. Minneapolis, MN.: U of Minnesota Press.

8. Garner D. The effects of starvation on behavior: Implications for dieting, disordered eating, and eating disorders, *Healthy Weight J* 1998;12:5:68-72.

9. Are (Were) You like me? *The Healthy Weigh* 1995;1:1:3.

10. Alexander-Mott L, and Lumsden DB. 1994. *Understanding eating disorders.* p290. Washington, DC: Taylor & Francis.

11. Bruch H. 1973. *Eating disorders: Obesity, anorexia nervosa and the person within.* New York: Basic Books.

12. Reiff DW, and Reiff KKL. Time spent thinking about food. *Healthy Weight J* 1998;12:6:84-86.
    Reiffs, *see Ch3:14*:p53,297.

13. Reiff, *see 12*:p245.

14. Berg F. Eating disorders — physical and mental effects. *Healthy Weight J* 1995;9:2:27-30.

15. Alexander-Mott, *see 10*:p290.

16. Reiff, *see 12:p312.*
    Alexander-Mott, *see 10*:p290.

17. Special Report, *see 1.*

18. Alexander-Mott, *see 10*:p290.

19. ANAD brochure. For more information, contact: Association of Anorexia Nervosa and Associated Disorders, PO Box 7, Highland Park, IL 60035; 847-831-3438; fax: 847-433-4632; email: and20@aol. com; website: members.aol.com/anad20/index.html.

20. *Parade Magazine* clipping, date missing.

21. Levine M. Prevalence of eating disor-

ders, some tentative facts. *EDAP*. Feb 1, 1996.
Also, National Association of Anorexia Nervosa and Associated Disorders.

22. Pawluck D, and Gorey K. Secular trends in the incidence of anorexia nervosa. *Int J Eating Disorders* 1998;23: 347-352.

23. Sesan R. 1994. Feminist inpatient treatment for eating disorders. In Feminist, *see Ch1:4*:p25.

24. Efron S. Eating disorders in Asia. *Los Angeles Times*. Oct. 21, 1997.

25. Hoek H. 1995. The distribution of eating disorders. In *Eating Disorders and Obesity*, ed. K Brownell and C Fairburn. p207-211. New York: Guilford Press.

26. Individual characteristics, environment affect risk of developing eating disorders. *Psychiatric News* July 17,1998: 13,20.

27. *J Consult & Clin Psychol* 1989; 57:2:215-221.

28. Fallon, *see Ch2:9*.

29. Smolak L, and Levine M. Toward an empirical basis for primary prevention of eating problems with elementary school children. *Eat Disorders* 1994;2:4:293-307.

30. Goodman E. Eating disorders: The Columbine for girls. *Boston Globe* 5/28/ 99.

31. McCabe, *see Ch3:20*.
Estes L, Crago M, and Shisslak C. Eating disorders prevention. *The Renfrew Perspective* 1996;2:1:3-5.
Fallon, *see Ch2:9*.
Berg, *see Ch1:1*.

32. Wilson, GT. 1995. *The controversy over dieting*. p87-92. New York: Guilford Press.

33. Position of the American Dietetic Association: *Nutrition intervention in the treatment of anorexia nervosa, bulimia nervosa, and binge eating*. ADA, Chicago.

34. Wooley S. 1996. Recognition of Sexual Abuse: Progress and Backlash. In *Sexual abuse and eating disorders*, eds. M Schwartz and L Cohn. New York: Brunner/Mazel.

35. Brewerton T. Sexual and physical assault are risk factors for bulimia nervosa. NEDO Newsletter 1994;7:4:1-5.

36. Schwartz M, L Cohn, eds. 1996. *Sexual abuse and eating disorders*. New York: Brunner/Mazel.

37. Berg F. Eating disorders affect mind and body. *Healthy Weight J* 1995;9:2: 27-30.
Berg, *see Ch1:3*:p57-58.

38. Davis C. 1996. *Body image and its influence. Progress in obesity research:7*, Angel A, et al, eds. p367-372. London: John Libbey & Co.

39. Kratina K. 1995. Exercise dependence. In *Nutrition Therapy: Advanced counseling skills*, K King Helm, and B Klawitte eds. In press.

40. Powers P, and Johnson C. Small victories. *Eating Disorders* 1996;4: 364-377.

41. Berning J, and Steen S. 1991. *Sports Nutr for the 90s*. p156-158. Gaithersburg, MD: Aspen.

42. Berg F. VLCD specialists warn against hazards. *HWJ/Obesity & Health* 1990;4:3:17-23.

43. Eating disorder suspected in death. *AP*. Boston. 7/11/97.

44. Garner D, Rosen LW, and Barry D. Eating disorders among athletes. Child and Adolescent Psychiatric Clinics of NA. *Sport Psychiatry* 1998;7:4: 839-857.

45. Berg F. Competitive bodybuilding. *Healthy Weight J* 1996;10:3:47-48.

46. Diagnostic criteria for eating disorders. 1994. *Diagnostic and Statistical Manual*, Fourth Edition. Washington, DC: American Psychiatric Association.

47. Fairburn G, Wilson GT, eds. 1993. *Binge Eating*. New York: Guilford.

48. Fairburn, *see 47*.

49. Binge eating. News briefs. *Healthy Weight J* 1996;10:4:66.
7th European Congress on Obesity. *I J Obesity* 1996;20(4):99.

50. Kaplan A, and Garfinkel P. 1993. *Medical issues and eating disorders*. New York: Brunner/Mazel.

Chapter 5

1. Kumanyika S. *Epidemiologic Reviews* 1987;9:31-50.

2. Kuczmarski RJ, Carroll MD, Flegal KM, and Troiano RP. Varying body mass index cutoff points to describe overweight prevalence among US adults: NHANES III (1988-1994). *Obesity Res* 1997;5:6:542-548.

3. NHLBI Guidelines, *see Ch1:5*:p23-26; 90-91.

4. Flegal KM, Carroll MD, Kuczmarski RJ,

and Johnson CL. Overweight and obesity in the United States: prevalence and trends, 1960-1994. *Int J Obes* 1998;22:39-47.

5. White LL, Ballew C, et al. Weight, body image, and weight control practices of Navajo Indians. *J Nutr* 1997; 127:2094-2098S.

6. *Contemporary Nutr* 1989;14:6.
   Obesity: prevention and managing the global epidemic: Report of a WHO consultation on obesity. WHO/NUT/NCD/98.1. 1998. Geneva, Switzerland: World Health Organization.

7. NHLBI Guidelines, *see Ch1:5.*

8. Kassirer JP, Angell M. Losing weight — an ill-fated New Year's resolution. *N Engl J Med* 1998;338:52-54.
   Berg F. Medical Journal Questions Obesity Treatment. *Healthy Weight J* 1998;12:3:36.

9. Gaesser, Glenn. 1996. *Big Fat Lies: The truth about your weight and your health.* New York: Ballantine Books.

10. Fontaine KR, Heo M, Cheskin LJ, and Allison DB. Body mass index, smoking, and mortality among older American women. *J Women's Health* 1998;7:1257-1261.

11. NHLBI Guidelines, *see Ch1:5*:p92S.

12. Fraser, *see Ch2:13*:p176-77, 178

13. Bjorntorp P. *Obesity Res* 1993;1:3: 206-222.
    Berg F. Risks focus on visceral obesity, may be stress linked. *HWJ/Obesity & Health* 1993;7:5:87-89.

14. Becque MD, K Hattori, et. al. *Em J Phys Anthro* 71;423-249.
    Berg F. 1993. *Health Risks of Obesity.* Hettinger, ND: Healthy Weight Journal.

15. Bouchard C, and Johnston F. 1988. *Fat distribution during growth and later health outcomes.* New York: Alan Liss.
    Berg, *see Ch5:14*:p43
    Berg F. Ethnic differences in fat patterning. *HWJ/International Obesity Newsletter* 1988;2:12:5.

16. A. Stunkard, and T. Wadden eds. 1993. *Obesity: Theory and Therapy.* p19. New York: Raven Press.
    Berg F. Measuring visceral fat by sagittal diameter. *HWJ/Obesity & Health* 1993;7:5:87.

17. *Int J Obesity* 1990;14:S2:62.

18. NHLBI Guidelines, *see Ch1:5.*

19. Mayer J. Genetic factors in human

obesity. PubEd workshop report, p27. *Ann NY Acad Sci* 1965;131:412-421.

20. West D, and York B. Dietary fat, genetic predisposition, and obesity. *Am J Clin Nutr* 1998;67(Suppl):505-512S.

21. Bouchard C, L Perusse, et al. Inheritance of the amount and distribution of human body fat. *Int J Obesity* 1988;12:205-215.
    Berg F. NAASO highlights. *HWJ/Obesity & Health* 1992:6:1:5.

22. Kumanyika, *see 1.*
    Wendorf M, and Goldfine I. *Diabetes* 1991;40:161-165.
    Berg F. Thrifty gene may set stage for obesity in blacks. *HWJ/Obesity & Health* 1991:5:1:6-7.
    Berg F. Former big game hunters succumb to diabetes. *HWJ/Obesity & Health* 1991;5:6:98.
    Berg F. Thrifty gene threatens the good life. *Healthy Weight J* 1995;9:4:64.

23. USDHHS. 1996. *Physical Activity and Health: A report of the Surgeon General.* CDC, National Center for Chronic Disease Prevention and Health Promotion, Atlanta, GA.

24. *N Engl J Med* 1991;324:739-745.

25. Is total fat consumption really decreasing? April 1998. *Nutrition Insights 5,* USDA Center for Nutrition Policy and Promotion.

26. Third report, *see Ch 2:12.*

27. Berg F. Fat intake: Is it responsible for rising obesity rates. Rethinking low-fat advice. *Healthy Weight J* 1998; 12:4:52-58,49,64.

28. Willett W. Is dietary fat a major determinant of body fat? *Am J Clin Nutr* 1998;67(Suppl):556-562S.

29. Willett, *see 28.*

30. Prentice A. Manipulation of dietary fat and energy density and subsequent effects. *Am J Clin Nutr* 1998;67(Suppl) :535-541S.

31. Kenney JJ. Should we reduce percent fat or calorie density? *Healthy Weight J* 1998;12:6:87-88.

32. *Restaurants, see Ch3:4.*

33. Is total fat, *see 25.*

34. Obarzanek E, G Schreiber, P Crawford, et al. Energy intake and physical activity in relation to indexes of body fat: the National Heart, Lung, and Blood Institute.

35. Fernstrom M. 1996. Psychiatric drugs and weight gain. In *Progress in obe-*

sity research 7th Ed., ed. Angel A, et al. p641-647. London: John Libbey & Co.

36. *Arch Gen Psychiatry* 1990;47:857-860.
37. *Nutr Review* 50:9:267-270.
    Suter P, Schutz Y, Jequier E. *N Engl J Med* 1992;326:983-987.
38. Rothblum ED. 1994. "I'll die for the revolution but don't ask me not to diet". In Feminist, *see Ch1:4*:p55.
39. Bennett W, and Gurin J. 1982. *The Dieter's Dilemma*. New York: Basic Books, Harper Collins.
40. Rossner S. et al. *Obesity Research* 1996;4:3:271-276.
41. *Intl J Obesity* 1994;18:2:45.
42. *Intl J Obesity* 1992;16:145-147.
43. *Intl J Obesity* 1996;20:526-532.
44. Kumanyika, *see Ch5:1*.
    Berg, *see 22*.
45. Filer LJ. Summary of the Workshop on Child and Adolescent Obesity, University of Critical Reviews in food. *Science and Nutrition* 1993:33:4/5:287-305.
46. *Nutrition During Pregnancy*. 1991. Food and Nutrition Board, National Academy of Sciences Institute of Medicine.
    Berg F. Weight gain in pregnancy. *HWJ/Obesity & Health* 1991;5:5:75-77, 72.
47. Nutrition, *see 46*.
48. Wing R, Matthews K, et al. *Arch Intern Med* 1991;151:97-102.
    Berg F. Weight gain in menopausal years. *Healthy Weight J* 1994;8:4:69-70.
49. *Tufts U Diet & Nutr Ltr* 1996;14:1:1.
50. Allison D. 1995. Report at North American Society for the Study of Obesity conference. Baton Rouge, La. NIH Obesity Research Center, NY.
51. *New Engl J Med* 11/2/95.
52. Astrup A, et al. Is obesity contagious? *Int J Obes* 1998;22:375-376.

Chapter 6
1. McAfee L. Discrimination in medical care. *Healthy Weight J* 1997;11:5:96-97.
2. LS Brown, and ED Rothblum, eds. 1989. *Overcoming Fear of Fat*. Binghamton, NY: Harrington Park Press/Haworth Press.
3. Goodman C. 1995. *The Invisible Woman: Confronting Weight Prejudice in America*. p4-6. Carlsbad, Calif.: Gurze Books.

4. *BBW* April 1994:19.
5. *Radiance* Magazine. Oakland, CA. Website: www.radiancemag-azine.com.
6. Cauthen L. Dealing with size discrimination in the workplace. *BBW* March 1998:44-47.
7. Cauthen, *see 6*.
8. McAfee, *see 1*:84.
9. McAfee, *see 1*:p96-97.
10. McAfee, *see 1*.
11. McAfee, *see 1*.
12. McAfee, *see 1*.
13. Fontaine K, et al. Body weight and health care among women. Also editorial: Yanovski S. Large patients and lack of preventive health care. *Arch Fam Med* 1998;7:381-385.
14. Adams C, et al. The relationship of obesity to the frequency of pelvic examinations: do physician and patient attitudes make a difference? *Women & Health* 1993;20:45-57.
15. Lubitz RM, et al. Is obesity a barrier to physician screening for cervical cancer? *Am J Med* 1995;98:491-496.
16. McAfee, *see 1*.
17. Sandow, Kathy. Health care from a large woman's perspective. *Healthy Weight J* 1993;7:4:75-76.
    Sandow, Kathy. Health care. *LifeSize, Newsletter of Women at Large*, S.A. Sept 1992:3-4. Women at Large, 12 Chancery Lane, Hawthorndene, South Australia 5051.
18. Olson C, et al. Overweight women delay medical care. *Arch Fam Med* 1994;3:888-892.
    McAfee L. Health care horror stories. *BBW* May 1998.
19. Smith S. Provide quality health care, not weight cycling. *Healthy Weight J* 1997;11:5:94-95.
20. McAfee, *see 1*.
21. McAfee, *see 1*.
22. *Nutrition News* 1988;51:2:5-7.
    Berg F. Weight-loss programs for children and adolescents, Criteria for evaluating clinical programs. *HWJ/Obesity & Health* 1989;3:10:78.
23. Goodman, *see 23*;pxi.
24. Dietz, William, and Scrimshaw, Nevin. *Potential advantages and disadvantages of human obesity*. Luxembourg: Social Aspects and Beach Publ.
25. Hall L. 1993. *Full Lives: Women who have freed themselves from food & weight obsession*. Carlsbad, CA.: Gurze

Books.

26. Brownell Kelly, C Fairburn, eds. 1995. *Eating Disorders and Obesity.* p417-421. New York: Guilford Press.

27. Stunkard A, and Wadden T. 1987. Psychopathology and obesity. In *Human Obesity*, ed. Wurtman T. p57. NY Academy of Sci.

28. *Report on Size Discrimination,* NEA, Adopted Oct. 7, 1994. For more information, contact: Mary Faber, NEA, 1201 16th St., NW, Washington, DC 20036-3290 (202-822-7700; Fax 202-822-7578).

29. Brownell, *see 26.*

30. *Healthy Eating Index, Table 10.* July 19, 1998. Center for Nutrition Policy and Promotion, United States Department of Agriculture; www.usda.gov. fcs.cnpp.htm.

31. Logue AW. 1991. *The Psychology of Eating and Drinking.* New York: W.H. Freeman and Co.

32. Berg F. Prader-Willi: A defect of insatiable appetite. *Healthy Weight J* 1996;10:6:110-111.

33. Barlow, *see ch 13, 11.*

34. Burgard D. Psychological theory seeks to define obesity. *HWJ/ Obesity & Health* 1993;7:2:25-27, 37.

Chapter 7

1. *Hunger 1996: Countries in Crisis.* 1995. Silver Spring, MD: Bread for World Institute.

2. Keesey RE. 1993. Physiological regulation of body energy: implications for obesity. In *Obesity: Theory and Therapy,* eds. AJ Stunkard, and T Wadden. p77-96. New York: Raven Press.

3. Keesey, *see 2.*

4. Stunkard, *see Ch3:3*:p38-39.

5. Bennett, *see Ch5:39.*

6. Keesey RE, 1980. A set point analysis of the regulation of body weight. In *Obesity,* ed. AJ Stunkard. p55. Philadelphia: W.B. Saunders Co.

7. *Am J Public Health* June 1988.
Berg F. VLCD and obesity surgery after 5 years. *HWJ/Obesity & Health* 1989;3:5:33-38.

8. Wadden TA, Stunkard A, and Liebschutz J. Three year follow-up of the treatment of obesity by very low calorie diet, behavior therapy, and their combination. *J Consult Clin Psych*

1988;5:6:925-928.

9. Weigle DS. Energy efficiency of reduced-obese men. In *Obesity in Europe 88,* eds. P Bjorntorp, and S Rossner. p359-364. London: John Libbey.
Keesey, *see 2*:p88

10. Keesey RE. A set-point model of body weight regulation. In *Eating Disorders and Obesity.* p46-50.

11. Garner DM, Vitousek KM, and Pike KM. 1997. Cognitive-behavioral therapy for anorexia nervosa. In *Handbook of Treatment for Eating Disorders,* second edition. DM Garner, PE Garfinkel, eds. p94-144. New York: Guilford Press.

12. Garner, *see Ch4:8.*

13. Keys, *see Ch4:7.*

14. Garner DM. Psychoeducational principles in the treatment of eating disorders. In Handbook, *see 11*:p145-174.

15. Keys, *see Ch4:7.*

16. Keys, *see Ch4:7*:p140-143.
Berg, *see Ch1:3*:p29-31.

17. Turnbull, Colin M. 1972. *The Mountain People.* Touchstone Edition, 1987. New York: Simon & Schuster.
Berg F. The starvation syndrome in Africa. *Healthy Weight J* 1998;12:5:73-75.

18. Kater, KJ. 1998. *Healthy Body Image: Teaching kids to eat and love their bodies too.* p121-123. Seattle, WA: Eating Disorders Awareness and Prevention.

19. Garner, *see Ch4:8.*

20. Andersen RE, Barlett SJ, Morgan GD, et al. Weight loss, psychological, and nutritional patterns in competitive male body builders. *Int J Eat Disord* 1995;18:49-57.

21. Bennett, *see Ch5:39.*

22. Guetzkow HS, and Bowman PH. 1946. *Men and Hunger.* p9. Elgin, Ill.: Brethren Publishing House.

Chapter 8

1. Klem M, et al. Individuals successful at long-term maintenance. *Am J Clin Nutr* 1997;66:239-246.

2. Methods for Voluntary Weight Loss and Control, Public Health Service, National Institutes of Health Technology Assessment Conference Statement, Mar 30-Apr 1, 1992.

3. Abstract, *Am Soc Clin Nutr* 1992.
J Bone Mineral Res 1994;9:4:459-463.
J Bone Mineral Res 1993;20:141-149.
Bone loss with weight loss. *Healthy Weight J* 1994;8:5:85-86.
Wardlaw G. Body weight influences osteoporosis risk. *Healthy Weight J* 1996;10:1:8-9, 12.
Berg F. Dieting and weight loss increase osteoporosis risk. *Healthy Weight J* 1996;10:1:10-12.
4. Allison DB, Zannolli R, Faith MS, et al. Weight loss increases and fat loss decreases all-cause mortality rate: results from two independent cohort studies. *I J Obesity* 1999;23:603-611.
5. Garner, *see Ch7:14.*
6. Keys, *see Ch4:7.*
7. Kassirer, *see Ch5:8.*
8. Berg, *see Ch1:3*:p34-38.
9. Levitsky D. Diet drugs gain popularity. *Healthy Weight J* 1997;11:1:8-12.
10. FDA discussion paper, Nov. 24, 1997; AP Washington, Nov. 25, 1997.
11. FDA committee backs another anti-obesity drug. AP, Bethesda, MD, May 15, 1997.
12. FDA, *see 10.*
13. FDA, *see 11.*
14. FDA News Release, Sept. 15, 1997.
Berg F. Redux, fen-phen withdrawn from market. *Healthy Weight J* 1997;11:6:105.
15. Berg F, Fen-phen tragedy triggers uproar. *Healthy Weight J* 1998;12:2:17, 32.
16. Graham D, and Green L. FDA. Further cases of valvular heart disease associated with fenfluramine-phentermine. *N Engl J Med* 1997;337:635.
Curfman G. Diet pills redux. *N Engl J Med* 1997;337:629-630.
Berg F. Heart valave damage implicates fen-phen. *Healthy Weight J* 1997;11:6:107.
17. FDA recomendations — find this on our website — Nov 13, 1997; another Sept 18. See also www.healthyweight network.com.
18. Say no to phen/pro. *Harvard Women's Health Watch* 1997;5:4:3.
19. Berg F. The case against PPA. *HWJ/Obesity & Health* 1991;5:1:9-12.
20. Berg, *see 19.*
21. Adolescents dieting. *JAMA* 191;266:2811-2812.
Berg F. Harmful weight loss practices are widespread among adolescents. *HWJ/Obesity & Health* 1992;6:4:69-72.
22. Dieting and purging behavior in black and white high school students. *JADA* 1992;92:3:306-312.
Berg, *see 21.*
23. Berg, *see 19.*
24. *Wis Rapids Daily Trib* Jan 27, 1994;5.
Berg F. Ephedrine strikes again. *Healthy Weight J* 1995;9:1:5.
Rosencrans K. Diet pills suspected in deaths. *HWJ/Obesity & Health* 1994;8:4:68.
Berg F. 1995. *Weight Loss Quackery and Fads*. p16. Hettinger, ND: Healthy Weight Journal.
25. *FDA Consumer* May 1995;3.
26. Berg F. Bee pollen "cures" truckers of obesity, tumors, radiation. *HWJ/Obesity & Health* 1991;5:2:30.
Rosencrans, *see 24.*
27. Berg F. Feds act against mix of scams. *Healthy Weight J* 1994;8:5:94.
28. Berg F. Slim America pulls in $9.5 million before it is closed down. *Healthy Weight J* 1998;12:3:45.
29. Berg, *see 24*:p3-6.
30. Mayer K. 1993. *Real Women Don't Diet*. p149. Silver Spring MD: Bartleby Press.
31. Berg, *see 21.*
Dieting and purging, *see 22.*
32. Baker D, and Sansone AR. 1994. *Overview of eating disorders*. NEDO.
33. Mehler P, and Weiner K. Frequently asked medical questions about eating disorder patients. *Eating Disorders,* 1994;2:1:22-30.
34. Kaplan, *see Ch4:50*:p101-122.
35. Berg F. Smoking cessation impacts weight. *Healthy Weight J* 1996;10:2:27-28.
36. *Girls smoking*. Youth Risk Behavior Surveillance — US, 1995. Morbidity and Mortality Weekly Report. CDC, US Public Health Service. Sept 27, 1996:45:SS-4.
37. *Addictive Behaviors* 2;1987.
Int J Eat Disorders May 1988;7:3:413-419.
Berg F. Setting goals for the New Year and new decade (editorial). *HWJ/Obesity & Health* 1988:2:1:1-4.
Berg F. Setting goals for 2000 A.D. *HWJ/Obesity & Health* 1988:2:1:1-4.
38. *New Engl J Med*

1995;333:1165-1170,1214-1216.

Berg, *see 35.*

39. Healthy People 2000, USDHHS, PHS, Sept. 1990;140.

40. Berg, *see Ch1:3*:p27-32.

Berg F. Potential side effects of very low calorie diets. *HWJ/Obesity & Health* 1990;4:3:21.

Keys, *see Ch4:7.*

Berg F. Starvation stages in weight loss patients similar to famine victims'. *HWJ/Obesity & Health* 1989;3:4: 27-30.

41. *I J Obesity* Nov 1989;13:2:19.

Berg, *see Ch4:42.*

42. *Obesity Research* 1993;1:1:51-56

Berg F. Linking gallstones with weight loss. *HWJ/Obesity & Health* 1993;7: 3:45.

43. Petersmarck K, and Smith P. 1989. *Toward safe weight loss — recommendations for adult weight loss programs in Michigan.* Michigan Health Council, Michigan Dept of Public Health.

Berg F. Potential, *see 40.*

44. Berg F. Three companies charged with false, deceptive claims. *HWJ/Obesity & Health* 1992;6:1:9,16.

Berg F. FTC charges false claims. *HWJ/ Obesity & Health* 1993;7:3:47.

45. Fraser, *see Ch2:13*:p141.

46. Sobal J. Group dieting, the stigma of obesity, and overweight adolescents. 1984. *In Obesity and the Family.* D Kallen and M Susman, eds. p9-20. New York: Haworth Press.

47. Berg, *see Ch1:3*:p44-49.

48. *Guidance for Treatment of Adult Obesity.* 1996. Shape Up America! and American Obesity Assoc.

49. *JAMA* 1989;261:10:1491-1494.

I J Obesity 1993;17:453-457.

Berg F. Surgery risks persist over time. *HWJ/Obesity & Health* 1993;7: 6:106.

50. *Surgery* 1985;98:700-707, 1990;107: 1:20-27.

Berg F. Surgical viewpoint. *HWJ/Obesity & Health* 1991;5:2:18-25.

51. Forse RA. Surgical management of obesity. *HWJ/Obesity & Health* 1991;5:2: 18-25.

52. Draft panel statement. NIH. March 27, 1991.

Berg F. NIH endorses stomach surgery. *HWJ/Obesity & Health* 1991;5:3:37.

53. Ernsberger P. Surgery risks outweigh its benefits. *HWJ/Obesity & Health* 1991; 5:2:21-25.

54. AP, Los Angeles, 8/25/97.

55. Hyperthermia and dehydration-related deaths in three collegiate wrestlers. *Morbidity, Mortality Weekly Report.* Centers of Disease Control and Prevention. Feb. 20, 1998;47:105-108.

Berg F. Deaths shock college wrestling. *Healthy Weight J* 1998;12:3:34.

56. Dieting, *see 22.*

Adolescents, *see 21.*

57. *See 22.*

58. Mehler, *see 33.*

59. Kaplan, *see 34.*

60. Mehler, *see 33.*

Kaplan, *see 34.*

61. Berg, *see 24.*

Berg F. 1997 Slim Chance Awards. *Healthy Weight J* 1997;11:1:7.

Chapter 9

1. *Recommended Dietary Allowances*, 10th Edition, p3,32-33. 1989. Food and Nutrition Board, National Research Council, National Academy Press, Washington, D.C.

2. Kantor LS. 1/22/99. *A dietary assessment of the US food supply.* USDA Economic Research Service, Center for Nutrition Information. CNI.

3. *Continuing Survey of Food Intakes by Individuals (CSFII),* What We Eat in America Survey. Dec 1998. US Department of Agriculture.

4. Recommended Dietary Allowances, *see 1.*

5. Third report, *see Ch 2:12.*

Briefel RL. 1997. *Personal communication.* USDHHS.

6. Muhlheim LS, Allison DB, Heshka S, et al. Do unsuccessful dieters intentionally underreport food intake? *Eat Disord* 1998;24:259-266.

7. *Dietary Reference Intakes for calcium, phosphorus, magnesium, vitamin D and fluoride.* 1997. Washington, DC. National Academy Press.

8. Third report, *see Ch 2:12.*

9. Looker AC, Dallman PR, Carrol MD, et al. Prevalence of iron deficiency in the U.S. *JAMA* 1997;277:973-976.

10. Shil M, Olson J, Shike M, eds. 1994. *Modern nutrition in health and disease.* p704. Pennsylvania: Lea & Fermiger.

The Surgeon General's Report on Nu-

trition and Health. 1988. US Dept. of Health and Human Services, Public Health Service.

Recommended Dietary Allowances, see 1.

11. Duyff RL. 1996. The American Dietetic Association's Complete Food and Nutrition Guide. Minneapolis, MN: Chronimed Publ.

Keen CL, and Gershwin ME. Zinc deficiency and immune function. Ann Rev Nutrition 1990;10:415-431.

Bogden JD, Oleske JM, Lavenhar MA, et al. Zinc and immunocompetence in elderly people. Am J Clin Nutr 1988;48:655-663.

12. What and where our children eat: 1994 Nationwide Survey results. USDA News release, Apr 18, 1996.

13. Jacobson MF. Liquid Candy: How soft drinks are harming Americans' health. Center for Science in the Public Interest. October 21, 1998. Online: www.cspinet.org/sodapop/liquid_candy.htm.

14. Nicklas T et al. Changes in meat consumption patterns of children from 1976 to 1988: The Bogalusa Heart Study. Nutr Research 1996;16:4: 591-601.

15. Continuing Survey, see Ch 9:3.

16. Very-low-fat diet is not associated with improved lipoprotein profiles in men. Am J of Clin Nutr 1999;69:411-418.

17. Nutrition Today Jan/Feb 1992;4.

18. Focus on women. European J of Clin Nutr 1993;47, 1994;3.

19. Nicklas T. Dietary studies of children: The Bogalusa Heart Study. JADA 1995;95:1127-1133.

20. Fogelholm M, et al. Energy balance and overweight in Finland. Int J Obesity 1996;20:1097-1104.

European Congress on Obesity, Barcelona, Spain. I J Obesity 1996;20(4):53.

21. Prentice A. Manipulation of dietary fat and energy density and subsequent effects. Am J Clin Nutr 1998;67(S): 535-541S.

22. Reiner S. CLA: Does fat have a silver lining? Priorities 1996;3:4:42-47.

23. Flatt, see Ch5:36.

24. Leonard W et al. Correlates of low serum lipid levels among the Evenki herders of Siberia. Am J of Human Biology 1994;6:329-338.

Waddington K. Hard work and reindeer steak. University of Guelph Research Spring/Summer 1994:27.

Leonard W. Energetics and population ecology of Siberian herders. Am J of Human Biology 1996;8:275-28.

Ho K-J et al. The Masai of East Africa: Some unique biological characteristics. Arch Pathol 91:387-410.

25. Ortega RM, et al. Influence of meat consumption in relation to various cardiovascular risk factors in the elderly. Rev Clin Esp 1994;194:3: 147-151.

26. Goldbohm RA, et al. A prospective cohort study on the relation between meat consumption and the risk of colon cancer. Cancer Res 1994;54:3: 718-723.

27. Eaton SB, and Konner M. Paleoplithic. New Engl J Med 1985;312:5:283-289.

28. Lawrie RA. Proteins as human food. Proceedings of the 16th Easter School in Agricultural Science.

Rona RJ, et al. Vegetarianism and growth in Urdu, Gujarati, and Punjabi children in Britain. J Epidemiol Community Health 1987;41:3:233-236.

29. Woolsey M. The eating disordered vegetarian. Healthy Weight J 1997;11: 2:32-34.

30. Jarvis W. Why I am not a vegetarian. Nutrition & Health Forum 1996;13:6: 57-64.

31. Whelan E. Smoking report. Priorities 1996;8:1:4-9.

32. Continuing Survey, see Ch 9:3.

33. Physical Activity, see Ch5:23.

34. Obesity, see Ch5:6:p48.

35. Haapanen N, et al.Association between leisure time physical activity and 10-year body mass change. I J Obesity 1997;21:288-296.

36. Miller WC. Exercise: Americans don't think it's worth it! HWJ/Obesity & Health 1994;8:2:29-31, 38.

37. Lutter JM. Obstacles to exercise for larger women. HWJ/Obesity & Health 1994;8:1:12-13.

38. Feltes L. Safety: The unspoken barrier to women's physical activity. Melpomene J 1997:16:3:9-11.

39. Kratina, see Ch4:39.

40. Glass J. Exercise benefits, risks and precautions for women. Healthy Weight J 1999;13:4:56.

41. Otis CL, Drinkwater B, Johnson M, et

al. ACSM Position Stand on the Female Athlete Triad. *Med Sci Sports Exer* 1997;29:5:i-ix.

42. Dwyer E, Silbiger D, and Ryan J. The red flags of over-training. *Shape* Apr 1996;122-123.

43. Frisch, Rose, ed. 1990. Adipose tissue and reproduction, Progress in reproductive biology. Basel, Switzerland: Karger.
Berg F. High body fat brings early puberty. *Healthy Weight J* 1990;4:74-76.

44. Loosli AR, and Ruud JS. Meatless diets in female athletes: A red flag. The *Physician and Sportsmedicine.* 1998;26:11:45-48,55.

45. Dwyer, *see 42.*

46. *Muscle & Fitness.* Feb 1996:137-138, 221-222.

47. Fraser L. *Mademoiselle.* March 1995: 194-197,228.

48. Berg, *see Ch4:45.*

Chapter 10

1. Fraser, Laura. 1994. *Losing it: America's obsession with weight and the industry that feeds on it.* New York: Penguin/Dutton.

2. JAMA, *see Ch1:9.*
Berg, *see Ch1:9.*

3. National Task Force on the Prevention and Treatment of Obesity. Drug Therapy. *J of the Am Med Assoc.* 1996;276:1907-1915.
Berg, *see Ch1:9.*

4. Ornstein, Charles. Fen-phen maker accused of funding journal articles; company defends input it had on published works. *The Dallas Morning News* 5/23/99.

5. Berg F. Witnesses charge diet drug is hazardous. *HWJ/Obesity & Health* 1991;5:1:9-12;
Sept 24, 1990, Congressional hearings, U.S. House of Representatives Small Business Subcommittee on Regulation, Business Opportunities and Energy.

6. NHLBI, *see Ch1:5.*

7. *Choosing a safe and successful weight-loss program.* WIN brochure, NIDDK.

8. National Task Force on the Prevention and Treatment of Obesity. Weight Cycling. *JAMA* 1994;272;15:11696-1202.
Berg F. Weight loss campaign heats up.

Healthy Weight J 1995;9:1:4, 11-12, 18-19.

9. *Weighing the Options.* 1995. Wash., DC: Natl Academy Press.
Berg F. Review: Weighing the Options. *Healthy Weight J* 1995;9:3:57-58.

10. *The Dietary Guidelines for Americans, 4th Edition.* 1995. Pueblo, CO: Consumer Information Center.
Berg F. New guidelines given for "healthy weight." *Healthy Weight J* 1996;10:3:44, 53-54, 57.

11. *Ann Int Med* 1993;119:681-687.

12. Miller, Wayne C. The history of dieting and its effectiveness. *Healthy Weight J* 1997;11:2:28-29.

13. Fraser, *see 1:*p12-13.

14. Berg, *see Ch1:7.*

15. Wolf A, and Colditz G. The cost of obesity. *PharmoEconomics* 1994;5:34-37.
Berg F. Obesity costs reach $45.8 billion. *Healthy Weight J* 1995;9:4:67-68.

16. Mundy, *see Ch1:2.*

17. Weintraub M. Long-term weight control study. *Clin Pharmacol Ther* 1992;51:642-646;
Weintraub M, et al. Long-term weight control study III. *Clin Pharmacol Ther* 1992;51:602-607.
Hirsch J. Comments on long-term weight loss. *Am J of Clin Nutr* 1994;60:658-659.

18. Levitsky, *see Ch8:9:*8-12, 18.

19. Berg F. Diet pill controversy embroils providers. *Healthy Weight J* 1997;11:1:4.

20. Berg F. What's the spin? *Healthy Weight J* 1997;11:2:24.

21. Abenhaim L, et al. Appetite-suppressant drugs and the risk of primary pulmonary hypertension. Intl Primary Pulmonary Hypertension Study. *N Engl J Med* 1996;335:609-616.

22. Manson JE, and Faich GA. Pharmacotherapy of obesity — do the benefits outweight risks? *N Engl J Med* 1996;335:659-660.

23. Levitsky, *see Ch8:9:*8-12, 18.

24. *New York Times* August 29, 1996.

25. FDA news release, Sept. 15, 1997
Berg, *see Ch8:14.*

26. Berg, *see Ch8:16.*

27. Connolly H, Crary J, et al. Valvular heart disease associated with fenfluramine-phentermine. *N Engl J Med* 1997;337:581-588.

28. Mundy, *see Ch1:2.*
29. FDA discussion paper, November 24, 1997.
    AP Washington, Nov. 25, 1997.
    Berg F. FDA approves Meridia. *Healthy Weight J* 1998;12:2:18.
30. NHLBI, *see Ch1:5.*
31. Berg F. NIH guidelines: an evaluation. *Healthy Weight J* 1999;13:2:26-29.
32. Bray G. In defense of a body mass index of 25 as the cut-off point for defining overweight. *Obesity Res* 1998;6:6:461-462.
33. Obesity, *see Ch5:6.*
34. American Heart Association Guidelines. *Healthy Weight J* 1997;11:6:108-110.
35. Coulston AM. Obesity as an epidemic: facing the challenge. *J Am Diet Assoc* 1998;98:10(S2):16-22.
36. *Deception and Fraud in the Diet Industry.* 1990. Hearing before the Subcommittee on Regulation, Business Opportunities and Energy, Committee on Small Business, House of Representatives. Chaired by Rep. Ron Wyden (D-Ore.) Washington, DC.
37. Berg F. FTC settles charges against weight loss companies. *Healthy Weight J* 1997;11:2:30-31.
38. Fraser, *see 1:*p103.
39. Methods, *see Ch8:2*
40. Yanovski SZ, Williamson DF, and Bain RP. Report of a NIH-CDC workshop on the feasibility of conducting a clinical trial on long term health effects of weight loss in obese persons. *Am J Clin Nutr* 1999:69:366-72.

Chapter 11

1. Berg F. Body mass index makes comparisons easier. *HWJ/Obesity & Health* 1991;5:1:8
2. Campfield LA. 1997. Role of pharmacological agents in the treatment of obesity. In *Overweight and weight management,* ed. S Dalton. p471-473. Gaithersberg, MD: Aspen Publ.
3. Vitality Leader's Kit, *see Ch1:11.*
4. Ornstein R, Sobel D. 1989. *Healthy Pleasures.* pg 163. New York: Addison-Wesley Publ. Co.
5. Ornstein, *see 4.*
6. Mossey JM, Shapiero E. Self-rated health: a predictor of mortality among the elderly. *Am J of Public Health*)82;72:800-807.
   ler W. Health promotion strategies

for obese patients. *Healthy Weight J* 1997:11:3:47-51.
    Barlow CE, Kohl HW III, Gibbens LW, and Blair SN. Physical fitness, mortality and obesity. *Int J Obesity* 1995;19:S41-S44.

Chapter 12

1. Hirschmann, *see Ch2:1.*
2. Ornstein, *see Ch11:4*
3. Tubesing, Donald A., and Tubesing, Nany Loving. 1983. *Seeking Your Healthy Balance.* Whole Person Assoc. 1702 E Jefferson St, Duluth MN 55812 (218-728-6807).
4. Berne, Eric. 1976. *Beyond games and scripts.* New York: Grove Press.
5. Maltz, Maxwell. 1976. *Psycho-cybernetics.* Hollywood, CA: Wilshire Book Co.
6. Maltz, *see 5.*
7. Carnegie, Dorothy. 1959. *Dale Carnegie's Scrapbook.* p 98. New York: Simon and Schuster.
8. Antony MM, Swinson RP. 1998. *When Perfect Isn't Good enough.* Oakland, CA: New Harbinger Publ.
9. Cash, Thomas. 1995. *What do you see when you look in the mirror? Helping yourself to a positive body image.* New York: Bantam Doubleday Dell Publ.
10. Freedman, Rita. 1988. *BodyLove: Learning to like our looks — and ourselves.* New York: Harper & Row, Publ.
11. Price, Deirdra. 1998. *Healing the Hungry Self.* New York: Penguin Putnam.
12. Miller, Timothy. 1998. *Wanting What You Have: A Self-Discovery Workbook.* Oakland, CA: New Harbinger Publ.
13. Alberti, Robert, and Emmonds, Michael. 1970. *Your Perfect Right.* San Luis Obispo: Impact Publ.
14. Phelps S, Austin N. 1975. *The Assertive Woman.* San Luis Obispo, CA: Impact Publ.
15. Hayes, Dayle. 1999. *Loving your body.* Billings, Mont.
16. Johnson, Carol. What kind of messages are we sending? *On a Positive Note* Spring 1999;1-3.
17. Vitality Leader's Kit, *see Ch1:11.*

Chapter 13

1. Johnston G. New vision for exercise.

HWJ/Obesity & Health 1992;6: 108-109.

2. Stolove, Jodi. Videos: *Chair Dancing.* Chair Dancing International, 2640 Del Mar Heights Rd, #183, Del Mar, CA 92014 (1-800-551-4FUN).

3. Lutter, *see Ch9:37.*

4. Fiatrone MA, O'Neill EF, Ryan ND, et al. Exercise training and nutitional supplementation for physical frailty in very elderly people. *N Engl J Med* 1994;330:1769-75.

5. Kayman Susan. *Am J Clin Nutr* 1990;52:800-807.

6. *Obesity Res* 1996;4:1S,7S. Klem ML, Wing RR, McGuire MT, et al. The National Weight Control Registry: A descriptive study of individuals successful at long-term maintenance of substantial weight loss. *Am J Clin Nutr* 1997;66:239-246.

7. *JADA* 1995;95:1414-1417. Berg F. Avoid weight loss focus. *Healthy Weight J* 1996;10:4:75.

8. NIH Technology Assessment Conference Panel. Methods for voluntary weight loss and control. *Ann Int Med* 1993;119:764-770.

9. Hammer Roger. Health and fitness benefits for the obese person. *Healthy Weight J* 1999;13:4:52-53, 57.

10. Hammer, *see 9.*

11. Lee CD, Jackson AS, Blair SN. US weight guidelines: is it also important to consider cardiorespiratory fitness? *Int J Obes* 1998;22:S2-7. Barlow, *see Ch11:7.*

12. Blair SN, Kohl HW, Barlow CE. Physical activity, physical fitness, and all-cause mortality in women: do women need to be active? *J Am Coll Nutr* 1993;12(4):368-371.

13. Tremblay A, Despres JP, Maheux J, et al. Normalization of the metabolic profile in obese women by exercise and a low fat diet. *Med Sci Sports Exerc* 1991;23:1326-1331.

14. Allison, *see Ch8:4.*

15. Andres R, Muller DC, Sorkin JD. Long-term effects of change in body weight on all-cause mortality: a review. *Ann Intern Med* 1993;119:737-743.

16. The great debate. *Remedy* Sep/Oct 1996:27-31.

17. Brownell KD, and Rodjin J. 1990. Exercise: your ticket to long-term success. In *The Weight Maintenance Survival Guide.* p 67-78. Dallas, TX: Brownell & Hager.

18. Miller WC. Practical Exercise for the Large Person. *Healthy Weight J* 1999:13:54-57.

19. American College of Sports Medicine. 1995. *Guidelines for Exercise Testing and Prescription, 5th ed.* p 216-219. Philadelphia, PA: Williams & Wilkins. American College of Sports Medicine. The recommended quantity and quality of exercise for developing and maintaining cardiorespiratory and muscular fitness, and flexibility in healthy adults. *Med Sci Sports Exerc.* 1998;30,975-991.

Chapter 14

1. Satter, *see Ch3:7.*

2. Omichiski L. Revised 1999, 1992. *You Count, Calories Don't.* Portage La Prairie, Manitoba: HUGS International, (www.hugs.com).

3. Siegel, Karen. Purposeful eating in the nondiet approach. *Healthy Weight J* 1997;11:52.

4. Kabatznick Ronna. 1998. *The Zen of Eating.* New York: Perigee Books, Berkley Publ.

5. Kratina, *see Ch3:6.*

6. *Food Insight* Mar/Apr 1998:3; Dietary Guidelines website: www.fcs.uga. edu/~selbon/appple/guides/choose.html.

7. *Dietary Guidelines for Americans.* 4th Edition, 1995. HG bulletin 232. USDA, Washington, DC.

8. Calcium supplements for the prevention of colorectal adenomas. *New Engl J of Med* 1998;340:101-107.

9. *1997 Dietary Reference Intakes (RDAs).* 1997. Institute of Medicine, National Academy of Sciences, Washington DC.

10. Recommended Dietary Allowances, *see Ch9:1.*

11. *Reaching consumers with meaningful health messages: Putting the Dietary Guidelines into action.* 1996. Dietary Guidelines Alliance.

Chapter 15

1. Kafer, Karen, RD, Director of Communications, Kellogg USA. Battle Creek, MI.

2. Johnson, Carol. 1995. *Self-Esteem Comes in All Sizes.* New York: Doubleday.

3. Jonas, Steven, and Konner, Linda. 1997. *Just the Weigh You Are.* Shelburne, VT: Chapters Publ.
4. Wooley S. *Radiance Magazine* Summer 1989:38-39. Oakland, Calif.
5. Camryn Manheim's memorable words in accepting her Emmy in the 1998 Emmy Awards are recorded on the educational video *Body Talk.* Available from: The Body Positive, 2417 Prospect St., #A, Berkeley, CA 94704 (510-841-9389).
6. *NAAFA Newsletter.* June/July 1998;28:9.
7. McBride, Angela Barron. 1989. Fat is generous, nurturing, warm. In *Overcoming Fear of Fat, see Ch6:2.*
8. Lee Gina. Fat people wear shorts. *Radiance* Spring 1995;42:14.
9. Lyons Pat, and Burgard Debby. 1988. *Great Shape.* p22. New York: Arbor House, Wm. Morrow.
10. Dworkin L Niquie. I Feel Fat and Ugly. *ANAD Working Together* Summer 1998:1,3.
11. Garcia Janet. Living Creatively in the Moment. *NEDO Newsletter* 1998; 32:11-12.
12. Martindale Lee. Say what's on your size-positive mind with Rump Parliament size-positive products. *Rump Parliament,* PO Box 181716, Dallas TX 75218.
Martindale Lee. Shooting from the rump. *Healthy Weight J* 1995;9:95.
13. Wann Marilyn. 1998. *Fat! So?* Berkeley, CA: Ten Speed Press.
14. *Nothing to Lose* video. Available from: Fat Lip Readers Theatre, PO Box 29963, Oakland, CA 94604.
15. Smith Sally. State of Movement Address. *NAAFA Newsletter* 1994;25:7-9; Smith S. Building bridges in the movement between past and future. *Healthy Weight J* 1995;9:3:53-54.
16. NAAFA Press release, Dec 1989.
17. Fishman Laurel. On-the-job Harassment. *BBW* March 1998:34, 75-76.
18. Cauthen, *see Ch6:6.*
Barlow, *see Ch11:7.*

Chapter 16

1. Pipher, *see Ch2:27.*
2. Pipher, *see Ch2:27.*
3. *EDAP Matters* Spring 1998:5.
EDAP website: http://members.aol.com/ edapinc/home.html.
4. Huon G. Health promotion and the prevention of dieting-induced disorders. *Eat Disorders* 1996;4:1:27-32.
5. News Release 4/30/99, University of Toronto.
6. Whelan, *see Ch9:31.*
7. Berg FM. Congress asked to take eating disorders seriously. *Healthy Weight J* 1998;12:41-44.

Chapter 17

1. Levine MP. 1999. Prevention of eating disorders, eating problems and negative body image. In *Controlling eating disorders with facts, advice and resources,* 2nd, ed. R Lemberg. p64-72. Phoenix, AZ: Oryx Press.
2. Johnson, Linda. 1999. *Prevention: Does it really work?* p3-99. Department of Public Instruction. Bismarck, N.D.
3. Piran N. The Last Word: Prevention of eating disorders: The struggle to chart new territories. *Eating Dis* 1998; 6:365-371.
4. Price RH, Cowen EL, Lorion RP, et al. dits. *14 ounces of prevention: A casebook for practitioners.* Washington, DC: American Psychological Association.
5. Latzer Y, and Shatz S. Comprehensive community prevention of disturbed attitudes to weight control: A three-level intervention program. *Eating Disorders* 1999;7:3-31.
6. Levine MP, and Piran N. 1999. Approaches to health promotion in the prevention of the eating disorders. *Unpublished manuscript,* Kenyon College, Gambier, OH.
Piran N. Prevention: Can early lessons lead to a delineation of an alternative model? Prevention with schoolchildren. *Eating Disorders* 1995;3:28-36.
7. Piran N. Eating disorders: A trial of prevention in a high risk school setting. *J Primary Prevention* 1999;20:75-90.
Piran N. On prevention and transformation. *The Renfrew Perspective* 1996;2:1:8-9.
Levine, *see 6.*
8. Levine MP, Piran N, Stoddard C. Mission more probable: Media literacy, activism and advocacy as primary prevention. 1999. In *Preventing Eating Disorders: A handbook of interventions and special challenges,* eds. N Piran, MP Levine, and C

Steiner-Adair. p 3-25. Philadelphia: Brunner/Mazel.

Levine MP, Piran N, Prevention of Eating Disorders: Reflections, conclusions and future directions. 1999. In *Preventing Eating Disorders: A handbook of interventions and special challenges,* eds. N Piran, MP Levine, and C Steiner-Adair. p319-329. Philadelphia: Brunner/Mazel.

9. Springer EA, Winzelberg AJ, Perkins R, et al. Effects of a body image curriculum for college students on improved body image. *Int J Eat Disord* 1999; 26:13-20.

10. Larkin, *see Ch2:25.*

11. Ikeda J, and Brainen-Rodriguez L. Physicians Learn to promote body satisfaction. *Healthy Weight J* 1999; 13:3:39-41.

The training kit Children and Weight: What Health Professionals Can Do About It is available by contacting Joanne Ikeda, jikeda@socrates. berkeley.edu (tel: 510-642-2790; fax: 510-642-0535)

12. Berg M, McAfee L, Summer N, et al. Weight-related diseases and conditions. *Healthy Weight J* 1997;11:5:89-92.

13. Levine, *see 1.*

14. Garner, DM, Reizes JM, Deutsch NL, et al. National Eating Disorders Screening Program. Presentation at the Academy for Eating Disorders 1999 annual meeting, June 11-12, 1999, San Diego CA.

15. Paul, Lynn. *Helping a friend with an eating disorder — What can you do?* Power Point presentation. Lynn Paul, MSU Extension, 101 Romney Hall, Bozeman, MT 59717 (406-994-5702; lpaul@montana.edu).

16. For information contact: Linda Omichinski, HUGS International. Box 102A, RR#, POrtage la Prairie, MB, Canada R1N 3A3 (204-428-3432; fax 204-428-5072) website: hugs.com.

17. Glass J. Exercise benefits, risks and precautions for women. *Healthy Weight J* 1999;13:58-60.

18. Miller WC. Exercise Prescription for the Large Person. *Healthy Weight J* 1999:13:54-57.

19. Glass, *see 17.*

Chapter 18
1. Berg, *see Ch1:3:*122-132.

2. Berg F. Connecticut law curbs diet claims. *Healthy Weight J* 1996; 10:6:109.
Connecticut law effective Oct.1, 1996 (SHB 5621; Pub Act 96-126). For information contact: Conn. Dept Consumer Protection, 165 Capitol Ave., Hartford CT 06106 (203-566-4499; fax 203-566-7630).

3. *Am J Clin Nutr* 1994;60:153-156.

Chart References

Chapter 4
1. *Diagnostic criteria for eating disorders.* Diagnostic and Statistical Manual, Fourth Edition, 1994. American Psychiatric Association, Washington, DC.

2. National Eating Disorders Orgnaization (NEDO), 6655 S Yale Ave, Tulsa, OK 74136.

Chapter 5
1. *NHLBI Guidelines: Clinical Guidelines on the Identification, Evaluation, and Treatment of Overweight and Obesity in Adults: The Evidence Report.* National Institutes of Health, National Heart, Lung, and Blood Institute. Preprint June 1998. Bethesda, MD.

2. NHLBI Guidelines, see 1.

Chapter 9
1. *Continuing Survey of Food Intakes by Individuals (CSFII), What We Eat in America Survey.* Dec 1998. US Department of Agriculture.

2. Continuing Survey, *see 1.*

3. Continuing Survey, *see 1.*

4. *Third report on nutrition monitoring in the US, Vol 1-2, Dec 1995.* National Center for Health Statistics, NHANES III, 1988-1991. Vol 1, p135. Life Sciences Research Office, Interagency Board for Nutrition Monitoring and Related Research, US Dept. of Health and Human Services, US Dept. Of Agriculture.

Chapter 11
1. Vitality Leader's Kit, 1994. Health Services and Promotion, Health and Welfare Canada. 4th Floor, Jeanne Mance Bldg, Ottawa, Ontario, Canada K1A 1B4 (613-957-8331).

Chapter 12
Hayes, Dayle. 1999. *Loving your body*. Revised. Hayes is an author, speaker and nutrition therapist, 3112 Farnam Street, Billings, MT, 59102. Phone: (406) 655-9082   Fax: (406) 656-0580 Email: EatWellMT@aol.com

Chapter 13
1. Glass J. Exercise benefits, risks and precautions for women. *Healthy Weight J* 1999;13:58-60.

Chapter 14
1. *Dietary Guidelines for Americans*. 4th Edition. 1995. HG bulletin 232. USDA, Washington, DC.

Chapter 15
1. Sheinin R. 1990. *Body shame: the shaming of women*. Rachel Sheinin is a past Assistant Programme Coordinator of the National Eating Disorder Information Centre. Bulletin. p1-3. To contact: NEDIC, 200 Elizabeth St., CW 1-328, Toronto, Ontario, Canada M5G 2C4.)
2. Sheinin R, *see 1*.
3. Johnson, CA. *Self-Esteem Comes in All Sizes*. 1995. NY: Doubleday. Carol Johnson, Gendale, Wisconsin, is a certified therapist, founder of Largely Positive, a support group for large women (and men), and editor of On a Positive Note newsletter.

Chapter 17
1. Ernsberger P. *Which path for the obese patient?* From a presentation at Texas Human Nutrition Conference, Feb. 1996, College Station. Paul Ernsberger, PhD, is Associate Professor of Medicine, Pharmacology and Neuroscience at Case Western Reserve School of Medicine, Cleveland, OH.
2. Garner DM, and Wooley SC. Confronting the failure of behavioral and dietary treatments for obesity. *Clin Psych Rev* 1991;11:729-780.
3. Weight cycling risks research:
   Lissner L, Odell P, D'Agostino D, and Stoke J, et al. Variability of body weight and health outcomes in the Framingham population. *New Engl J Med* 1991;324:1839-44.
   Lissner L, Bengtsson C, Lapidus L, et al. Body weight variability and mortality in the Gothenburg prospective studies of men and women. *Obesity in Europe 88* 1989:55-58.
   Abstract, 34th Annual Conference on Cardiovascular Disease Epidemiology and Prevention, March 16-19, 1994.
   Brownell K, and Rodin J. Medical, metabolic, and psychological effects of weight cycling. *Arch Intern Med* 1994;154;1325-1330.
   Lu H, et al. Long-term weight cycling in female Wistar rats. *Obes Res* 1995;3:521-530.
   Berg F. Harvard alums risk heart disease by always dieting. *Healthy Weight J* 1994;8:3:52.
   Berg F. Weight cycling. *HWJ/Obesity & Health* 1989;3:10:73.
4. Mortality with weight loss research:
   NIH Technology assessment conference: Methods for voluntary weight loss and control. Conference report: program and abstracts. March 30-April 1, 1992.
   Andres R, Muller DC, Sorkin JD. Long-term effects of change in body weight on all-cause mortality: a review. *Ann Intern Med* 1993;119:737-743.
   Williamson DF, Pamuk E, Thun M, et al. Prospective study of intentional weight loss and mortality in never-smoking overweight US white women aged 40-64 years. *Am J Epidemiol* 1995;141:1128-1141.
   Williamson DF, Pamuk E, Thun M, et al. Prospective study of intentional weight loss and mortality in never-smoking overweight US men aged 40-64 years. *Obes Res* 1997;5 (Suppl 1):S94.
5. Fat loss vs lean loss research:
   Allison DB, Zannolli R, Faith MS, et al. Weight loss increases and fat loss decreases all-cause mortality rate: results from two independent cohort studies. *I J Obesity* 1999;23:603-611.
   Allison DB, Faith MS, Heo M, et al. Hypotesis concerning U-shaped relation between body mass index and mortality. *Am J Epidemiol* 1997;146:339-349.
   Segal JC, Verschuren WMM, VanLeer EM, et al. Overweight, underweight and mortality. *J Clin Inves* 1987;80:1050-1055.
   Van Itallie TB, Yang MU. Diets and weight loss. *New Engl J Med* 1977;297:1158-1161.

Index

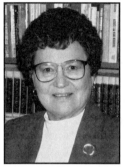
An internationally known authority on eating and weight, FRANCES M. BERG, M.S., LN, is a licensed nutritionist, family wellness specialist, and Adjunct Professor at the University of North Dakota School of Medicine. As the editor and founder of *Healthy Weight Journal,* Berg has reported eating and weight-related research for over 16 years to health professionals and educators worldwide.

The author of ten books and a weekly column, *Healthy Living,* published in more than 50 newspapers, she has presented at numerous national and international conferences, and been a guest on national television, including Oprah, Leeza and Inside Edition. Her master's degree in family social science and anthropology is from the University of Minnesota, and she holds a Family and Consumer Science degree from Montana State University.

Francie Berg serves as National Coordinator of the Task Force on Weight Loss Abuse, National Council Against Health Fraud, and on advisory boards working with prevention of childhood obesity, eating disorders, and quality health care for people of all sizes. She is a member of the Society for Nutrition Education (Chair of Weight Realities Division), the Academy for Eating Disorders, the North American Association for the Study of Obesity, the National Association to Advance Fat Acceptance, and the Society for the Study of Ingestive Behavior. She has four children and lives with her husband Bert, a veterinarian, in Hettinger, North Dakota.

A personal note

A question I'm often asked is: Why did you write this book? The easy answer is that I was growing more and more concerned as I read the appalling research on kids' eating problems, and as I watched that research personified in the gaunt, vacant-looking girls I was seeing everywhere at high school basketball games, hanging out in malls, in school hallways, wherever kids gather.

Someone has to do it, I kept thinking uneasily. Someone needs to tell parents and teachers what's happening, and why we can't do this to our kids. But no one did. And when I'd tell other writers in the field of my concerns, they'd say, it's you. But I didn't want to take a year out of my already busy life.

The first book on children and teens addressed what I consider the most acute concern of all — our children. This book on women naturally followed as it became clear to me that women are the key to ending this appalling thinness obsession that has gripped the modern world.

There were personal reasons, too. I'd experienced acute pain in the seasonal dieting of our two wrestling sons. Both were champion high school wrestlers in the lower weights, and every wrestling parent knows what that means: they cut weight, cut food and even cut water to "make weight" for each match.

Still, this isn't the complete answer. In Vancouver a Canadian dietitian told me, "We need to know where you're coming from, it will help us process our own feelings. We can accept others, but it's not easy to accept ourselves."

So yes, there's more. I can understand the desperation to lose weight, because I recall only too well how, as an overweight teenager, I lived through the miseries of gazing into the mirror wishing I could pull off a hunk here, and here, of watching my best resolutions dissolve into uncontrolled eating binges.

Then by a lucky accident I lost my excess weight. I was on my first job out of college, living alone, trying each new diet that came along. I'd begin the diet with enthusiasm and high hopes — and always lose weight. But as the excitement faded the pounds returned. The diets made no real changes in my life, except they kept me thinking about food and weight and hunger. I skipped meals and filled up on snack foods. I fasted and binged by turns.

The lucky accident came when I happened to acquire a roommate with amazingly simple and sensible eating habits. Unlike my other friends, Carol didn't diet. She didn't even talk about dieting. She didn't need to, I told myself — she was slender and athletic.

Carol insisted straight off that we eat three meals each day beginning with a good breakfast. She couldn't mean scrambled eggs, toast and cereal? She did. I was dismayed. Breakfast was the one meal I could and did skip with ease.

Reluctantly I gave in, sure I'd gain weight fast. (At the same time, I knew she was right. As a nutrition educator, I taught the value of balanced meals. I just didn't apply it to myself.)

Nonetheless, Carol won me over. At noon we fixed quick hot food, such as soup and toasted cheese sandwiches. Our evening meals were based solidly on meat, potatoes, vegetables, salad, bread and milk. I couldn't get Carol to understand that I'd certainly fatten up on such fare. She'd just look at me in mild surprise and say, "Well sure, we have to eat potatoes. We need to keep up our strength."

No more eating on the run, reading as I ate, rushing back to work, hunger unsatisfied. Carol insisted we sit at the table and enjoy the food. Meals became a relaxing and pleasant time.

A couple of months passed before I happened to step on a scale. What a surprise. The scale was wrong, I thought. How could I have shed 10 pounds without so much as a struggle? But it was no mistake. My clothes began fitting easier. Soon I bought them in a smaller size.

Surprisingly, I wasn't caught up in the fervor of losing weight as I had been in the past. I was busy, active and having fun. My stomach was satisfied and my days were filled. Food just wasn't very important in my life anymore. Even my precise weight wasn't important. The pounds slipped off rather slowly, but in a natural, painless and lasting way. That year I lost another 10 pounds and some months later another 10. My weight stabilized at about 125 pounds — the very point I'd struggled so long and hopelessly to reach. All those years of agonized dieting, frustration and despair had accomplished exactly nothing. It was only when I forgot about eating and turned my energy toward other areas of living that I shed my excess weight in a lasting way.

The weight stayed off naturally until my fourth baby was born. I tried a couple of diets, then decided to recreate that earlier experience: gradually change some bad habits and let the weight come off as it may. I returned to eating normally, dropped those "Mommy habits" I'd acquired — nibbling when fixing a meal, clearing up, unloading groceries, skipping meals because I "wasn't hungry." I began running a couple of miles a day, which I'd always loved, and which has been a continuing pleasure. This time I used a contract system and records to keep track of habit changes, and again over the course of a year the extra weight came off.

Then midlife came along, and with it 15 pounds or so. Research tells me this is normal. Nearly all women gain some weight (and it tends to settle around the middle). By this time I was reading sad studies about the bitter fights many women put up against this, even into their 70's or 80's, and I recalled my aunt at 86, 120 pounds, wondering how to rid herself of that tummy roll.

Should I double my activity, then? No. That could make a difference, but it's not worth it. I enjoy my life, just as it is. If this weight gain is normal, maybe there's a good reason. And there is. A little extra weight is protective against the fragile bones and osteoporosis that many women suffer at midlife, especially if they're thin or dieting. Research suggests it may be protective in other ways, too. So I'm happy to regard it as natural and protective — and a good time to buy some new clothes.

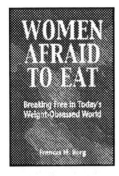
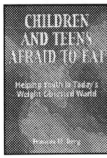

Children and Teens Afraid to Eat

REVIEWS

BERG SERVES UP A FEAST of facts on four major problems: dysfunctional eating, eating disorders, size prejudice, and overweight. The book contains advice for parents but emphasizes that social change is needed in schools, organized sports, and federal policies that focus too narrowly on antiobesity. Berg's book is a valuable consciousness raiser. Recommended for public libraries for both parents and concerned professionals.

—LIBRARY JOURNAL

A COMPELLING CASE ... The discussion on how to help overweight children and children with eating disorders is very well written, featuring excellent tables that highlight practical tips for parents and nutrition educators. ... The last two chapters are probably the most powerful. ... Anyone who works in the area of weight control and disordered eating will want a copy of this book on his or her shelf.

— JOURNAL OF THE AMERICAN DIETETIC ASSOCIATION

A GROUND-BREAKING BOOK about an issue in our culture that is affecting almost every child in ways that range from detrimental to disastrous. ... We need a national awareness of an intolerable situation that will not self-correct. *Afraid to Eat* needs to be read, discussed, argued about, and acted upon.

— ACADEMY FOR EATING DISORDERS NEWSLETTER

I CAN'T RECOMMEND THIS BOOK STRONGLY ENOUGH! Ms. Berg writes with compassion while exposing and dispelling many prejudicial beliefs. ... One of the best messages that this book expresses is the basic human right to be treated as an individual.

— JOURNAL OF FAMILY LIFE

AN EXTRAORDINARY contribution to both professionals and the public. *Afraid to Eat* identifies the cultural, social, physiological, emotional and spiritual issues facing kids today and how these issues collide, resulting in a generation of kids afraid to eat. Ms. Berg is an award winning writer and has a gift for gathering and clearly explaining how these forces influence our children relationally and developmentally.

— PULSE, Dietitians in Sports, Cardiovascular and Wellness

BERG STATES IT IS A MAJOR HEALTH CRISIS when more than two-thirds

of high school girls are dieting ... nearly one-fourth are overweight and subject to discrimination, hazardous weight loss attempts and related health risks, and more than one-tenth have potentially fatal eating disorders.
— ROCHESTER TIMES UNION, Rochester, N.Y.

A MUCH NEEDED BOOK ... Berg dares to speak out on behalf of parents, educators, health professionals, and all members of society. The news (on nutrient deficiencies) should be alarming, but the media's attention is fixated on obesity fear rather than long-term health. ... This is an issue that should touch our hearts deeply, make us angry, and give us motivation to bring about change. Inspires the reader to action.
— EATING DISORDERS: Journal of Treatment & Prevention

THERE'S A SILENT EPIDEMIC so large and extreme, it could only happen in this weight-obsessed culture: children's fear of eating. The good news is that *Healthy Weight Journal* editor Berg is out to change these attitudes. Her call to action is loud, clear, and above all, provides the framework for change. Anyone involved in shaping the eating habits of the young must read this book, especially parents and teachers.
— CHOICE, American Library Association

AN INDISPENSABLE RESOURCE ... Her jewel of a book is a wake-up call to health education professionals to address all aspects of the problem. ... This is not light reading. But it is extremely interesting.
— BBW: Big Beautiful Woman

WHAT CAN WE DO to combat destructive influences and feelings about weight? ... Setting a nutritionally-sound example, encouraging regular exercise, questioning advertising and role model images and focusing on accepting kids for who they are, rather than what they look like, Berg says.
— THE NEW YORK POST

A GOOD BLEND OF FACT and research with personal experiences. ... A resource for parents, teachers, coaches and health professionals.
— PEDIATRIC NUTRITION

BEST OF ALL, Berg provides many practical solutions to the problems she addresses. This is more than a penetrating analysis of a major public health problem; it is also a how-to book of solutions.
— NATIONAL COUNCIL AGAINST HEALTH FRAUD NEWSLETTER